The M. D. Anderson Surgical Oncology Handbook

M. D. Anderson Cancer Center
Department of Surgical Oncology
Houston

David H. Berger, M.D.

Barry W. Feig, M.D.

George M. Fuhrman, M.D.

Editors

Foreword by **Charles M. Balch, M.D.**
Head, Division of Surgery and Anesthesiology
University of Texas M. D. Anderson Cancer Center
Houston

Little, Brown and Company
Boston   New York   Toronto   London

First Edition

Library of Congress Cataloging-in-Publication Data

The M. D. Anderson surgical oncology handbook / M. D. Anderson
    Cancer Center Department of Surgical Oncology / edited by David H.
    Berger, Barry W. Feig, George M. Fuhrman.
        p.   cm.
    Includes bibliographical references and index.
    ISBN 0-316-56431-1
    1. Cancer--Surgery--Handbooks, manuals, etc.   I. Berger,
David H., 1959–   .   II. Feig, Barry W., 1959–   .   III. Fuhrman,
        George M.
    [DNLM: 1. Neoplasms--surgery--handbooks. QZ 39 M111 1994]
RD651.M17   1994
616.99'4059--dc20
DNLM/DLC
for Library of Congress   94-3421
                                                                  CIP

Printed in the United States of America

RRD-VA

Editorial: Nancy E. Chorpenning
Production Editor: Marie A. Salter
Copyeditor: Elizabeth Willingham
Indexer: Alexandra Nickerson
Production Supervisor: Michael Burggren
Composition and Production: Silverchair Science + Communications
Cover Designer: Michael Burggren

To our wives, Adrianne, Barbara, and Laura,
for their support, enthusiasm, and patience
through our many years of training

Contents

Foreword

Surgical residents and fellows will find this an invaluable book to keep in a handy location, for it provides practical, up-to-date information about oncology care of the surgical patient. It was written by surgical oncology fellows for an audience of their peers. Each chapter outlines the essential elements of the diagnosis, staging, and clinical management of the solid tumors treated in surgical practice. It emphasizes the importance of multidisciplinary treatment planning, which is essential to the surgeon in counseling cancer patients.

The surgeon's role in cancer care has expanded and diversified greatly because of new information about the natural history of cancer, earlier detection of many cancers, and the increased availability of effective systemic therapy regimens. Cancer therapy has evolved to the point that multidisciplinary approaches are the standard treatment for most cancer patients, even those with early-stage disease. The surgeon today must possess a broad set of clinical skills to participate as an effective partner in a multidisciplinary cancer care team and to ensure that the full range of diagnostic and treatment options are considered in the management of each patient's cancer. If the surgeon is to retain the primary coordinating role in cancer management, he or she must fully understand all modalities of oncology therapy and know how to deploy them to benefit patients. This role as coordinator of therapy demands knowledge about the indications, risks, and benefits of adjuvant chemotherapy, hormonal therapy, and radiation therapy.

Determining the most appropriate treatment plan for a surgical patient with cancer is one of the most difficult decision-making processes in clinical medicine. The biological presentations of many cancers are varied, the treatment options and sequences are numerous, and patients' differing perceptions of "quality of life" are diverse. All these considerations have to be incorporated into an organized treatment plan. This surgical oncology handbook will help readers formulate these plans for their cancer patients.

Surgical oncology is a rapidly growing surgical specialty that reflects our advancing understanding of cancer biology and treatment. The surgical oncology fellows at the M. D. Anderson Cancer Center join me in dedicating this book to the cancer patients we serve. We hope it will be a valuable companion to the reader's daily rounds and study.

Charles M. Balch, M.D.

Preface

The M. D. Anderson Surgical Oncology Handbook is the first attempt to document the philosophies of the Department of Surgical Oncology at the M. D. Anderson Cancer Center. The purpose of this book is to outline basic management approaches based on our experience with common surgical oncologic problems at M. D. Anderson. It provides the established surgical oncology principles for treating cancer as it involves each organ system in the body. It also points out controversial treatment issues.

This book was written by current and former surgical oncology fellows for surgical house staff and surgical oncology trainees. The authors are a varied group of individuals from a wide variety of training programs who have spent at least 2 years at the M. D. Anderson Cancer Center studying only surgical oncology. The variety of authors allowed us to present the current opinions and practices of the M. D. Anderson Department of Surgical Oncology along with other opinions and treatment options practiced in our diversified general surgical training. Although there is no "senior" well-known name associated with the book, the authors represent 160 total years of surgical training; we have not become dogmatic and unyielding in our medical practices, however.

The handbook is not meant to encompass all aspects of oncology in minute detail. Rather, it is an attempt to address the commonly encountered as well as the controversial issues in surgical oncology. While other texts present their opinions and approaches as firmly established, we have tried to point out where controversy resides and to show our approach as well as other accepted approaches to these problems.

We are indebted to Melissa Burkett of the Department of Scientific Publications at M. D. Anderson for her skillful and tireless editorial work. In addition, we would particularly like to thank the attending surgical staff of the M. D. Anderson Cancer Center for their assistance with the content of the book as well as their devoted teaching in the hospital clinics, wards, and operating rooms.

D.H.B.
B.W.F.
G.M.F.

Contributing Authors

Stephen Archer, M.D.
Fellow, Department of Surgical Oncology, University of
Texas M. D. Anderson Cancer Center, Houston
1. Noninvasive Breast Cancer

John R. Austin, M.D.
Assistant Professor, Department of Head and Neck
Surgery, University of Texas Medical School at Houston;
Assistant Surgeon, Department of Head and Neck Surgery,
University of Texas M. D. Anderson Cancer Center, Houston
6. Carcinoma of the Head and Neck

George Barnes, Jr., M.D.
Assistant Professor of Surgery, Morehouse School of
Medicine, Atlanta
15. Carcinoma of the Thyroid and Parathyroid Glands

Derrick J. Beech, M.D.
Junior Faculty Associate, University of Texas
M. D. Anderson Cancer Center, Houston
19. Oncologic Surgical Emergencies

David H. Berger, M.D.
Assistant Professor of Surgery, Medical College of
Pennsylvania, Philadelphia
2. Invasive Breast Cancer
12. Pancreatic Adenocarcinoma

Elizabeth A. Blair, M.D.
Fellow, Department of Head and Neck Surgery, University
of Texas M. D. Anderson Cancer Center, Houston
15. Carcinoma of the Thyroid and Parathyroid Glands

Robert L. Coleman, M.D.
Assistant Professor of Obstetrics and Gynecology and
Director, Gynecologic Oncology, Creighton University
School of Medicine, Omaha, Nebraska
18. Gynecologic Oncology

James C. Cusack, Jr., M.D.
Junior Faculty Associate, Department of Surgical Oncology,
University of Texas M. D. Anderson Cancer Center, Houston
9. Small-Bowel Malignancies and Carcinoid Tumors

Mark G. Delworth, M.D.
Fellow, Department of Urology, University of Texas
M. D. Anderson Cancer Center, Houston
17. Genitourinary Cancer

Colin P. N. Dinney, M.D.
Assistant Professor, Department of Urology, University of
Texas Medical School at Houston; Assistant Urologist,
Department of Urology, University of Texas M. D. Anderson
Cancer Center, Houston
17. Genitourinary Cancer

Barry W. Feig, M.D.
Assistant Professor, Departments of Surgical Oncology,
Anesthesiology, and Critical Care, University of Texas
M. D. Anderson Cancer Center, Houston
2. Invasive Breast Cancer
12. Pancreatic Adenocarcinoma

George M. Fuhrman, M.D.
Staff Surgeon and Director of Residency Training,
Ochsner Clinic, New Orleans
12. Pancreatic Adenocarcinoma

Haim Gutman, M.D.
Fellow, Department of Surgical Oncology, University of
Texas M. D. Anderson Cancer Center, Houston
10. Cancer of the Colon, Rectum, and Anus

Alton V. Hallum, III, M.D.
Assistant Professor, Department of Obstetrics and
Gynecology, University of Arizona School of Medicine and
Department of Gynecologic Oncology, Arizona Cancer
Center, Tuscon, Arizona
18. Gynecologic Oncology

Keith M. Heaton, M.D.
Research Fellow, Department of Surgical Oncology,
University of Texas M. D. Anderson Cancer Center, Houston
4. Nonmelanoma Skin Cancer

Thelma Hurd, M.D.
Assistant Professor of Surgery, University of Texas
Southwestern Medical School, Dallas
10. Cancer of the Colon, Rectum, and Anus

Steven D. Leach, M.D.
Junior Faculty Associate, Department of Surgical Oncology,
University of Texas M. D. Anderson Cancer Center, Houston
2. Invasive Breast Cancer

Jeffrey E. Lee, M.D.
Assistant Professor, Department of Surgical Oncology,
University of Texas M. D. Anderson Cancer Center, Houston
3. Melanoma

Phillip B. Ley, M.D., R.Ph.
Junior Faculty Associate, Department of Surgical Oncology,
University of Texas M. D. Anderson Cancer Center, Houston
21. Pharmacotherapy of Cancer

Andrew M. Lowy, M.D.
Junior Faculty Associate, Department of Surgical Oncology,
University of Texas M. D. Anderson Cancer Center, Houston
19. Oncologic Surgical Emergencies

Sarkis H. Meterissian, M.D.C.M.
Assistant Professor, Department of Surgery, McGill
University Faculty of Medicine; Assistant Surgeon,
Department of Surgical Oncology, Royal Victoria Hospital,
Montreal
5. Bone and Soft-Tissue Sarcoma

Paul T. Morris, M.D.
Junior Faculty Associate, Department of Thoracic and
Cardiovascular Surgery, University of Texas M. D.
Anderson Cancer Center, Houston
7. Thoracic Carcinoma

James A. Reilly, Jr., M.D.
Clinical Assistant Professor, Department of General
Surgery, University of Nebraska Medical Center,
Omaha, Nebraska
16. Hematologic Malignancies and Splenic Tumors

Charles A. Staley, M.D.
Junior Faculty Associate, Department of Surgical Oncology,
University of Texas M. D. Anderson Cancer Center, Houston
8. Gastric Carcinoma

Kenneth K. Tanabe, M.D.
Assistant Professor, Department of Surgery, Harvard
Medical School; Assistant in Surgery, Massachusetts
General Hospital, Boston
5. Bone and Soft-Tissue Sarcoma

Paula M. Termuhlen, M.D.
Resident, Department of General Surgery, University of
Texas Medical School at Houston, Houston
20. Nutrition in Cancer Patients

Bruce Toporoff, M.D.
Assistant Professor, Department of Surgery, Tulane
University School of Medicine and Cardiothoracic Surgery
Division, Tulane University Medical Center Hospital, New
Orleans
7. Thoracic Carcinoma

Douglas S. Tyler, M.D.
Assistant Professor of Surgery, Duke University School of
Medicine; Chief, Department of General Surgery, Veterans
Administration Hospital, Durham, North Carolina
9. Small-Bowel Malignancies and Carcinoid Tumors
*13. Pancreatic Endocrine Tumors and Multiple Endocrine
Neoplasia*
14. Adrenal Tumors

David J. Winchester, M.D.
Clinical Assistant Professor, Department of Surgery,
Northwestern University Medical School, Chicago
1. Noninvasive Breast Cancer

Judy Wolf, M.D.
Junior Faculty Associate, Department of Gynecologic
Oncology, University of Texas M. D. Anderson Cancer
Center, Houston
18. Gynecologic Oncology

Alan M. Yahanda, M.D.
Junior Faculty Associate, Department of Surgical Oncology,
University of Texas M. D. Anderson Cancer Center, Houston
11. Hepatobiliary Cancers

The M. D. Anderson Surgical Oncology Handbook

Noninvasive Breast Cancer

Stephen Archer and David J. Winchester

Noninvasive breast cancer includes two separate entities: ductal carcinoma in situ (DCIS) and lobular carcinoma in situ (LCIS). DCIS and LCIS are defined as a proliferation of neoplastic epithelial cells confined to the mammary ducts or lobules, respectively, without demonstrable evidence of invasion through the basement membrane. Because they are noninvasive, DCIS and LCIS offer no risk of metastatic spread. The term *minimal breast cancer*, once used to encompass in situ lesions and invasive cancers less than 5 mm in diameter, has been abandoned because the treatment strategies for each are entirely different.

Ductal Carcinoma In Situ

EPIDEMIOLOGY

Since the introduction of routine screening mammography, the incidence of DCIS has increased threefold from that observed in older series, when DCIS presented as a palpable lesion. In the United States, the incidence is now 10–20 per 100,000 woman-years, with the ratio of DCIS to LCIS being 4:1. The prevalence of DCIS has risen as the quality and sensitivity of mammography have improved, and DCIS currently accounts for 20–44% of all new screening-detected breast neoplasias.

The median age reported for patients with DCIS is 47–63 years—no different from that reported for patients with invasive carcinoma. Some studies suggest a trend toward a lower median age in patients with screening-detected DCIS. Similarly, the frequency of a positive family history of DCIS among first-degree relatives (10–35%) is no different from that reported for invasive carcinoma. In epidemiologic terms, therefore, DCIS behaves like invasive malignancy and is presumed to have the same risk factors.

PATHOLOGY

Histologic Subtypes

DCIS is thought to arise from duct epithelium in the region of the terminal lobular-ductal unit and represents one stage in a continuum between atypical ductal hyperplasia (ADH) and invasive carcinoma. DCIS comprises a heterogeneous group of lesions with variable histologic architecture, cellular characteristics, and clinical behavior. Malignant cells proliferate to obliterate the ductal lumen, and there may be an associated inflammatory reaction, stromal response, or lymphoid infiltration surrounding the duct.

DCIS is generally classified as one of five subtypes based on differing architectural pattern and nuclear features: comedo, solid, cribriform, micropapillary, and papillary. Cribriform, comedo, and micropapillary are the most common subtypes, although two or more patterns coexist in up to 50% of cases.

Comedo DCIS is characterized by large cells with pleomorphic nuclei, numerous mitoses, and prominent central necrosis with variable calcification. The biological aggressiveness of this lesion is evidenced by its high proliferative rate in thymidine labeling studies, overexpression of the *c-erb* B-2 oncogene in almost all cases, and high frequency of aneuploidy as determined by flow cytometry. It is important to note that comedo DCIS is more often associated with microinvasion compared with other subtypes, implying a short intraductal growth phase. There is a direct relationship between the size of DCIS lesions and the likelihood of occult invasive carcinoma. Lesions that are excised and measure less than 25 mm in histologic diameter do not commonly demonstrate microinvasion. In fact, 80% of microinvasion has been observed in DCIS lesions more than 45 mm in diameter.

Noncomedo forms of DCIS are composed of cells of variable size, with monomorphic nuclei, few mitoses, and a low proliferative rate. The architecture is variable, and coagulative necrosis is minimal or absent. In the *solid* subtype, the duct is completely filled with malignant cells, whereas the *cribriform* subtype exhibits small uniform cells growing in a fenestrated pattern. These two subtypes are histologically the least aggressive, often of limited extent, and generally not associated with microinvasion. *Papillary* DCIS is characterized by large intraluminal projections with fibrovascular cores, whereas *micropapillary* DCIS is characterized by tufts that are smaller and lack fibrovascular cores. Micropapillary DCIS tends to be a more extensive lesion and is multicentric, uncommonly associated with microinvasion, and presumed to have a long intraductal growth phase. Estrogen receptors have been demonstrated in DCIS, but their correlation with clinical outcome is unknown.

Pathologic Differential Diagnosis

The pathologic differential diagnosis of DCIS includes severe epitheliosis, ADH, LCIS, and DCIS with microinvasion. In severe epitheliosis, both epithelial and myoepithelial cells proliferate. ADH differs from DCIS only by degree of cellular atypia and is most often confused with noncomedo DCIS. LCIS can be confused with solid-type noncomedo DCIS because DCIS may extend into lobules and LCIS may involve extralobular ducts. Furthermore, DCIS and LCIS may coexist. The diagnosis of microinvasion can be difficult, with severe periductal fibrosis causing duct distortion commonly mistaken for microinvasion.

Multifocality and Microinvasion

Multifocality is generally considered to be present when separate DCIS foci more than 5 mm apart occur in the same breast quadrant; it has been noted in 20% of cases. Multicentricity is defined as the occurrence of DCIS outside the index quadrant, although it is unclear whether it indicates truly independent tumors or contiguous spread of tumor through ducts. Series of mastectomy patients with extensive DCIS note true multicentricity in one-third of cases, often with subclinical nipple involvement.

In contrast, most screening-detected DCIS is of limited extent and unassociated with multicentricity or microinvasion. When present, multicentricity is more commonly associated with micropapillary and papillary DCIS. Comedo DCIS can also demonstrate multicentricity.

The term *extensive intraductal component* (EIC) was defined by the Joint Center for Radiation Therapy as a lesion with at least 25% of the primary mass consisting of DCIS as well as the presence of DCIS extending beyond the infiltrating tumor margin or in sections of grossly normal adjacent breast tissue. They determined that EIC was a risk factor for local failure in patients treated with breast conservation. Subsequent studies have suggested that in select groups of patients with microscopically free margins, EIC can be treated with segmental mastectomy and radiotherapy.

DIAGNOSIS

Clinical Presentation

In the past, patients with DCIS presented with a palpable mass, nipple discharge, or Paget's disease of the nipple, or DCIS was an incidental finding in an otherwise benign biopsy specimen. Most of these lesions were large, and up to 25% demonstrated associated foci of invasive disease. The presence of microinvasion and a 10% incidence of axillary metastasis led to the same treatment being recommended for DCIS as for invasive breast cancer. Now that screening mammography is a routine procedure, palpable or symptomatic DCIS with microinvasion and lymph node metastasis is rarely encountered, leading to a rethinking of treatment strategies.

Mammographic Features

Approximately 80% of DCIS lesions are detectable by screening mammography (oblique and craniocaudal views) because of associated intraductal microcalcifications. Suspicious abnormalities can be further characterized using magnification and spot compression views. Current mammographic techniques can detect DCIS lesions as small as 2 mm.

The classic mammographic feature of DCIS is clustered microcalcifications, defined as five or more calcifications, each less than 1 mm in diameter, within an area of 1 cm³. The microcalcifications are made up of calcified intraluminal cellular debris, adjacent necrotic cells, or cellular secretions. Most DCIS lesions arise from terminal ducts, and hence the microcalcifications typically assume a linear or branching pattern. Note that these features are not specific for DCIS because benign lesions, such as those caused by fibroadenosis, often demonstrate a pattern of microcalcifications similar to that of DCIS. Consequently, only 25% of biopsied mammographic abnormalities will be neoplastic. Therefore it is not possible to differentiate invasive carcinoma from DCIS on the basis of mammography alone.

Diagnostic Biopsy

Because the majority of DCIS lesions are nonpalpable abnormalities detected by mammography, needle localization is required to direct a diagnostic biopsy. At the University of Texas M. D. Anderson Cancer Center, microcalcifications are excised after needle localization, whereas nonpalpable mammographic masses that can be visualized using ultrasonography undergo fine-needle aspiration and are excised only if the cytologic findings are positive, suspicious, or nondiagnostic. Reports on stereotactic core biopsy, a newer technique, indicate that it is also an accurate diagnostic modality.

All diagnostic biopsies should be performed with the assumption that the mammographic abnormality is malignant. Therefore the goal should be to excise the abnormality completely with 1-cm macroscopically clear margins.

Natural History

The natural history of DCIS is incompletely understood because most cases in the past were treated by mastectomy. The best estimation of invasive potential has been obtained from a retrospective review of large biopsy series in which small numbers of DCIS lesions were inadvertently treated by excisional biopsy only. These studies indicate that, over a period of 10–20 years, 25–30% of patients will develop invasive cancer. These studies are clearly biased because the biopsy may have altered the natural history, the lesions were often incidentally found to be low-grade noncomedo DCIS, and the extent and pathologic margins of the lesions were unknown. The majority of invasive recurrences occurred in the same quadrant as the original biopsy. It has been postulated that up to half of invasive recurrences arise from residual invasive foci in the breast not seen on the original biopsy, with the remainder arising from progression of residual DCIS to invasive carcinoma.

The risk to the contralateral breast in patients with DCIS is the same as that in patients with invasive carcinoma. Contralateral DCIS is seen in about 10% of patients followed for 10–20 years after mastectomy for DCIS.

TREATMENT

Little information exists regarding the optimal treatment of the breast in patients with DCIS detected by screening mammography. The present options for treatment of the breast alone are total mastectomy, with consideration of immediate breast reconstruction; segmental mastectomy alone; or segmental mastectomy with postoperative radiotherapy. There is no consensus regarding selection criteria for these different treatments. Still, there is general agreement that axillary dissection is not required for DCIS. The lone exception would be for the uncommonly large (>3 cm), palpable tumors for which the risk of microinvasion with subsequent lymph node metastasis is significant. Patients with DCIS have an excellent long-term prognosis, with reported 5-year overall survival rates of 95–100%, independent of whether the breast was treated by conservative surgery or mastectomy.

Total Mastectomy

The rationale for total mastectomy for DCIS has been the high frequency of multicentricity, the occasional development of occult invasive carcinoma in other quadrants, the likelihood of residual DCIS even after wide local excision, the incidence of local recurrence after wide local excision and radiotherapy, and the potential for the remaining normal ducts to undergo neoplastic change. Mastectomy is an effective treatment for DCIS but is disfiguring and unnecessary for many patients. Mastectomy is, however, recommended for most patients with multicentric lesions. When total mastectomy is considered as a treatment option, immediate breast reconstruction should also be considered.

Segmental Mastectomy

The goal of segmental mastectomy is to excise the mammographic abnormality or palpable mass with pathologically negative margins of 1 cm but maintain optimal cosmesis of the breast. The majority of patients with DCIS detected by screening mammography would be candidates for breast-conserving treatment if tumor size were the sole criterion for determining therapy. The major controversial issue surrounding local excision is when to combine it with irradiation of the breast to reduce local recurrence. Studies of segmental mastectomy alone are difficult to interpret because they have short follow-up, limited patient numbers, differences in surgical technique, lack of interpretation of pathologic margins, and different criteria for patient selection. The rate of invasive local recurrence rates varies widely from 3 to 34%, with higher rates noted in series with symptomatic DCIS. The fact that almost all recurrences occur in the operative field implies that multicentricity plays only a minimal role. Approximately 90% of the patients in these studies who developed a local recurrence after segmental mastectomy were rendered disease-free by total mastectomy. However, the follow-up is too short to comment on the long-term survival of patients who develop local recurrences.

Segmental Mastectomy and Radiotherapy

The rationale for combining postoperative radiotherapy with segmental mastectomy is to prevent local recurrence in the residual breast tissue as a result of residual or multicentric disease. The radiation ports are usually directed to the breast only as tangential opposed fields of megavoltage photons; some institutions support administering a boost dose to the tumor bed as well. The results of several nonrandomized studies support the use of a boost dose, with an overall 50% reduction in local recurrence rates reported, a reduction similar in magnitude to that reported for invasive carcinoma. These studies, however, are limited by small patient numbers, short follow-up, and lack of definition of margins or the extent or indication of grade of disease being treated.

The National Surgical Adjuvant Breast and Bowel Project (NSABP) protocol B-17 compared segmental mastectomy with segmental mastectomy and postoperative radiotherapy. In this prospective randomized study, with a mean follow-up of 43 months, there was a significant disease-free survival advantage for women receiving postoperative radiotherapy. Follow-up was relatively short for determining whether radiotherapy prevents or merely delays the development of recurrent disease.

Unfortunately, no subset analysis of the NSABP B-17 protocol was performed to evaluate whether certain low-risk groups, such as those with small, well-differentiated noncomedo DCIS, could be spared radiotherapy. Segmental mastectomy without radiotherapy is appropriate treatment for patients wanting to avoid radiotherapy, with localized DCIS, and a histology not associated with multifocality or multicentricity. The surgeon must be certain to achieve a negative-margin excision.

There is an increased risk of local recurrence when positive margins, larger lesions, comedo histology, or nipple discharge is present. The fact that local recurrences tend to be of the same histologic subtype suggests that incomplete excision may be the major determinant of local recurrence, which is further evidence supporting the need for negative margins of excision for DCIS. Studies suggest that comedo histology is an independent predictor of local recurrence, although there are several studies that have failed to show this difference. There is a suggestion in studies of conservatively treated patients with DCIS that the comedo subtype may be associated with a shorter interval to local recurrence than noncomedo DCIS.

Adjuvant tamoxifen NSABP protocol B-24 and a British trial will examine the role of tamoxifen in preventing local recurrence as well as the development of metachronous contralateral primary breast cancer. The rationale for these two trials and a third chemoprevention trial (NSABP P1), initiated in 1992, is that patients randomized to receive tamoxifen in NSABP-B14 had a reduced incidence of local recurrence and contralateral breast carcinoma.

MANAGEMENT

The present schema for managing DCIS at M. D. Anderson is outlined in Fig. 1-1.

SURVEILLANCE

Follow-up of patients after conservative surgery with or without radiotherapy involves twice-yearly physical examination and annual mammography for 5 years, with annual physical examination and mammogram thereafter.

Lobular Carcinoma In Situ

LCIS was first recognized as a distinct histologic entity in 1941. During the era that followed, the treatment for LCIS was radical mastectomy, the same as that for invasive carcinoma. Haagensen is credited with altering the treatment philosophy for LCIS. In his review of 211 cases, he noted a 17% incidence of subsequent invasive carcinoma in women diagnosed as having LCIS who were followed by observation only instead of undergoing surgery. The risk of developing a subsequent carcinoma was equal for both breasts, and only six women died of breast cancer. Haagensen concluded that close observation for LCIS allowed for early detection of subsequent malignancy, with associated high cure rates. Haagensen's rationale for observation as a treatment philosophy for LCIS was based on his view that patients with LCIS were at increased risk for developing invasive breast cancer, but that the LCIS itself did not differentiate into a malignancy.

EPIDEMIOLOGY

The true incidence and prevalence of LCIS are difficult to estimate because it is diagnosed as a purely incidental finding. LCIS is not detectable by palpation, gross pathologic examination, or mammography. The incidence of LCIS has risen dramatically in recent years as a result of the increased use of screening mammography and therefore increased number of biopsies of mammographically detected non-LCIS breast abnormalities.

LCIS occurs most commonly in premenopausal women. Ninety percent of the women in Haagensen's series were premenopausal, and most studies have reported mean ages between 45 and 50 years. Estrogens are hypothesized to play an important role in the pathogenesis of LCIS. Postmenopausal regression of LCIS has been noted and may explain the decreased incidence in the elderly. The theory

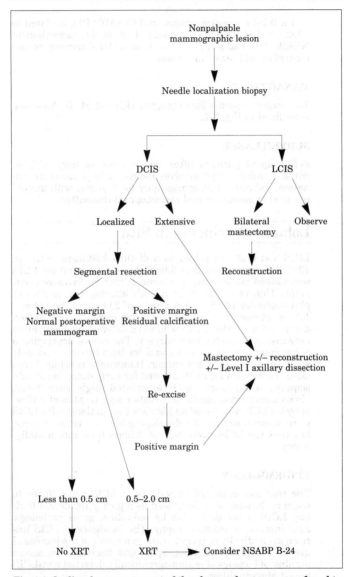

Fig. 1-1. Outline for management of the abnormal mammogram found to be noninvasive breast cancer (nonpalpable lesion). (DCIS = ductal carcinoma in situ; LCIS = lobular carcinoma in situ; XRT = radiotherapy.)

that LCIS represents a marker of increased risk for invasive breast carcinoma is supported by the fact that the mean age at diagnosis precedes that for invasive cancer by 10–15 years.

When the diagnosis of LCIS is established, there is a 0–6% chance that the patient has a synchronous invasive breast lesion. The risk of developing a subsequent invasive lesion has been estimated to be 0.5% per year of follow-up. The invasive malignancies seen in women with LCIS are ductal carcinomas in 60–70% of cases. This provides further evidence supporting the theory that LCIS does not differentiate into invasive carcinoma; if it did, a larger percentage of patients would develop invasive lobular carcinoma. The tumors that develop in women with LCIS are no more aggressive than invasive breast carcinomas not associated with LCIS.

PATHOLOGY

LCIS is characterized by an intraepithelial proliferation of the terminal lobular-ductal unit. The cells are slightly larger and paler than the cells normally lining the acini, but the lobular architecture is maintained. The cells have a homogeneous morphology and do not display prominent chromatin. There is a normal cytoplasm to nucleus ratio, with infrequent mitoses and no necrosis. The basement membrane is not penetrated by any of the proliferating cells.

The diagnosis of LCIS involves the differentiation of LCIS from other forms of benign disease and from invasive lesions. In the absence of the well-defined regularity described for LCIS, *atypical lobular hyperplasia* becomes the designated pathologic term. Papillomatosis in the terminal ducts may have the appearance of LCIS but lacks the characteristic involvement of the acini. DCIS may extend retrograde into the acini but has a more characteristic anaplastic cell morphology. The distinction of LCIS from invasive lobular carcinoma is based on LCIS's lack of penetration of the basement membrane.

Numerous studies have documented the multifocal and multicentric nature of LCIS. If diligently searched for, multiple foci can be located elsewhere in the breast in almost all cases. In addition, LCIS is identified in the contralateral breast in 50–90% of cases. Thus, the presence of LCIS reflects a phenotypic manifestation of a generalized abnormality present throughout both breasts. As a result, the treatment of LCIS should be directed not at the index lesion but at both breasts.

DIAGNOSIS

Clinical Presentation

Because LCIS is not detectable by physical examination or mammography, it is most commonly diagnosed as an incidental finding in a breast biopsy specimen. Therefore the clinical presentation of patients with LCIS is identical to that of patients requiring breast biopsy for fibroadenoma, benign duct disease, DCIS, and invasive breast cancer.

TREATMENT

There are two treatment options for women with LCIS. Most patients should be followed by close observation, as recommended by Haagensen. The only surgical procedure that removes all tissue at risk for developing subsequent invasive disease is bilateral mastectomy. Since there is no risk of regional metastasis, axillary dissection is not required. Breast reconstruction should be considered at the time of mastectomy. Contralateral mirror-image breast biopsy, a procedure often advocated for LCIS, has fallen out of favor because an ipsilateral mastectomy and a negative mirror-image biopsy do not eliminate the need for close observation of the residual breast tissue.

Adjuvant therapy for LCIS is not indicated. However, because LCIS is a marker of high risk for the development of invasive breast cancer, patients with LCIS may be included in the NSABP chemoprevention trial (NSABP P-1). This trial is designed to evaluate the ability of tamoxifen to reduce the incidence of breast carcinoma in high-risk patients.

Selected References

Alpers CE, Wellings SR. The prevalence of carcinoma in situ in normal and cancer-associated breasts. *Hum Pathol* 16:796, 1985.

Bornstein BA, Recht A, Connolly JL, et al. Results of treating ductal carcinoma-in-situ of the breast with conservative surgery and radiation therapy. *Cancer* 67:7, 1991.

Fisher BF, Constantino J, Redmond C, et al. Lumpectomy compared with lumpectomy and radiation therapy for the treatment of intraductal breast cancer. *N Engl J Med* 328:1581, 1993.

Fisher ER, Leeming R, Anderson S, et al. Conservative management of intraductal carcinoma (DCIS) of the breast. Collaborating NSABP Investigators. *J Surg Oncol* 47:139, 1991.

Frykberg ER, Bland KI. In situ breast carcinoma. *Adv Surg* 26:29, 1993.

Haagensen CD, Lane N, Lattes R, et al. Lobular neoplasia (so-called lobular carcinoma *in situ*) of the breast. *Cancer* 42:737, 1978.

Holland R, Connolly JL, Gelman R, et al. The presence of an extensive intraductal component following a limited excision correlates with the prominent residual disease in the remainder of the breast. *J Clin Oncol* 8:113 1990.

Holland R, Hendriks JH, Verbeek AM, et al. Extent, distribution, and mammographic/histological correlations of breast ductal carcinoma-in-situ. *Lancet* 335:519, 1990.

Lagios MD, Margolin FR, Westdahl PR, et al. Mammographically detected duct carcinoma-in-situ. Frequency of local
recurrence following tylectomy and prognostic effect of
nuclear grade on local recurrence. *Cancer* 63:618, 1989.

Page DL, Dupont WD, Rogers LW, et al. Intraductal carcinoma
of the breast. Follow-up after biopsy only. *Cancer* 49:751,
1982.

Page DL, Kidd TE Jr., Dupont WD, et al. Lobular neoplasia of
the breast: Higher risk for subsequent invasive cancer predicted by more extensive disease. *Hum Pathol* 22:1232, 1991.

Price P, Sinnett HD, Gusterson B, et al. Duct carcinoma-in-situ:
Predictors of local recurrence and progression in patients
treated by surgery alone. *Br J Cancer* 61:869, 1990.

Recht A, Danoff BS, Solin LJ, et al. Intraductal carcinoma of the
breast: Results of treatment with excisional biopsy and irradiation. *J Clin Oncol* 3:1339, 1985.

Salvadori B, Bartoli C, Zurrida S, et al. Risk of invasive cancer
in women with lobular carcinoma *in situ* of the breast. *Eur J
Cancer* 27:35, 1991.

Schwartz GF, Finkel GC, Garcia JC, et al. Subclinical ductal carcinoma in situ of the breast. *Cancer* 70:2468, 1992.

Solin LJ, Fowble BL, Schultz JY, et al. Definitive irradiation for
intraductal carcinoma of the breast. *Int J Radiat Oncol Biol
Phys* 19: 843, 1990.

Stotter AT, McNeese M, Oswald MJ, et al. The role of limited
surgery with irradiation in primary treatment of ductal in-
situ breast cancer. *Int J Radiat Oncol Biol Phys* 18:283, 1990.

Van Dongen JA, Holland R, Peterse JL, et al. Ductal carcinoma
in-situ of the breast; Second EORTC Consensus Meeting. *Eur
J Cancer* 28:626, 1992.

Walt AJ, Simon M, Swanson M. The Continuing dilemma of lobular carcinoma in situ. *Arch Surg* 127:904, 1992.

Zafrani B, Fourquet A, Vilcoq JR, et al. Conservative management of intraductal breast carcinoma with tumorectomy and
radiation therapy. *Cancer* 57:1299, 1986.

Invasive Breast Cancer

Steven D. Leach, Barry W. Feig, and
David H. Berger

Epidemiology

Breast cancer has become a leading health concern in the
United States: 12% of American women will be diagnosed
with breast cancer during their lifetimes, and 3.5% will die
of the disease. Breast cancer incidence rates have been
steadily increasing since the start of data collection in the
1930s. In Connecticut, which has one of the oldest cancer
registries in the country, the incidence of breast cancer rose
by 1.2% per year from 1940 to 1982. According to the
National Cancer Institute Surveillance, Epidemiology, and
End Results Program (SEER), the incidence of breast cancer
increased by 33% from 1973 to 1988. Because the breast cancer incidence rate increased by only 3% from 1973 to 1980,
the majority of the increase occurred during the 1980s, indicating that this dramatic rise may be related to the increased
use of mammographic screening during that time. If screening, and therefore increased detection, is responsible for the
dramatic rise in incidence, a plateau should occur over the
next few years.

Breast cancer is the leading cause of death among American
women 40–55 years of age. The incidence of breast cancer
increases rapidly during the fourth decade of life and
becomes substantial before age 50. After menopause, the
incidence continues to rise but at a much slower rate. In
spite of an increasing incidence, the mortality from breast
cancer has remained relatively stable over the past several
decades. This may be due to either a shift towards a more
benign form of the disease, earlier detection of disease, or
advances in treatment. Among women younger than 50
years of age, breast cancer mortality has declined by 12%,
while it has increased by 5% among women 50 years of age
and older.

Risk Factors

The most important risk factor for the development of breast
cancer is sex. The female to male ratio for breast cancer is
100:1. We therefore focus on risk factors related to the development of breast cancer in women.

Age is another important risk factor for the development of
breast cancer. The risk that breast cancer will develop in a
white American woman in a single year increases from
1:5,900 at age 30 to 1:290 at age 80.

Any *family history* of breast cancer increases a woman's risk
of developing breast cancer. However, in most cases the

increased risk is negligible. A more important increase in risk is associated with the presence of breast cancer in a first-degree relative. For a 30-year-old woman with a sister who had bilateral breast cancer before age 50, the cumulative probability of developing breast cancer by age 70 is 55%. This cumulative probability decreases to 8% for a woman whose sister developed unilateral breast cancer after age 50. The overall risk depends on the number of relatives with cancer, their ages at diagnosis, and whether the disease was unilateral or bilateral.

There has recently been a great deal of research into potential *genetic lesions* responsible for the increased risk associated with familial breast cancer. Women with Li-Fraumeni syndrome, a rare disorder in which patients have a germline mutation in the tumor suppressor gene *P53*, invariably develop breast carcinoma in addition to other types of tumors. Evidence suggests that a gene located on chromosome 17q known as BRCA-1 is responsible for early-onset (familial) breast cancer. Women who have inherited germline mutations in this gene have a cumulative probability of developing breast cancer approaching 100%. However, it is important to remember that genetic breast cancer accounts for less than 3% of all breast cancers.

Prior breast cancer is a significant risk factor for the development of cancer in the contralateral breast, with an incidence of 0.5–1.0% per year of follow-up.

Benign breast disease itself is not a risk factor for the subsequent development of breast cancer. Only patients with a proliferative histologic pattern and *atypical hyperplasia* are at substantially increased risk of developing breast cancer. Their relative risk is 4.4 when compared to patients without atypical hyperplasia.

A number of *endogenous endocrine factors* have been implicated as risk factors in breast cancer, including age at menarche, age at menopause, parity, and age at first full-term pregnancy. The cumulative duration of menstruation also may be important. Women who menstruate for more than 30 years are at increased risk compared with women who menstruate for fewer than 30 years. The risk of breast cancer for women who experience menopause after age 55 is twice that of women who experience menopause prior to age 44. Although age at menarche is important, age at onset of regular menses may be even more critical. Women who have regular ovulatory cycles before age 13 have a fourfold increased risk compared with women whose menarche occurred after age 13 and who had a 5-year delay to the development of regular cycles. Age at first birth has a greater impact on risk than the number of pregnancies, with a woman who had her first child before age 19 having half the risk of a nulliparous woman. Interestingly, women who have their first child between 30 and 34 years of age have the same risk as nulliparous women, whereas women who have their first child after age 35 have an increased risk compared with nulliparous women. These observations indicate that the hormonal milieu at different times in a woman's life may impact on her risk of breast cancer.

Exogenous hormone use has been associated with an increased risk of breast cancer. The use of postmenopausal estrogen replacement appears to increase the risk of breast cancer by about 40%. The increased risk among current users is concentrated among older women who have been taking them for a long time. There does not appear to be an increased risk of breast cancer in women who have stopped taking estrogen supplements. Additionally, when all potential causes of death are taken into account (i.e., acute myocardial infarction and stroke), estrogen therapy appears to decrease the overall mortality rate among older women. There has been no statistically significant increase in breast cancer risk with the use of oral contraceptives. However, prolonged use (longer than 10 years) may be associated with an increased risk of breast cancer in women younger than 45 years of age.

Although exposure to *ionizing radiation* between ages 13 and 30 can substantially increase the risk of breast cancer, exposure to clinically significant levels is rare.

Obesity is not an important risk factor for breast cancer. Among premenopausal women, obesity is associated with a decreased incidence of breast cancer. In postmenopausal women, there is a clinically unimportant association of obesity with breast cancer. Despite the fact that a high-fat diet promotes mammary tumors in animals, only weak or nonexistent associations have been observed in human studies.

Alcohol consumption, even at the level of one drink per day, has been associated with an increased risk of breast cancer. At least one study suggests that alcohol consumed before age 30 is more important in determining a woman's risk than is alcohol consumed later in life.

Pathology

Invasive carcinomas of the breast tend to be histologically heterogeneous tumors. Overwhelmingly, these tumors are adenocarcinomas that arise from the terminal ducts. There are five common histologic variants of mammary adenocarcinoma.

1. *Infiltrating ductal carcinoma* accounts for 75% of all breast cancers. This lesion is characterized by the absence of special histologic features. The lesion is hard when palpated and gritty when transected. It is often associated with various degrees of fibrotic response. Often there is associated ductal carcinoma in situ (DCIS) within the specimen. Infiltrating ductal carcinomas commonly metastasize to axillary lymph nodes. The prognosis for patients with these

tumors is poorer than that for patients with some of the special histologic subtypes. Distant metastases are found most often in the bones, lungs, liver, and brain.

2. *Infiltrating lobular carcinoma* is seen in 5–10% of breast cancer cases. Clinically this lesion often presents as an area of ill-defined thickening within the breast. Microscopically, small cells in a single-file arrangement are seen. Infiltrating lobular cancers have a tendency to grow around ducts and lobules. Multicentricity is observed more frequently in infiltrating lobular carcinoma than in infiltrating ductal carcinoma. The prognosis for lobular carcinoma is similar to that of infiltrating ductal carcinoma. Lobular carcinoma is known to metastasize to unusual sites, such as meninges and serosal surfaces, more often than do other forms of breast cancer.

3. *Tubular carcinoma* accounts for only 2% of all breast carcinomas. The diagnosis of tubular carcinoma is made only when more than 75% of the tumor demonstrates tubule formation. Axillary nodal metastases are uncommon with this type of tumor. The prognosis for patients with tubular carcinoma is considerably better than that for patients with other types of breast cancer.

4. *Medullary carcinoma* accounts for 5–7% of tumors. Grossly, medullary carcinomas are well circumscribed. Histologically, they are characterized by poorly differentiated nuclei, syncytial growth pattern, a well-circumscribed border, intense infiltration with small lymphocytes and plasma cells, and little or no DCIS. The prognosis for patients with medullary carcinoma is favorable only if all of these characteristics are present.

5. *Mucinous or colloid carcinoma* constitutes approximately 3% of all breast cancers. It is characterized by an abundant accumulation of extracellular mucin surrounding clusters of tumor cells. Colloid carcinoma is slow-growing and tends to be bulky. If a breast carcinoma is predominantly mucinous, the prognosis is favorable.

There are several rarer special histologic types of breast malignancy, including papillary, apocrine, secretory, squamous cell, spindle cell, cystosarcoma phylloides, and carcinosarcoma. Infiltrating ductal carcinomas will occasionally have small areas containing one or more of these special histologic types. Tumors with these mixed histologies behave similarly to pure infiltrating ductal cancers.

Staging

Typically breast cancer is staged using the American Joint Committee on Cancer (AJCC) guidelines. The TNM classifications and stage groupings for breast cancer are summarized in Table 2-1.

Table 2-1. Current AJCC TNM classification and stage grouping for breast carcinoma

TNM classification		Stage grouping			
Primary tumor (T)					
TX	Primary tumor cannot be assessed	Stage 0	Tis	N0	M0
T0	No evidence of primary tumor	Stage I	T1	N0	M0
Tis	Carcinoma in situ	Stage IIa	T0	N1	M0
T1	Tumor ≤2 cm in greatest dimension		T1	N1	M0
			T2	N0	M0
T2	Tumor >2 cm but <5 cm	Stage IIb	T2	N1	M0
T3	Tumor >5 cm		T3	N0	M0
T4	Tumor of any size with direct extension to chest wall or skin; includes inflammatory carcinoma	Stage IIIa	T0	N2	M0
			T1	N2	M0
			T2	N2	M0
			T3	N1, 2	M0
Regional lymph nodes (N)					
NX	Regional lymph nodes cannot be assessed	Stage IIIb	T4	Any N	M0
N0	No regional lymph node metastases		Any T	N3	M0
N1	Metastasis to movable ipsilateral axillary lymph node(s)	Stage IV	Any T	Any N	M1
N2	Metastases to ipsilateral axillary lymph nodes fixed to one another or to other structures				
N3	Metastasis to ipsilateral internal mammary lymph nodes				
Distant metastasis (M)					
MX	Presence of distant metastasis cannot be assessed				
M0	No distant metastasis				
M1	Distant metastasis (includes ipsilateral supraclavicular node(s)				

Diagnosis

HISTORY AND PHYSICAL EXAMINATION

The way breast cancer is diagnosed has undergone a dramatic evolution since the mid-1980s. Traditionally, 50–75% of all breast cancers were detected by self-examination. Subsequent to the widespread availability of mammographic screening programs, there has been a shift towards the diagnosis of clinically occult, nonpalpable lesions. In spite of this trend, evaluation of the woman with potential breast cancer continues to be based on a careful history and physical examination.

The history is directed at assessing cancer risk as well as establishing the presence or absence of symptoms potentially related to breast disease. It should include the age of menarche, menopausal status, previous pregnancy, and use of oral contraceptives or postmenopausal replacement estrogens. A prior personal history of breast cancer is of obvious importance. In addition, careful documentation of a family history of breast cancer in first-degree relatives (i.e., mother or sister) should be sought.

In addition to determining cancer risk, the history should establish the presence or absence of specific symptoms potentially referable to breast cancer. It is worthwhile to inquire about breast pain and nipple discharge, although these symptoms are more commonly associated with benign processes, including fibrocystic disease and intraductal papilloma. Malaise, boney pain, and weight loss may all be indicators of metastatic disease.

Physical examination of patients with potential breast cancer must constantly take into consideration the comfort and emotional well-being of the patient. Adequate privacy measures and good lighting are mandatory. Examination is initiated by careful visual inspection with the patient sitting upright. Nipple changes, gross asymmetry, and obvious masses are all noted. The skin must be carefully inspected for subtle changes; these can range from slight dimpling to the more dramatic peau d'orange appearance associated with locally advanced or inflammatory breast cancer.

Following careful inspection, and with the patient still sitting, the supraclavicular fossae are examined for potential nodal disease. Both axillae are then carefully palpated. If palpable, nodes should be characterized as to their number, size, and whether they are mobile or fixed. Examination of the axilla always includes palpation of the axillary tail of the breast; assessment of this area is often overlooked once the patient is placed in a supine position.

Palpation of the breast parenchyma itself is accomplished with the patient in a supine position and the ipsilateral arm placed over the head. The subareolar tissues and each quadrant of both breasts are systematically palpated. Dominant masses are noted with respect to their size, shape, location, consistency, and mobility. With experience, the examiner can begin to predict that the spherical, rubbery, movable mass occurring in a 25-year-old woman will prove to be a fibroadenoma, and that the less circumscribed, firm, fixed lesion in a 50-year-old patient will likely prove malignant.

When subjected to critical analysis, however, physical examination often proves to be inadequate in differentiating benign from malignant breast masses. Various series have identified a 20–40% error rate, even among experienced examiners. Given this rate of inaccuracy, any persistent dominant breast mass occurring in a patient older than age 30 requires additional evaluation.

EVALUATION OF THE PALPABLE BREAST MASS

The choice of initial evaluation following the detection of a dominant breast mass should be individualized for each patient according to age, perceived cancer risk, and characteristics of the lesion in question. For most patients, mammographic evaluation is an important initial step. Mammography in this setting serves two purposes: (1) the risk of malignancy for the palpable lesion is further assessed, and (2) both breasts are screened for nonpalpable lesions. Bilateral synchronous cancers occur in about 3% of all cases; at least half of these lesions are nonpalpable.

For a palpable lesion, mammography may demonstrate the stellate or spiculated appearance typical of malignancy. Calcifications, nipple changes, and axillary adenopathy also may be visualized. Together, the presence or absence of these mammographic findings can predict malignancy with an overall accuracy of 70–80%. Mammography is least accurate in younger patients with dense breasts; it is rarely applied in patients under the age of 30.

Following mammographic evaluation, palpable masses suspected to be malignant should undergo fine-needle aspiration. Some clinicians advocate needle aspiration at the time of initial evaluation, prior to mammography. For most patients, we prefer to delay fine-needle aspiration until after mammographic examination is completed, as a needle puncture hematoma will occasionally confuse future radiographic evaluation. For young patients with dense breasts in whom mammography is not contemplated, needle aspiration remains an ideal primary mode of evaluation.

Fine-needle aspiration with a 22-gauge needle allows for accurate differentiation between cystic and solid masses (mammography is typically not useful in this regard) and also provides material for cytologic examination. Benign breast cysts typically yield nonbloody fluid and become nonpalpable after aspiration. Only bloody fluid need be submitted for cytologic analysis. In several large series, the incidence of malignancy among breast cysts is typically 1%; this is limited almost exclusively to those cysts that yield bloody fluid or have a residual mass following aspiration. Aspiration is often curative; only one in five breast cysts will recur following aspiration, and the majority of these are obliterated with a second drainage.

For solid lesions, several passes through the lesion with the syringe under constant negative pressure will typically yield ample material for cytologic evaluation. The material is evacuated onto a microscopic slide and immediately fixed in 95% ethanol. Multiple reports have demonstrated this technique to be simple, safe, and accurate in evaluating benign and malignant breast masses. Accuracy rates typically approach 90% and may allow benign lesions to be carefully followed without open biopsy. For lesions interpreted as malignant, fine-needle aspiration is unable to differentiate between in situ and invasive carcinoma. Most clinicians would defer definitive treatment plans until after confirmation by open biopsy.

Although physical examination, mammography, and fine-needle aspiration all carry significant error rates when used as single modalities, the combination of these three investigations has proven extremely accurate in predicting whether a palpable lesion is benign or malignant. In one combined review, the false-negative rate when all three evaluations indicated a benign lesion was only 3 out of 457 (0.7%); when all three evaluations predicted malignancy, the false-positive rate was 1 out of 239 (0.4%). For lesions with equivocal or contradictory results, open biopsy remains mandatory.

EVALUATION OF NONPALPABLE LESIONS

Because of the increasing availability of mammographic screening programs, there has been a rapid increase in the diagnosis of nonpalpable breast cancer in the United States. Analysis of SEER data demonstrated a 213% increase in the age-adjusted incidence of DCIS among white women between the years 1983 and 1989, and a 140% increase in the incidence of node-negative invasive lesions smaller than 1 cm in diameter. During this same period, cancers larger than 2 cm in diameter or associated with distant metastases have undergone a substantial decrease in incidence. Although these changes in the relative incidence of early and late lesions have not yet translated into changes in SEER breast cancer mortality, other studies have demonstrated the efficacy of screening mammography in preventing deaths from breast cancer. Among screened populations, breast cancer mortality appears to be reduced by approximately 30–40%, although the benefit of screening patients younger than age 50 remains controversial. Currently, the American Cancer Society recommends yearly screening mammography and clinical breast examination for all women 50 years and older.

Mammographic signs of malignancy can be divided into two main categories: microcalcifications and density changes. Microcalcifications can be either clustered or scattered; density changes include discrete masses, architectural distortions, and asymmetries. Mammographic findings most predictive of malignancy include spiculated masses with associated architectural distortion, clustered microcalcifications in a linear or branching array, or the combination of microcalcifications with a mass. For nonpalpable lesions, the mammographic prediction of malignancy is associated with a 15–30% risk of biopsy-documented cancer.

Once screening mammography demonstrates a suspicious lesion, further evaluation is mandated. For lesions interpreted as "probably benign" (well-defined, solitary masses), careful counseling and repeat mammography in 6 months may be undertaken in low-risk patients. For appropriate lesions, additional examination using ultrasonography may identify a subset of cystic lesions that will not require biopsy. For most suspicious lesions, breast biopsy is required. In some centers, mammography-guided stereotactic breast biopsy has emerged as a useful technique for nonpalpable lesions. Similarly, ultrasound-guided fine-needle aspiration may be used in this setting. Ultrasound-guided biopsy is not useful in the evaluation of microcalcifications; these are typically not sonographically visible. In spite of these newer techniques, in most centers excisional breast biopsy following needle localization remains the evaluation of choice for nonpalpable lesions identified by screening mammography.

BREAST BIOPSY TECHNIQUE

For either palpable or nonpalpable lesions, planning an optimal biopsy mandates careful consideration of at least three issues. First, the biopsy site may require future re-excision, even under a strategy of breast conservation. Second, the biopsy site must be incorporated into a future mastectomy incision should this form of treatment be chosen. Third, the biopsy must be constructed in a cosmetically optimal manner. *All* breast biopsies should be performed with the assumption that the target lesion is malignant.

Biopsies are typically performed in an outpatient setting using local anesthesia. In general, curvilinear incisions placed parallel to Langer's lines should be used. Radial scars are generally avoided, except in the extreme medial aspect of the breast where mastectomy incisions become radially oriented; lesions in the inner-lower quadrant are often best approached through a radial incision. Circumareolar incisions have obvious cosmetic advantage but carry the potential disadvantage of leading to sacrifice of areolar tissue should re-excision be required for any reason. While a modest amount of peripheral "tunneling" is acceptable to maintain an incision within a potential mastectomy scar, extreme tunneling to the periphery of the breast from a central peri-areolar incision makes it virtually impossible to identify the tumor bed should re-excision be required, and also exposes an inordinate amount of breast tissue to potential contamination by tumor cells. In patients in whom breast conservation with axillary dissection is contemplated, the biopsy site should *not* be contiguous with the axillary incision; separating these incisions may prevent tumor seeding of a previously negative axilla and avoid the need to irradiate a dissected axilla.

The excisional breast biopsy should serve both diagnostic and local treatment purposes. Dissection should be performed sharply with little or no application of electrocautery, as steroid hormone receptors are heat labile. For palpable lesions, the placement of clamps on the tumor to facilitate the dissection should be avoided; this can lead to tumor disruption and dissemination of malignant cells. Instead, a figure-of-eight traction suture may be applied. The entire mass and a surrounding 1-cm rim of normal tissue should be excised. In so doing, the excisional biopsy will fulfill the requirements for "lumpectomy" and allow subsequent re-excision to be avoided.

For nonpalpable lesions, preoperative needle localization with a self-retaining hook-wire is required. This procedure requires careful communication between radiologist and surgeon. For most lesions, the localizing needle is placed under mammographic guidance into the breast via the shortest direct path to the lesion. The self-retaining wire is placed through the needle, and the needle is removed. Postlocalization mammograms are then reviewed. Biopsy is undertaken with excision of a core of target breast tissue surrounding the wire tip. For superficial lesions, an ellipse of skin at the point of wire insertion may be removed en bloc with the underlying breast tissue. Postexcision specimen mammograms are essential to confirm successful biopsy.

Once the biopsy specimen has been excised, careful handling is critical. The surgeon should meticulously note the orientation of the excised breast tissue and hand-deliver the specimen to the pathology department. The lateral, medial, superior, inferior, superficial, and deep margins should be inked in a color-coded manner. For palpable lesions, material should be processed for receptor analysis and flow cytometry. Tissue to be assayed for steroid hormones should be rapidly frozen, as both estrogen and progesterone receptor concentrations have been shown to decline rapidly with warm ischemic time.

Closure of the biopsy incision must involve meticulous hemostasis. Deep parenchymal sutures often cause cosmetically unpleasing distortion of the residual breast and should be avoided. Drains are generally not used. The skin is closed with a subcuticular suture, and a light dressing is placed. Breast support is mandatory for the first 48 hours postoperatively.

Pretreatment Evaluation

Once the diagnosis of breast cancer has been made, appropriate treatment planning involves some evaluation for the possibility of metastatic disease. For patients with stage I or stage II breast cancer, this is typically limited to complete history and physical examination, a chest radiograph, and evaluation of serum liver chemistries. The routine use of bone scans in asymptomatic patients with early-stage breast cancer carries an extremely low yield; several series have demonstrated only a 2% incidence of positive scans in this setting. In contrast, up to 25% of asymptomatic patients with apparent stage III cancer demonstrate positive bone scans; routine scanning in this population appears worthwhile. In the absence of elevated serum liver chemistries or palpable hepatomegaly, liver imaging is similarly not routinely applied in the preoperative evaluation of patients with early-stage disease.

Treatment

Many of the current recommendations regarding therapy for invasive breast cancer have been influenced by the results of randomized, prospective clinical trials performed by the National Surgical Adjuvant Breast and Bowel Project (NSABP). A selected summary of these trials is presented in Table 2-2.

MICROINVASIVE BREAST CANCER

The diagnosis of microinvasive breast cancer has increased with the use of routine screening mammography. The incidence of this disease is difficult to determine because of overlap in the pathologic definition of microinvasion. The most accurate description is that of DCIS with limited microscopic stromal invasion below the basement membrane in one or several ducts, but not invading more than 10% of the surface of the histologic sections examined. Five to ten percent of patients with noninvasive breast cancer will be noted to have an area of microinvasion present on careful pathologic examination. The significance of the finding of a microscopic focal area of invasion is uncertain. The presence of lymph node metastasis associated with this diagnosis has been documented in 0–10% of all cases. Not surprisingly, those authors finding a low incidence of microinvasion deem an axillary lymph node dissection unnecessary for these patients. Most authors would agree that an axillary dissection is warranted in patients with an anticipated risk of lymph node metastasis of 10% or more, in order to accurately stage these patients.

At the University of Texas M. D. Anderson Cancer Center, we do not base the decision to perform an axillary dissection solely on the finding of a focal area of microinvasion. Other prognostic factors that need to be assessed are age, histology, hormone receptor status, and family history. An informed decision based on the risks and benefits of an axillary dissection is then made by the patient and physician. In most cases, patients with a single focus of microinvasion are adequately treated by simple excision.

Table 2-2. Selected summary of NSABP therapeutic trials for invasive breast cancer

Trial	Treatments	Outcome
NSABP B-04	Total mastectomy vs. total mastectomy with XRT vs. radical mastectomy	No difference in disease-free or overall survival
NSABP B-06	Total mastectomy vs. lumpectomy vs. lumpectomy with XRT	No difference in disease-free or overall survival; addition of XRT to lumpectomy reduced local recurrence rate from 39% to 10%
NSABP B-13	Surgery alone vs. surgery plus adjuvant chemotherapy in node-negative patients with ER-negative tumors	Improved disease-free survival for adjuvant chemotherapy group
NSABP B-14	Surgery alone vs. surgery plus adjuvant tamoxifen in node-negative patients with ER-positive tumors	Improved disease-free survival for adjuvant tamoxifen group
NSABP B-21	Adjuvant tamoxifen vs. tamoxifen plus XRT vs. placebo plus XRT for locally excised node-negative tumors <1 cm in diameter	Ongoing

ER = estrogen receptor; XRT = radiotherapy.

EARLY-STAGE BREAST CANCER (T1–T2, N0–N1)

About 75% of patients with breast cancer present with tumors less than 5 cm in diameter and no evidence of fixed or matted nodes. These patients with early-stage breast cancer are generally treated by one of three surgical options: (1) breast conservation surgery with irradiation, (2) modified radical mastectomy, or (3) modified radical mastectomy with either immediate or delayed reconstruction. With careful patient selection, the goal of maintaining either a conserved or reconstructed breast can be achieved in the majority of cases.

Breast Conservation versus Mastectomy

It is now clear that many patients with breast cancer can be effectively treated with breast conservation. Since 1970, seven different prospective randomized trials comparing breast conservation strategies to radical or modified radical mastectomy have failed to demonstrate any survival benefit to the more aggressive approach. Among these trials, the two most widely known were conducted by Veronesi, et al., at the National Cancer Institute in Milan, Italy, and by Fisher, et al., in conjunction with the NSABP in the United States. The Milan trial was limited to patients with stage I breast cancer (tumor <2 cm, negative axillary nodes) and compared radical mastectomy to a breast conservation strategy involving quadrantectomy, axillary dissection, and radiotherapy. No differences in local control, disease-free survival, or overall survival have been noted.

NSABP trial B-06 examined an expanded patient population that included women with primary tumors up to 4 cm in diameter and either N0 or N1 nodal status. Patients were randomized to one of three treatment strategies: modified radical mastectomy, lumpectomy with axillary dissection and radiotherapy, or lumpectomy and axillary dissection alone. Histologically negative margins were required in the breast conservation groups. Again, there were no differences in disease-free survival or overall survival among the three groups. Local recurrence, however, was markedly reduced by the addition of radiotherapy to lumpectomy and axillary dissection (10% versus 39% at 8 years). These results upheld breast conservation as appropriate treatment for patients with stage I or stage II breast cancer and made it clear that radiotherapy is required as an integral part of any breast conservation strategy. At the M. D. Anderson Cancer Center, we typically initiate radiotherapy 2–3 weeks following surgery. A dose of 50 Gy is given through tangential ports using computerized dosimetry.

Although it is clear that breast conservation is equal to mastectomy for patients with stage I or II disease, the decision to embark on a treatment strategy involving breast conservation must be individualized for each patient. Numerous factors contribute to this decision. The patient's motivation and commitment to breast conservation must be strong, as daily outpatient radiation treatments over 5–6 weeks are required. The patient also must be willing to accept the risk of a 10% local recurrence rate within the conserved breast.

Other factors contributing to the choice between mastectomy and breast conservation surgery include the size of the breast, tumor size, tumor histology, and patient age. For extremely small breasts, the cosmetic result may be unacceptable following local excision, especially for larger lesions. For large pendulous breasts, lack of uniformity in radiation dosing may result in unattractive fibrosis and retraction. Patients with either extreme may benefit from a strategy of mastectomy and reconstruction, occasionally coupled with surgical augmentation or reduction of the contralateral breast. Patients with larger tumors also might be best served by mastectomy. At this point, there are no data to suggest that T3 lesions are adequately treated by breast conservation. From a purely practical point of view, local excision of such lesions rarely results in a cosmetically acceptable result. The ability of preoperative chemotherapy to downstage these tumors to the point where breast conservation may be undertaken remains an intriguing approach.

A number of attempts have been made to identify patients with a high rate of local recurrence following breast conservation based on the histology of the primary tumor. To date, there have been no documented differences in local recurrence among the various histologic subtypes. There is a suggestion, however, that invasive tumors with an extensive intraductal component carry an increased risk of local recurrence following breast conservation surgery. This risk is amplified for patients less than age 35. For patients younger than 35 with an extensive intraductal component, the local recurrence rate exceeds 50% at 10 years. Such patients should be counseled to undergo mastectomy and reconstruction.

Axillary Dissection

A substantial portion of patients with breast cancer present with axillary nodal metastases, even in the setting of a clinically N0 axilla. In one series, 17% of patients with clinically T1N0 disease had histologically positive nodes; this figure rose to 27% for patients with clinically T2N0 disease. For either breast conservation surgery or modified radical mastectomy, axillary dissection remains an important component and a source of significant potential morbidity. It is clear that axillary dissection contributes little to overall survival but remains important for staging and local control.

The contribution of axillary dissection to local control is small but measurable. In NSABP trial B-04 comparing radical mastectomy to simple mastectomy with and without radiation, 40% of patients with clinically negative axillae were found to have positive nodes at the time of radical mastectomy, and 1% of these patients eventually failed in the axilla. In patients with unoperated axillae, 18% (65 out of 365) eventually developed clinical adenopathy requiring delayed axillary dissection. Four of these patients eventually failed in the axilla in spite of delayed dissection. No survival disadvantage was seen for patients undergoing delayed versus immediate axillary dissection. Radiation was less effective than axillary dissection in preventing eventual failure in the axilla; this was especially true for patients with clinically positive nodes.

In addition to contributing to local control, axillary dissection provides important staging and prognostic information. As noted above, clinical staging of the axilla remains relatively inaccurate. However, nodal status remains a major predictor of outcome. For all patients with node-negative cancer, at least a 70% 10-year survival rate may be anticipated. This drops to 40% for patients with 1–3 positive nodes, and less than 20% for patients with 4–10 positive nodes. Micrometastatic disease (<2 mm in diameter) carries a better prognosis than macrometastatic disease. Independent of its contribution to subsequent treatment decisions, axillary dissection thus provides important prognostic information for the woman with breast cancer. As discussed below with regard to adjuvant chemotherapy, the contribution of axillary dissection to subsequent treatment planning is currently in flux.

We currently recommend axillary dissection for all patients undergoing either breast conservation surgery or mastectomy for T1 or T2 lesions. As discussed below, exceptions to this policy may include patients for whom adjuvant therapy will be offered regardless of nodal status. For patients undergoing breast conservation, axillary dissection should be performed via a separate axillary incision that does not extend anterior to the pectoralis fold. To provide adequate prognostic information, at least 10 lymph nodes should be examined. The technique of axillary "sampling" is poorly defined and provides an uncertain yield of nodes. More formal axillary dissection should be directed towards en bloc removal of level I and level II nodal tissue. The addition of level III nodes to the dissection often requires division or resection of the pectoralis minor muscle and is of little benefit with respect to staging; only 1% of all patients show level III involvement in the absence of level I or II disease. On the other hand, level III dissections carry a substantially higher risk of subsequent lymphedema, especially if radiotherapy is used. The level I and II axillary dissection should preserve the long thoracic and thoracodorsal nerves and avoid stripping of the axillary vein. A closed-suction drain is placed and removed during the first outpatient visit.

Breast Reconstruction

For patients not undergoing breast conservation, breast reconstruction should be considered a standard component of cancer therapy. Reconstruction may involve autologous tissue, synthetic implants, or a combination of both. While satisfactory results can be obtained with either immediate or delayed reconstruction, we favor immediate reconstruction for the majority of patients. Immediate reconstruction carries a substantial psychological benefit for many women and often allows for a better cosmetic result. The initiation of adjuvant chemotherapy is not significantly delayed, and concerns that local recurrence may go undetected in a reconstructed breast are not well founded, especially for T1 and T2 lesions.

In our institution, 50% of all patients treated with mastectomy undergo immediate reconstruction; while the method of reconstruction is individualized for each patient, either traditional or free transverse rectus abdominus myocutaneous (TRAM) flaps are most commonly used. Contralateral augmentation or reduction may be performed to maximize symmetry. For premenopausal women with a perceived high risk for a contralateral second primary lesion, simultaneous contralateral mastectomy with bilateral free TRAM flap reconstruction is increasingly used. We typically perform a skin-sparing mastectomy in patients undergoing immediate breast reconstruction; the preservation of breast skin brings a more natural contour to the reconstructed breast. To date, no increased risk of local recurrence has been observed for patients treated with skin-sparing techniques.

While breast mass reconstruction may be undertaken immediately following mastectomy, nipple reconstruction is typically delayed 6–12 weeks to allow time for the reconstructed breast to remodel and attain its final shape and position. Only then can appropriate nipple position be determined. The nipple is formed by raising local skin flaps using local anesthesia; pigment is provided using tattooing techniques.

Adjuvant Chemotherapy: Node-Positive Patients

For both node-positive and node-negative patients, decisions regarding adjuvant chemotherapy must be individualized. Multiple factors must be considered, including patient age, overall health status, tumor size, estrogen receptor expression, nodal status, and various other prognostic features including ploidy, S-phase fraction, c-erb B-2 oncogene amplification, and cathepsin D expression. General guidelines regarding the use of adjuvant chemotherapy are presented in Table 2-3.

The first clear demonstrations that adjuvant chemotherapy was beneficial in a subset of women with breast cancer were provided by the NSABP in the United States and by the National Cancer Institute in Italy during the mid-1970s. In the Milan trial, surgery plus postoperative cyclophosphamide, methotrexate, and 5-fluorouracil (CMF) delivered over 12 monthly cycles was demonstrated to be superior to surgical therapy alone in a population of node-positive patients. Examination of the 15-year results from this trial show a 10% improvement in both relapse-free and overall survival among treated patients. Subsequent trials have demonstrated a benefit for both pre- and postmenopausal patients and shown that six treatment cycles are as effective as 12. Additional studies evaluating doxorubicin-based therapy in the adjuvant setting have demonstrated an inconsistent advantage over CMF. The sequential administration of four cycles of doxorubicin followed by eight courses of CMF may provide some additional benefit, especially in patients with four or more positive nodes.

Initially applied to patients with advanced or recurrent disease, high-dose chemotherapy with autologous bone marrow transplantation is now also being applied in the adjuvant setting. Early disease-free survival rates are encouraging; long-term results are lacking. These regimens are usually

Table 2-3. Adjuvant chemotherapy recommendations for patients with invasive breast carcinoma based on tumor size, estrogen receptor (ER) expression, and nodal status

Tumor size	ER status	Nodal status	Recommended adjuvant therapy
≤1 cm	+/–	–	No adjuvant therapy required, especially for tumors with other favorable prognostic features (i.e., ploidy, S-phase, *c-erb* B-2, cathepsin D expression)
>1 cm	+	–	For women ≥ 50 yr, tamoxifen 10 mg bid; for women <50 yr, either cytotoxic chemotherapy (i.e., CMF vs. FAC) or tamoxifen as above
	–	–	Cytotoxic chemotherapy
Any size	+	+	For women ≥ 50 yr tamoxifen 10 mg bid × 5 yr; for women < 50 yr, cytotoxic chemotherapy +/– tamoxifen
	–	+	Cytotoxic chemotherapy

CMF = cyclophosphamide, methotrexate, and 5-fluorouracil;
FAC = 5-fluorouracil, doxorubicin, and cyclophosphamide.

reserved for patients with an anticipated high rate of recurrence (i.e., ≥10 positive lymph nodes).

For patients with positive estrogen receptors, adjuvant therapy with tamoxifen may be considered. Among women with positive lymph nodes, the use of tamoxifen as a single adjuvant agent is typically limited to postmenopausal patients. The efficacy of antiestrogen therapy in the adjuvant setting has been demonstrated by several clinical trials, with the largest study published in 1987 from the Scottish Cancer Trials Office. In this study, 1,323 patients were randomized to receive either adjuvant tamoxifen (20 mg/day for 5 years) or observation alone following primary surgical treatment by mastectomy. Both pre- and postmenopausal patients were enrolled, and estrogen receptor positivity was not required. When patients in the observation group had a recurrence, tamoxifen therapy was initiated; this feature allowed comparison of the benefit of adjuvant tamoxifen versus tamoxifen initiated at the time of clinical relapse. Overall, there was a 24% incidence of disease recurrence in the tamoxifen group compared with 38% in the observation group. An improvement in total survival was also noted among patients receiving adjuvant tamoxifen. Subgroup analysis according to menopausal, nodal, and estrogen receptor status demonstrated a benefit for each group examined, although the beneficial effect of adjuvant tamoxifen was most pronounced for postmenopausal, node-positive patients with estrogen receptor levels exceeding 100 fmol/mg. This trial confirmed the efficacy of adjuvant tamoxifen and further identified this strategy to be superior to a strategy of delayed tamoxifen initiated at the time of clinical relapse. Subsequent meta-analysis examining 28 different trials involving adjuvant tamoxifen confirmed a 16% reduction in the risk of death for women treated with tamoxifen. This benefit was limited to women older than age 50.

Adjuvant Chemotherapy: Node-Negative Patients

During the 1980s, attention turned toward the possibility that adjuvant chemotherapy might benefit node-negative patients. In 1989, four reports were published in a single issue of the *New England Journal of Medicine* that addressed the potential benefit of adjuvant therapy in node-negative patients. Among these, NSABP trial B-13 reported on 679 node-negative patients with estrogen receptor–negative tumors who were randomized to receive either surgery alone or surgery followed by adjuvant therapy involving methotrexate, 5-fluorouracil, and leucovorin. The group receiving adjuvant therapy demonstrated an improvement in disease-free survival compared to the group treated with surgery alone (80% versus 71% at 4 years) but no improvement in overall survival. Other studies, including a Milan trial, an Intergroup trial, and the Ludwig V trial, have demonstrated a similar small benefit to adjuvant chemotherapy in node-negative patients.

Following the publication of these trials, much controversy has ensued regarding the necessity of adjuvant therapy for all patients with node-negative disease. Clearly, the majority of patients do not require additional therapy, and recent work has been directed at identifying the subgroup of node-negative patients most likely to benefit. Toward this end, tumor size, nuclear grade, steroid receptor status, DNA ploidy, S-phase fraction, *c-erb* B-2 oncogene amplification, and cathepsin D expression have all been identified as prognostic variables that may assist in stratifying node-negative patients regarding the necessity of adjuvant therapy. Patients with diploid tumors that are smaller than 1 cm in diameter, have a low nuclear grade, and have a low S-phase fraction as determined by flow cytometry can expect a disease-free survival rate approaching 90% even without additional therapy. We currently do not recommend adjuvant cytotoxic therapy for this select low-risk group.

For node-negative patients whose tumors express estrogen receptors, adjuvant treatment with tamoxifen remains an attractive alternative. NSABP protocol B-14 examined the effectiveness of tamoxifen in both premenopausal and postmenopausal node-negative patients. Overall, there was an absolute 6% increase in the disease-free survival rate among tamoxifen-treated patients at 4 years. No difference in overall survival rate was noted. Tamoxifen significantly reduced the rate of both local and distant failure as well as local recurrence following lumpectomy and radiotherapy. Of note, there was a 45% reduction in the incidence of contralateral breast cancer for tamoxifen-treated women; this finding has stimulated interest in the possibility that tamoxifen may be effective in the primary chemoprevention of breast cancer. The NSABP has embarked on a randomized trial of tamoxifen chemoprevention in women 60 years and older, as well as in women aged 35–59 with a perceived high risk for breast cancer based on family history and other factors. The results from this trial should be available in 1999.

Tamoxifen therapy is generally well tolerated; treatment-limiting adverse effects develop in less than 5% of all patients. Concerns regarding an increased incidence of endometrial cancer and thromboembolic events in women taking tamoxifen may be offset by beneficial effects on bone density and serum cholesterol, as well as an overall reduction in cardiovascular mortality. For these reasons, many practitioners recommend adjuvant tamoxifen therapy even for low-risk node-negative patients.

The merits of combining cytotoxic and hormonal therapies remain to be established. While several trials have suggested a potential benefit to combination therapy, data remain inconclusive. NSABP protocol B-20 randomized patients with node-negative invasive breast cancer to receive either adjuvant tamoxifen alone or tamoxifen combined with one of two cytotoxic chemotherapy regimens. The results of this trial await long-term follow-up.

LOCALLY ADVANCED BREAST CANCER

Locally advanced breast cancer encompasses tumors with a broad range of biological behavior. It is generally thought to include tumors that are large and/or have extensive regional lymph node involvement without evidence of distant metastatic disease on initial presentation. These patients are classified as having stage III disease according to the AJCC system. Approximately 10–20% of all breast cancer patients have stage III disease, which includes T3 tumors with N1, N2, or N3 disease, T4 tumors with any N stage, or any T stage with N2 or N3 regional lymph node involvement. Stage III disease is further subdivided into stage IIIa and stage IIIb (see Table 2-1). Approximately 25–30% of stage III breast cancers are inoperable at the time of diagnosis.

Because of the advanced stage of disease at diagnosis, many locally advanced breast cancers are discovered by the patient or her spouse. The remainder are discovered during routine physical examination. On occasion, a discrete mass may not be present; rather, there is a diffuse infiltration of the breast tissue. These patients present with a breast that is asymmetric, immobile, and different in consistency from the contralateral breast. Seventy-five percent of stage III patients will have clinically palpable axillary or supraclavicular lymph nodes at the time of diagnosis. This clinical finding is confirmed on pathologic examination in 66–90% of patients.

Of those patients with positive nodes, 50% will have more than four nodes involved by tumor. When appropriate staging is performed, 20% of stage III patients will have distant metastases at presentation. Distant metastases are also the most frequent form of treatment failure, usually appearing within 2 years of the initial diagnosis.

Both fine-needle aspiration and core needle biopsy can be used to confirm the suspicion of breast cancer in these patients. These procedures usually are easily performed because of the large tumor size at presentation.

The Halsted radical mastectomy was initially thought to be the treatment of choice for locally advanced breast cancer. However, it was found early on to be inadequate treatment both in terms of local control and long-term survival. In 1942, Haagensen reported a 53% local failure rate and a 0% 5–year survival rate in a group of 1,135 stage III breast cancer patients.

The failure of surgery alone to control stage III breast cancer led to the use of radiotherapy as a single-agent treatment modality in this group of patients. However, the results with radiation therapy were in, some cases, inferior to those seen with surgery alone. The 5-year survival and local recurrence rates seen with radiation therapy alone were 10–30% and 25–70%, respectively.

The subsequent combination of surgery and radiotherapy for locally advanced breast cancer also resulted in poor results. The lack of efficacy in using a combination of two local treatment modalities confirmed the fact that stage III breast cancer is a systemic disease. Although there was a slight improvement in local recurrence, 5-year survival was unchanged, as patients continued to succumb to distant metastases.

In the early 1970s, systemic combination chemotherapy was added to the local treatments for advanced breast cancer. Initial protocols were designed to administer the chemotherapy following local treatment. However, this sequence of treatment does not allow for any assessment of the efficacy of the chemotherapy, as all measurable disease is removed prior to administration of the drugs. This has led to the current practice of administering induction chemotherapy prior to any local treatment. This affords several advantages, including reduction of the initial tumor burden before surgery, the ability to treat the potential systemic disease without delay, and the ability to assess the response of the tumor to the treatment being rendered.

Several centers have reported experience with combined modality therapy for locally advanced disease. Although the protocols differ among institutions with respect to the specific chemotherapy regimens and the type of local treatment, all of the studies have used induction chemotherapy followed by local treatment (surgery and/or radiotherapy) with a subsequent period of adjuvant chemotherapy. Based on these reports, it has now become the standard of care to treat patients with locally advanced breast cancer using this "sandwich" approach. Chemotherapy should consist of a doxorubicin-based regimen for six cycles followed by surgery. Following surgery, adjuvant chemotherapy should precede radiotherapy to avoid interrupting the treatment of systemic disease since distant metastases are the most frequent form of treatment failure. The role of adjuvant hormonal therapy in this group of patients is still under investigation.

INFLAMMATORY BREAST CANCER

Inflammatory breast cancer is a rare, virulent form of locally advanced breast cancer. It represents 1–4% of all breast cancers and presents as erythema, warmth, and edema of the breast. Pain is also present in approximately one-half of these patients. These physical findings are often confused with an infectious process, resulting in frequent delays in diagnosis and treatment. Tumor emboli are seen in the subdermal lymphatics on microscopic examination. Biopsy for diagnosis should include a segment of involved skin since there is usually no dominant mass palpable on physical examination.

Inflammatory carcinoma, like other forms of locally advanced breast cancer, is a systemic disease. This was manifest in the poor outcome seen when local therapy was used as the only treatment modality. Median survival was less than 2 years, with 5-year survival rates around 5%.

The use of multimodality therapy in these patients has improved local control and survival compared with local therapy alone. At M. D. Anderson, improvements in disease-free and overall survival rates were noted with several different chemotherapy regimens combined with surgery and/or radiotherapy when compared with previous local treatment modalities.

FOLLOW-UP AFTER PRIMARY TREATMENT OF INVASIVE BREAST CANCER

Following primary therapy for invasive breast cancer, patients must be made aware of the long-term risk for recurrent or metastatic disease. While most series report the majority of recurrences occurring within the first 5 years following primary therapy, recurrences more than 20 years following primary therapy have been reported.

For each patient with breast cancer, follow-up evaluation should be individualized based on the treatments applied, the perceived risk of disease recurrence, and specific patient needs. Despite the availability of multiple biochemical and radiographic tests, periodic history-taking and physical examination remain the most effective modalities for detecting recurrent disease. Numerous studies have demonstrated that 65–85% of all breast cancer recurrences may be detected by history and physical examination alone.

For patients who have undergone breast conservation therapy, follow-up examination should be undertaken every 3–6 months for the first 2 years, and annually thereafter. Monthly self–breast examination is also required. Mammography is obtained 6 months following the completion of therapy to allow for surgical and radiation changes to stabilize, and then on a yearly basis. For patients who have undergone mastectomy, a contralateral mammogram is obtained yearly. For both groups, further evaluation should be limited to yearly serum biochemical evaluation and a chest radiograph. The routine use of bone scans, skeletal surveys, and computed tomography scans of the abdomen and brain yields an extremely low rate of occult metastases in otherwise asymptomatic patients and is not cost-effective for patients with early-stage breast cancer.

LOCALLY RECURRENT BREAST CANCER

The time course, significance, and prognosis of locally recurrent breast cancer vary dramatically for patients undergoing breast conservation versus those undergoing mastectomy. Local recurrence in the conserved breast typically occurs over a protracted time period and is rarely associated with systemic metastases. Local recurrence following lumpectomy remains curable in the majority of cases; 60–70% of patients suffering local recurrence will remain disease-free 5 years after salvage mastectomy.

In contrast, local chest wall recurrence following mastectomy typically occurs within the first 2 years after surgery, is frequently associated with distant metastases, and predicts eventual death from breast cancer for the majority of patients. One-third of patients with chest wall recurrence will have distant metastatic disease concurrent with their local recurrence; within 1 year, half will demonstrate distant disease. The median survival in this setting is 2–3 years.

Patients with apparently isolated local recurrence can often be treated without systemic cytotoxic chemotherapy. These patients should undergo complete restaging following the detection of recurrence; for patients with purely local recurrence, treatment with surgical excision combined with radiotherapy provides better local control than either modality used alone.

METASTATIC BREAST CANCER

Metastatic breast cancer generally cannot be cured; the median survival following the detection of metastases is 2 years. Treatment in this setting is purely palliative, although significant prolongation of survival can be obtained with appropriate therapy. For patients with overt metastases, the decision to treat with either systemic chemotherapy or hormonal therapy rests on several issues: patient age, physiologic status, disease-free interval, estrogen receptor status of the primary tumor, rapidity of metastatic growth, and whether the metastatic disease is skeletal or visceral. In selected patients who have isolated skeletal, pericardial, or pleural disease following a substantial disease-free interval (i.e., >2 years), radiotherapy with or without hormonal manipulation is often the most attractive strategy. In patients with a shorter disease-free interval and rapidly growing visceral (i.e., liver, lung, central nervous system) metastases, cytotoxic chemotherapy is usually required. While doxorubicin remains the single agent with the highest response rate for advanced breast cancer, an actual benefit in terms of overall survival compared to non–doxorubicin-containing regimens remains difficult to establish. Most patients are initially treated with CMF, with doxorubicin reserved for disease progression. In selected patients with good performance status, high-dose chemotherapy with autologous stem cell rescue using hematologic growth factor support represents a promising new treatment strategy. Response rates exceed 50%, and 1-year survival rates of 60% are reported. Long-term data are unavailable. At present, it remains unclear which chemotherapeutic agents are best used under such a strategy as well as which subsets of patients are most likely to benefit.

BREAST CANCER AND PREGNANCY

The incidence of breast cancer detected during pregnancy is 2 per 10,000 gestations, accounting for 2.8% of all breast malignancies. The diagnosis of breast cancer is typically more difficult in the gravid female because of several factors, including a low level of suspicion based on generally young patient age, the relative frequency of nodular changes in the breast during pregnancy, and the fact that increased breast density during pregnancy renders mammographic imaging less accurate. For these reasons, the diagnosis of breast cancer during pregnancy is frequently delayed. This feature, rather than specific differences in the biology of breast cancer among gravid and nongravid females, likely explains the relatively poor prognosis for women with breast cancer detected during pregnancy. When matched for tumor stage, pregnant women with breast cancer appear to have a prognosis no worse than nonpregnant patients.

Because of the inaccuracy of mammography in this setting, all persistent, suspicious breast masses discovered during pregnancy should undergo evaluation either by fine-needle aspiration or excisional biopsy. Excisional biopsy under local anesthesia represents a safe procedure at any time during pregnancy. Once a diagnosis of malignancy is established, subsequent treatment decisions are influenced by their timing with respect to the specific trimester of pregnancy. For women who want to complete their pregnancies, the goal should be curative treatment of the breast cancer without injury to the fetus. It is important to note that numerous studies have demonstrated that termination of pregnancy in hopes of minimizing hormonal stimulation of the tumor has no benefit to maternal survival.

Surgical treatment of gestational breast cancer is generally conducted in a manner identical to nongestational breast cancer. There is no evidence that extraabdominal surgical procedures are associated with premature labor, or that the typically used anesthetic agents are teratogenic. For women desiring modified radical mastectomy as primary therapy, this can be undertaken at any point during pregnancy without undue risk to mother or fetus. For cancer detected during the third trimester, delays in primary treatment of up to 4 weeks to allow for delivery prior to surgery appear to be acceptable. If modified radical mastectomy is undertaken during pregnancy, breast reconstruction should not be done simultaneously; a symmetric result is impossible until the postpartum appearance of the contralateral breast is known.

For women desiring breast conservation, treatment is complicated by the fact that radiotherapy is contraindicated during pregnancy. For cancers detected during the third trimester, lumpectomy and axillary dissection can safely be performed using general anesthesia, with radiotherapy delayed until after delivery. Longer delays may be detrimental to maternal outcome, although the time limit within which radiotherapy must be carried out to minimize the risk of local recurrence is not known.

It may be necessary to administer cytotoxic adjuvant chemotherapy during pregnancy, raising fears of congenital malformations. Most series have demonstrated no increased risk of fetal malformation for chemotherapy administered during the second and third trimesters. In contrast, chemotherapy administration during the first trimester is associated with an increased incidence of spontaneous abortion and congenital malformation, especially when methotrexate is used.

CYSTOSARCOMA PHYLLOIDES

Cystosarcoma phylloides represents an uncommon group of neoplasms, accounting for only 0.3–0.9% of all breast tumors. The term *cystosarcoma* is antiquated nomenclature that has generated great confusion regarding this diagnosis. Phylloides tumors may actually be either benign or malignant and exhibit a wide spectrum of metastatic potential. Features suggesting malignancy include large tumor size, stromal atypia, an infiltrating margin, and frequent mitoses. Nevertheless, the clinical course is often difficult to predict based on histologic appearance alone. When metastases do occur, common sites include the lung, bone, and mediastinum.

Women with phylloides tumors present at a median age of 50 years. These tumors are typically quite large, with a mean diameter of 4–5 cm. Given the fact that phylloides tumors are mammographically indistinguishable from fibroadenomas, the decision to perform excisional biopsy is usually based on large tumor size, a history of rapid growth, and the age of the patient.

Appropriate treatment for phylloides tumors remains complete surgical excision. The decision to perform wide local excision versus total mastectomy has traditionally been based on the size of the lesion and the potential for malignancy based on histologic appearance. In one series, the incidence of subsequent recurrence was 4% for histologically benign lesions, and 37% for tumors considered histologically malignant. Local recurrences are typically salvageable by way of total mastectomy and have no impact on overall survival. As for ductal carcinoma, it would therefore appear that breast conservation should be considered for many patients with phylloides tumors. For all phylloides tumors, the incidence of axillary nodal metastases is less than 1%, obviating the need for lymphadenectomy. To date, no role for radiotherapy, chemotherapy, or hormonal therapy has been established for this disease.

Selected References

Abner AL, Recht A, Eberlein T, et al. Prognosis following salvage mastectomy for recurrence in the breast after conservative surgery and radiation therapy for early-stage breast cancer. *J Clin Oncol* 11:44, 1993.

Balch CM, Singletary SE, Bland KI. Clinical decision-making in early breast cancer. *Ann Surg* 217:207, 1993.

Barnovon Y, Wallack MK. Management of the pregnant patient with carcinoma of the breast. *Surg Gynecol Obstet* 171:347, 1990.

Deckers PJ. Axillary dissection in breast cancer: When, why, how much, and for how long? *J Surg Oncol* 48:217, 1991.

Early Breast Cancer Trialists' Collaborative Group. Effects of adjuvant tamoxifen and of cytotoxic therapy on mortality in early breast cancer: An overview of 61 randomized trials among 28,896 women. *N Engl J Med* 319:1681, 1988.

Fisher B, Constantino J, Redmond C, et al. A randomized clinical trial evaluating tamoxifen in the treatment of patients with node-negative breast cancer who have estrogen-receptor-positive tumors. *N Engl J Med* 320:479, 1989.

Fisher B, Redmond C, Dimitrov NV, et al. A randomized clinical trial evaluating sequential methotrexate and fluorouracil in the treatment of patients with node-negative breast cancer who have estrogen-receptor-negative tumors. *N Engl J Med* 320:473, 1989.

Fisher B, Redmond C, Fisher ER, et al. Ten-year results of a randomized clinical trial comparing radical mastectomy and total mastectomy with or without radiation. *N Engl J Med* 312:674, 1985.

Fisher B, Redmond C, Poisson R, et al. Eight-year results of a randomized clinical trial comparing total mastectomy and lumpectomy with or without irradiation in the treatment of breast Cancer. *N Engl J Med* 320:822, 1989.

Harris JR, Lippman ME, Veronesi U, et al. Breast cancer. *N Engl J Med* 327:319, 390, 473, 1992.

Henderson IC. Risk factors for breast cancer development. *Cancer* 71(6)(Supp):2128, 1993.

Hortobagyi GN, Buzdar AU. Locally Advanced Breast Cancer: A Review Including the M. D. Anderson Experience. In J Ragaz J, IM Ariel (eds), *High Risk Breast Cancer*. Berlin: Springer-Verlag, 1991.

Margolese R, Poisson R, Shibata H, et al. The technique of segmental mastectomy (lumpectomy) and axillary dissection: A syllabus from the NSABP workshops. *Surgery* 102:828, 1987.

McGuire WL, Clark GM. Prognostic factors and treatment decisions in axillary node-negative breast cancer. *N Engl J Med* 326:1756, 1992.

Salvadori B, Cusumano F, Del Bo R, et al. Surgical treatment of phylloides tumors of the breast. *Cancer* 63:2532, 1989.

Melanoma

Jeffrey E. Lee

Epidemiology

Although melanoma is a relatively uncommon malignancy worldwide, its incidence is increasing dramatically—150% since 1971. Melanoma incidence is similar in men and women and increases from the age of 10 years to the fifth decade. In the United States, incidence varies from 4 to 26 per 100,000, increasing at lower latitudes. Approximately 1 in 123 whites alive today will develop melanoma in their lifetimes; lifetime risk is expected to be 1 in 90 by the year 2000. Melanoma occurs primarily in whites, although other races are also affected. There have been changes in the distribution and stage of melanoma at diagnosis over the past 30 years, with an increase in thinner lesions. The majority of melanomas seen at many institutions now measure less than 1 mm thick.

Risk Factors

1. *Previous melanoma*: The risk of developing a second melanoma in a patient who has had a melanoma is 3–5%.

2. *Fair complexion*: Fair or red hair, light skin, blue eyes, and a propensity to sunburn are associated with an increased risk of melanoma.

3. *Sunlight exposure*: Occasional or recreational exposure to sunlight, especially a history of blistering sunburn, has been associated with an increased risk of melanoma. The effects of sunlight have been attributed to exposure to ultraviolet B (UVB) radiation.

4. *Benign nevi*: Though a benign nevus is most likely not a precursor of melanoma, the presence of large numbers of nevi has been consistently associated with an increased risk of melanoma.

5. *Family history*: See genetic predisposition below.

6. *Genetic predisposition*: Specific genetic alterations have been implicated in the pathogenesis of melanoma. At least four distinct genes, located on chromosomes 1p, 6q, 7, and 9, may play a role in melanoma. A tumor suppressor gene located on chromosome 9p21 is probably involved in familial and possibly sporadic melanoma.

7. *Familial atypical mole and melanoma syndrome* (FAM-M): Previously known as dysplastic nevus syndrome, FAM-M is characterized by the presence of large numbers of atypical moles (dysplastic nevi) that represent a distinct clinico-pathologic type of melanocytic lesion. They can be precursors of melanoma as well as markers of increased melanoma risk. The actual frequency of an atypical mole progressing to melanoma is small. After identification of FAM-M, patients

should be followed closely and family members should be screened.

Pathology

There are four major melanoma growth patterns:

1. *Superficial spreading melanoma* (SSM) constitutes the majority of melanomas (about 70%).

2. *Nodular melanoma* (NM) is the second most common growth pattern (15–30%). NMs are more aggressive tumors than SSMs.

3. *Lentigo maligna melanoma* (LMM) does not have the same propensity to metastasize as do other histologies. LMMs constitute a small percentage of melanomas (4–10%) and are typically located on the face in older white women.

4. *Acral lentiginous melanoma* (ALM) occurs on the palms (palmar) or soles (plantar) or beneath the nail beds (subungual), although not all palmar, plantar, and subungual melanomas are ALMs. ALMs occur in only 2–8% of white patients with melanoma but in a substantially higher proportion (35–60%) of darker-skinned patients. ALMs are the most aggressive histologic type.

Clinical Presentation

Clinical features of melanoma include variegated color, raised surface, irregular perimeter, and ulceration. Any pigmented lesion that undergoes a change in size, configuration, or color should be biopsied.

When a patient presents with a lesion suspicious for melanoma, a thorough physical examination must be performed with particular emphasis on the skin, all nodal basins, and the subcutaneous tissue. Chest radiograph and liver function studies should be obtained. Further evaluation is based on pathologic findings. We discourage routine extensive evaluation with computed tomography or bone scan since their yield in the absence of symptoms, abnormal laboratory findings, or an abnormal chest radiograph is very low in patients with primary melanoma.

Biopsy

The choice of biopsy technique varies according to the anatomic site, size, and shape of the lesion. Definitive therapy must be considered in choosing a biopsy technique. Either an excisional biopsy or an incisional biopsy using a scalpel or punch is acceptable. An excisional biopsy allows the pathologist to more accurately determine the thickness of the lesion. For excisional biopsies, a narrow margin of normal-appearing skin (1–3 mm) is taken with the specimen. An elliptical incision is used to facilitate closure. The biopsy incision should be oriented to facilitate later wide local excision (e.g., longitudinally on extremities). We reserve punch biopsy for lesions that are large, are located on anatomic areas where maximum preservation of surrounding skin is important, or can be completely excised with a 6-mm punch biopsy. Punch biopsies should be performed at the most raised or darkest area of the lesion. Full-thickness skin must be included.

Shave biopsies are contraindicated if a diagnosis of melanoma is considered. Fine-needle aspiration biopsy may be used to document nodal and extranodal melanoma metastases but should not be used to diagnose primary melanomas. We send all pigmented lesions for permanent-section examination only and perform definitive surgery at a later time.

Markers of melanocytic cells can be useful in confirming the diagnosis of melanoma. Two widely used markers are S-100 and HMB-45. S-100 is expressed by more than 90% of melanomas but also by several other tumors and some normal tissues. HMB-45 is more specific for melanocytic cells but is not always positive in metastatic melanoma.

Staging

Collaboration between the American Joint Committee on Cancer (AJCC) and the Union Internationale Contre le Cancer (UICC) has resulted in the current clinical staging system for melanoma (Table 3-1).

Two methods have been used in microstaging the primary melanoma. Breslow microstaging determines the thickness of the lesion using an ocular micrometer to measure the total vertical height of the melanoma from the granular layer to the area of deepest penetration. Clark microstaging defines levels of invasion reflecting increasing depth of penetration into the dermis. Discrepancies between the Clark level and the Breslow thickness occur frequently. For localized primary melanoma, the Breslow thickness is the single most significant prognostic factor.

Significant prognostic factors not included in the AJCC staging system include ulceration, sex, and the anatomic location of the primary lesion. Ulceration, male sex, and location on the trunk or head are all associated with a worse prognosis.

Management of Local Disease

Local control of a primary melanoma requires wide excision of the tumor or biopsy site down to the deep fascia with a margin of normal-appearing skin. Risk of local recurrence correlates more with tumor thickness than with margins of surgical excision. It is rational to excise melanomas using surgical margins that vary according to tumor thickness.

Table 3-1. AJCC-UICC melanoma staging system*

Stage	Criteria	
I	pT1	Primary melanoma ≤0.75 mm thick and/or Clark's level II; no nodal or systemic metastases (N0, M0)
	pT2	Primary melanoma 0.76–1.50 mm thick and/or Clark's level III (N0, M0)
II	pT3	Primary melanoma 1.51–4.00 mm thick and/or Clark's level IV (N0, M0)
	pT4	Primary melanoma >4 mm thick and/or Clark's level V and/or satellites within 2 cm of the primary tumor (N0, M0)
III		Regional lymph node and/or in-transit metastases; any pT, N1(regional nodes ≤3 cm) or N2 (regional nodes >3 cm), M0
IV		Systemic metastases; any pT, any N, M1 (distant metastases)

*The AJCC Melanoma Committee recommends that when there is a discrepancy between tumor thickness and Clark's level, the pT category be based on the less favorable finding.
Source: OH Beahrs, DE Henson, RVP Hutter, et al (eds). *Manual for Staging of Cancer* (4th ed). Philadelphia: Lippincott, 1992.

MARGINS

The first randomized study involving surgical margins for melanomas less than 2 mm thick was reported by the World Health Organization (WHO) Melanoma Group. In an update of the study of 612 evaluable patients randomly assigned to receive a 1-cm or 3-cm margin of excision, there were no local recurrences among patients with melanomas thinner than 1 mm. There were four local recurrences in the 100 patients with melanomas 1–2 mm thick, and all four patients had received 1-cm margin excisions. There was no statistically significant difference in survival between the 1-cm and 3-cm surgical margin goups. These results demonstrate that a narrow excision margin for thin (<1 mm) melanomas is safe.

A multi-institutional prospective randomized trial from France compared a 5-cm margin with a 2-cm margin in 319 patients with melanomas 2 mm or less in thickness. There were no differences in local recurrence rate or survival.

A randomized prospective study conducted by the Intergroup Melanoma Committee evaluated 2-cm versus 4-cm radial margins of excision for intermediate-thickness melanomas (1–4 mm). There was no difference in local recurrence rate between the 2-cm or 4-cm margin groups. Of note is that 46% of the 4-cm group required skin grafts, whereas only 11% of the 2-cm group did ($p<.001$). These data strongly support the use of a 2-cm margin for intermediate-thickness lesions.

General recommendations for margins are as follows:

1. *Thin melanomas* (<1 mm thick) have a minimal risk of local recurrence. Wide excision with a 1-cm margin of normal-appearing skin is recommended.

2. *Intermediate-thickness melanomas* (1–4 mm thick) have an increased risk of local recurrence. A 2-cm margin can be safely used.

3. *Thick melanomas* (>4 mm thick) have a risk of local recurrence that may exceed 10–20%. A 3-cm margin is probably safe.

CLOSURE

If there is any question about the ability to achieve suitable wound closure, a plastic or reconstructive surgeon should be consulted preoperatively. Options for closure include primary closure, skin grafting, and local and distant flaps.

Primary closure is the method of choice for most lesions, but it should be avoided when it distorts the appearance of a mobile facial feature or when it interferes with function. Many defects can be closed using an advancement flap, undermining the skin and subcutaneous tissues to permit primary closure. Primary closure usually requires that the longitudinal axis of an elliptical incision be at least three times the short axis. Closure of the wound edges is usually performed in two layers: closure of the subcutaneous tissue using interrupted 3-0 undyed absorbable suture and subcuticular closure of the dermis using 4-0 monofilament absorbable suture.

Application of a *skin graft* is one of the simplest reconstructive methods. Split-thickness skin grafts (STSGs) are the most commonly used. For lower extremity primary lesions, STSGs should be harvested from the extremity opposite the melanoma. A full-thickness skin graft (FTSG) can provide a result that is both durable and of high aesthetic quality. The most common use of the FTSG has been on the face, where aesthetic considerations are most significant. Donor sites for FTSGs to the face should be chosen from locations that are likely to match the color of the face, such as the postauricular or preauricular skin or the supraclavicular portion of the neck.

Local flaps offer a number of advantages for reconstruction of defects that cannot be closed primarily, especially on the distal extremities and the head and neck. Color match is excellent, durability of the skin is essentially normal, and normal sensation is usually preserved. Transposition flaps and rotation flaps of many varieties have been successfully used.

Distant flaps should be used when sufficient tissue for a local flap is not available and when a skin graft would not provide adequate wound coverage. Myocutaneous flaps and free flaps can be used. Discussion of such complex methods is beyond the scope of this chapter, but these techniques are familiar to plastic and reconstructive surgeons.

SPECIAL ANATOMIC SITES

Fingers and Toes

A melanoma located on the skin of a digit or beneath the fingernail should be removed by a digital amputation, saving as much of the digit as possible. In general, amputations are performed at the middle interphalangeal joint of the fingers or proximal to the distal joint of the thumb. More proximal amputations are not associated with a prolongation of survival. For a melanoma located on a toe, an amputation of the entire digit at the metatarsal-phalangeal joint is indicated. Lesions arising between two toes often require the amputation of both surrounding toes. Over three-fourths of subungual melanomas involve either the great toe or the thumb.

Sole of the Foot

Excision of a melanoma on the plantar surface often produces a sizable defect in a weight-bearing area. If possible, a portion of the heel or ball of the plantar surface should be retained to bear the greatest burden of pressure. Where possible, deep fascia over the extensor tendons should be preserved as a base for skin coverage. Rotation flaps or myocutaneous free flaps are recommended for coverage of weight-bearing areas.

Face

Facial lesions usually cannot be excised with more than a 1-cm margin because of adjacent vital structures. The tumor diameter, thickness of the melanoma, and its exact location on the face must all be considered when determining margin width.

Breast

Wide local excision with primary closure is the treatment of choice for melanoma on the skin of the breast; mastectomy is not generally recommended. As with any trunk lesion, lymphoscintigraphy (see below) should be performed before considering prophylactic node dissection.

SPECIAL CLINICAL SITUATIONS

Giant Congenital Nevi

Decisions about the management of giant congenital nevi are difficult since such lesions are often so extensive that prophylactic surgical excision is not possible. When the location and size of a lesion permit prophylactic excision, it is recommended that it be done before the age of 2 years.

Mucosal Melanoma

Patients with true mucosal melanoma, including melanoma of the mucosa of the head and neck, vagina, and anal canal, have a poor prognosis regardless of surgical therapy. We generally do not recommend an aggressive surgical approach to patients with clinically localized disease. We reserve extended resection for bulky or recurrent tumors and favor therapeutic over elective lymph node dissection (see below). In particular, we recommend local excision of anal melanomas over abdominoperineal resection (APR). APR is associated with a much higher morbidity, leaves the patient with a permanent colostomy, offers no survival advantage, and does not treat at-risk inguinal nodes unless combined with groin dissection. Adjuvant radiotherapy may be considered for patients with mucosal melanoma in an attempt to decrease locoregional recurrence.

Desmoplastic Melanoma

Desmoplastic or neurotropic melanoma is a rare variant of melanoma. Desmoplastic melanomas have a propensity for perineural invasion and infiltration of the blood vessel adventitia. These tumors often recur locally. Frozen-section examination must be performed to ensure that excision margins are free of tumor. Adjuvant radiotherapy may decrease the risk of local recurrence.

Pregnancy

The precise influence of pregnancy or hormonal manipulation on the clinical course of malignant melanoma has not been defined. There is no conclusive evidence that concurrent pregnancy has an adverse effect on the clinical course of melanoma. Several large studies report no difference in outcome between gravid and nongravid patients with primary melanoma. Surgery is the treatment of choice in pregnant patients with early-stage melanoma. There is no proof that abortion of the pregnancy protects the mother from subsequent development of metastases. Although there are differing opinions on planning a pregnancy after a diagnosis of melanoma, the weight of evidence does not demonstrate an increased risk for developing metastatic disease with pregnancy. Furthermore, several studies have found no association between oral contraceptive use and survival in melanoma.

General recommendations for managing melanoma during pregnancy are as follows:

  1. The ultimate decision about continuing or terminating a pregnancy should be left to the patient and family.

2. A patient who presents with a primary melanoma during pregnancy should be evaluated with the minimum number of diagnostic tests.

3. The primary melanoma should be excised under appropriate anesthesia. Elective lymph node dissection should not be performed. However, therapeutic dissection of regional lymph nodes should be considered.

4. In pregnant patients with systemic metastases, the decision to abort or continue the pregnancy must be made on a case by case basis. Systemic chemotherapy during the second and third trimesters does not usually cause abnormalities in fetal development, unless alkylating agents are used.

5. If the mother had melanoma during pregnancy, the placenta should be examined histologically for evidence of metastasis at the time of delivery. Additionally, the child should be monitored carefully for metastatic disease during the first 6–12 months of life.

6. Women of child-bearing age who have melanoma should probably not become pregnant or take oral contraceptives for 2 years after their treatment. Those 2 years represent the period of greatest risk for relapse with metastases. Conversely, however, should pregnancy occur during this time, abortion of the pregnancy is not necessary.

Management of Local Recurrence and In-Transit Disease

The overall risk of local recurrence is low—3% in a collected series of 3,520 patients. Local recurrence usually develops within 5 years after primary melanoma excision. Local recurrence implies a poor prognosis and often portends distant metastases. In a study of 95 patients with local recurrences, the median survival was 3 years, with a 10-year survival rate of only 20%.

In-transit metastases are located between the primary melanoma and the first major regional nodal basin. The incidence of in-transit metastases is 2–3%. Regional nodal metastases occur in about two-thirds of patients with in-transit metastases.

Comparison studies of treatment alternatives for local recurrences and in-transit disease have not been performed. Options include surgical excision, regional chemotherapy using isolated limb perfusion, and radiotherapy.

A single local recurrence in a patient whose primary melanoma had favorable prognostic features can be excised and no further treatment given. However, patients with multiple local recurrences, with local recurrence and poor prognostic features of the primary melanoma, or with in-transit metastases should be considered for regional treatment. Regional treatment options include isolated limb perfusion and radiotherapy using a high-dose fraction technique.

Rarely, amputation may be necessary for extensive or deeply infiltrative lesions involving the foot, hand, arm, or leg.

Melphalan is the most active single agent for use in hyperthermic isolated limb perfusion. Complete response rates average 40% in patients with measurable disease. Recent nonrandomized studies of hyperthermic regional limb perfusion by Leinard, et al., have reported a high complete response rate (90%) using a combination of melphalan, tumor necrosis factor-alpha (TNF-α), and interferon-gamma. Hyperthermic isolated limb perfusion continues to be associated with significant regional toxicity, including arterial thrombosis, sometimes requiring major amputation. Systemic toxicity, including hypotension and adult respiratory distress syndrome, is seen with the addition of TNF-α to the regimen. The treatment requires a high degree of technical expertise and carries significant risk of major complications, including limb loss. The procedure should therefore be performed only in centers that have experience with the technique, preferably in the setting of a clinical trial. At present, there is little evidence to justify the use of prophylactic perfusion except as part of a clinical trial.

Management of Regional Disease

Regional lymph nodes are the most common site of metastatic melanoma. Effective palliation and sometimes cure can be achieved in patients with regional metastases. Fine-needle aspiration can often yield a diagnosis in patients who develop clinically enlarged regional nodes. Open biopsy is sometimes warranted. If, by clinical examination, the index of suspicion for metastases is high, definitive surgical treatment can be performed without open biopsy.

Surgical excision of nodal metastases is the only effective treatment to achieve local disease control and cure. In patients with clinical stage III disease, a biopsy or partial lymphadenectomy results in lower survival rates compared with a complete lymphadenectomy. Incomplete lymph node dissection is unacceptable.

Lymphatic drainage on the trunk can be multidirectional and unpredictable. A study of lymphatic drainage revealed that up to 59% of patients undergoing dissections for head and neck or trunk melanomas would have had misdirected operations if their operation was based on classic anatomic studies. These findings strongly support the use of lymphoscintigraphy in these patients.

CUTANEOUS LYMPHOSCINTIGRAPHY

In many patients, cutaneous lymphoscintigraphy using a radionuclide injected into the primary site can accurately define the location of nodes that are the primary drainage sites for melanoma located anywhere on the trunk. The most popular tracer is ^{99m}Tc-labeled human serum albumin.

Scans can only be accurately performed prior to a wide local excision. It is not uncommon for two or more nodal basins to be identified by these scans.

IMMEDIATE VERSUS DELAYED LYMPH NODE DISSECTION

Some surgeons prefer to perform lymphadenectomy only for clinically demonstrable metastatic nodes. This type of excision has been termed *therapeutic or delayed lymph node dissection*. Other surgeons choose to excise the nodes even when they appear normal in patients who are at increased risk of developing nodal metastases. This excision has been termed *immediate, prophylactic,* or *elective lymph node dissection* (ELND).

ELND has the theoretic advantage of treating melanoma nodal metastases at a relatively early stage in the natural history of the disease. Its disadvantage is that some patients undergo surgery when they do not have nodal metastases. Thus, an advantage of delayed lymphadenectomy is that only patients with demonstrable metastases undergo major operations. The disadvantage of delayed lymphadenectomy is that delay of treatment until lymph node metastases are clinically palpable results in the majority of patients having distant micrometastases at the time of lymphadenectomy. Chances for cure are therefore likely to be diminished.

Tumor thickness is the best (but not only) predictor of regional and distant metastases and therefore the most important (but not sole) guide in selecting who might benefit from an ELND. Thin melanomas (<1 mm) are generally localized and are associated with a 95% or greater cure rate following wide local excision. ELND does not benefit these patients. Intermediate-thickness melanomas (1–4 mm) confer an increased risk (up to 60%) of occult regional metastases but a relatively low risk (<20%) of distant metastases. Patients with these lesions might benefit from ELND. Thick melanomas (>4 mm) carry a high risk for regional nodal micrometastases (>60%) as well as a high risk (>70%) of occult distant disease at the time of initial presentation. In fact, the risk of distant microscopic metastases is so high in these patients that it negates any potentially curative benefit of a regional operation. Therefore, regional lymph node dissection in patients with thick primary melanomas should generally be deferred until nodal metastases become clinically evident. Alternatively, some surgeons prefer to perform ELND as "expectant palliation" in patients with thick melanomas to avoid the chance (about 30%) of having to perform a second operation for lymph node metastases.

Two prospective trials to evaluate ELND in the treatment of stage I and II melanoma have been reported: an international cooperative study conducted by the WHO Melanoma Group and a study at the Mayo Clinic. These studies clearly demonstrated that not all patients benefit from ELND. Both studies included melanomas of all thicknesses and did not specifically address the potential benefit of ELND for the subgroup of intermediate-thickness melanomas described above.

Three nonrandomized studies involving melanomas from all anatomic sites showed significantly improved survival for a subgroup of patients with intermediate-thickness melanomas. Two prospective randomized trials of lymphadenectomy are currently ongoing in patients with intermediate-thickness melanomas. Results of these trials should be available within the next few years and should provide extremely important information regarding the role of ELND. Until these are completed, it is justified to consider ELND in select intermediate-thickness melanoma patients for whom the benefit appears sufficiently high and the morbidity sufficiently low.

Our general guidelines for ELND are as follows: (1) women with extremity melanomas 1.5–4.0 mm thick and (2) men with extremity melanomas and men and women with melanomas located on the trunk or head and neck area as thin as 1 mm. Other factors, such as the presence of tumor ulceration, the patient's sex and age, and the operative risk are all considered when making the decision to perform ELND. When more than one nodal basin is identified to be at risk by cutaneous lymphoscintigraphy, an ELND of two nodal basins (e.g., bilateral axillary dissection for trunk melanomas) may be warranted in select cases. Removing more than two nodal basins or performing a bilateral cervical or inguinal dissection as an ELND is generally not indicated.

CUTANEOUS LYMPHATIC MAPPING AND SENTINEL NODE BIOPSY

Morton has reported a technique to accurately identify the presence of nodal metastases within regional basins. At the time of wide excision a vital blue dye (patent blue V or isosulfan blue) is injected intradermally at the primary melanoma or biopsy site. Exploration of the draining nodal basin (aided by prior lymphoscintigraphy) allows the lymphatic channels and the first draining (or "sentinel") lymph node to be identified by a blue color. More than 80% of the time, a sentinel node can be identified. This node is removed and subjected to frozen-section examination for evidence of metastasis. When a metastasis is identified, a therapeutic lymphadenectomy is performed. In the study by Morton, et al., all patients underwent lymphadenectomy following sentinel node excision. In only two cases was tumor found in other nodes within the basin when no tumor was found in the sentinel node (a 5% false-negative rate). This technique may accurately identify patients who harbor micrometastatic disease and spare patients who do not the morbidity of a lymphadenectomy. Our preliminary results in more than 100 patients treated at the University of Texas M. D. Anderson Cancer Center support the accuracy of this technique. Confirmation of the effectiveness of this technique could make the practice of ELND a "selective" one.

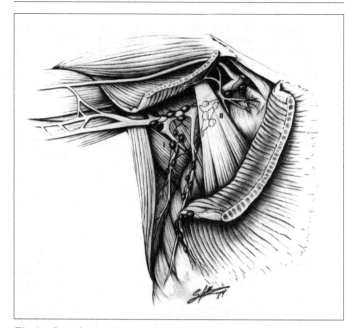

Fig. 3-1. Lymphatic anatomy of the axilla demonstrating the three groups of axillary lymph nodes defined by their relationship to the pectoralis minor muscle. The highest axillary nodes (level III) medial to the pectoralis minor muscle should be included in an axillary lymph node dissection for melanoma. (From CM Balch, GW Milton, HM Shaw, S-J Soong [eds]. *Cutaneous Melanoma*. Philadelphia: Lippincott, 1985.)

AXILLARY NODE DISSECTION

General

A complete operation including level III nodes must be performed (Fig. 3-1). The arm, shoulder, and chest are prepped into the surgical field.

Incision

We use a horizontal S-shaped incision beginning anteriorly along the superior portion of the pectoralis major muscle, traversing the axilla over the fourth rib, and extending inferiorly along the anterior border of the latissimus dorsi muscle.

Skin Flaps

Skin flaps are raised anteriorly to the midclavicular line, inferiorly to the sixth rib, posteriorly to the anterior border of the latissimus dorsi, and superiorly to just below the pectoralis major insertion. The medial side of the latissimus dorsi is dissected free from the specimen, exposing the thoracodorsal vessels and nerve. The lateral edge of dissection then proceeds cephalad beneath the axillary vein. These maneuvers allow the remainder of the dissection to proceed from medial to lateral. The fatty and lymphatic tissue over the pectoralis major is dissected free around to its undersurface, where the pectoralis minor is encountered. The interpectoral groove is exposed.

Lymph Node Dissection

The medial pectoral nerve is preserved. The interpectoral nodes are dissected free. Exposure of the upper axilla is obtained by bringing the patient's arm over the chest by adduction and internal rotation. If nodes are bulky, the pectoralis minor may need to be removed. Dissection proceeds from the apex of the axilla inferolaterally. The upper axillary lymph node dissection should be sufficiently complete so that the thoracic outlet beneath the clavicle, Halsted's ligament, and the subclavius muscle can be visualized (Fig. 3-2). Fatty and lymphatic tissues are dissected downward over the brachial plexus and axillary artery until the axillary vein is exposed. The apex of the dissected specimen is tagged. Dissection then continues until the thoracodorsal vessels and the long thoracic and thoracodorsal nerves are identified. The fatty tissue between the two nerves is separated from the subscapularis muscle. The specimen is removed from the lateral chest wall. The intercostobrachial nerve is sacrificed. The specimen is swept off the latissimus dorsi and the serratus anterior muscles.

Wound Closure

One 10-mm closed suction catheter is placed percutaneously through the inferior flap into the axilla. An additional catheter may be inserted through the inferior flap and placed over the pectoralis major. Skin is closed with interrupted 3-0 undyed absorbable sutures and running 4-0 subcuticular undyed absorbable sutures.

Postoperative Management

Wound catheter suction drainage is continued until output is less than 40 ml per day. By the tenth day, the suction catheters are removed, regardless of the amount of drainage, to avoid infection. Any subsequent collections of serum are treated by needle aspiration. Mobilization of the arm is discouraged during the first 7–10 days after surgery. Over the ensuing 4 weeks, gradual mobilization of the arm is encouraged. The complication rate for axillary lymph node dissection is low. The most frequent complication is wound seroma.

GROIN DISSECTION

General

The patient is placed in a slight frog-leg position.

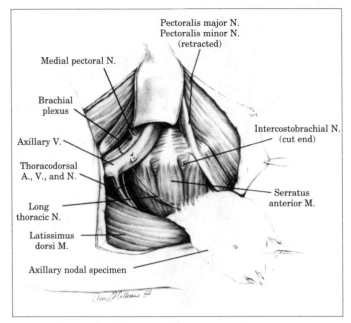

Fig. 3-2. Access to the upper axilla. The arm is draped so that it can be brought over the chest wall during the operation. This facilitates retraction of the pectoralis muscles upward to reveal level III axillary lymph nodes. (From CM Balch, GW Milton, HM Shaw, S-J Soong [eds]. *Cutaneous Melanoma.* **Philadelphia: Lippincott, 1985.)**

Incision

A reverse lazy "S" incision is made from superomedial to the anterior superior iliac spine, vertically down to the inguinal crease, obliquely across the crease, and then vertically down to the apex of the femoral triangle.

Skin Flaps

The limits of the skin flaps are medially to the pubic tubercle and the midbody of the adductor magnus muscle, laterally to the lateral edge of the sartorius muscle, superiorly to above the inguinal ligament, and inferiorly to the apex of the femoral triangle. Some surgeons incorporate an ellipse of skin with the specimen. We do this only when there are enlarged superficial lymph nodes; otherwise, we prefer to trim the skin edges back to healthy tissue at the completion of the procedure.

Lymph Node Dissection

Dissection is carried down to the muscular fascia superiorly (Fig. 3-3). All fatty, node-bearing tissue is swept down to the inguinal ligament and off the external oblique fascia.

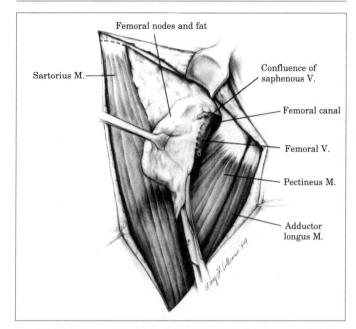

Fig. 3-3. Technique of inguinal lymph node dissection. (From CM Balch, GW Milton, HM Shaw, S-J Soong [eds]. *Cutaneous Melanoma.* Philadelphia: Lippincott, 1985.)

Medially, the spermatic cord or round ligament is exposed and nodal tissue swept laterally. Nodal tissue is swept off the adductor fascia to the femoral vein. At the apex of the femoral triangle, the saphenous vein is divided. Laterally, nodal tissue is dissected off the sartorius and femoral nerves medial to the femoral artery. The sensory branches of the femoral nerve that penetrate the specimen are sacrificed, while deeper motor branches are preserved. Dissecting in the plane of the femoral vessels, the nodal tissue is elevated up to the level of the fossa ovalis, where the saphenous vein is suture ligated at its junction with the femoral vein. The specimen is dissected to beneath the inguinal ligament, where it is divided. Cloquet's node (the lowest iliac node) is sent as a separate specimen for frozen-section examination (Fig. 3-4).

Sartorius Muscle Transposition

The sartorius muscle is disconnected at its insertion on the anterior superior iliac spine (Fig. 3-5). The lateral femoral cutaneous nerve is preserved. The proximal two or three neurovascular bundles to the sartorius are divided to facilitate transposition. The muscle is placed over the femoral vessels and tacked to the inguinal ligament, fascia of the adductor, and vastus muscle groups.

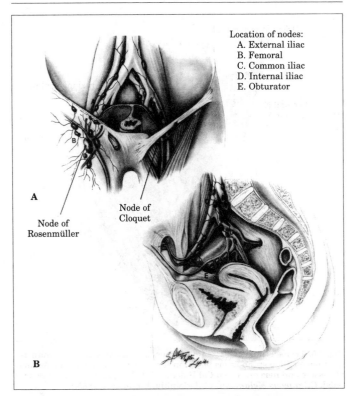

Fig. 3-4. A. Lymphatic anatomy of the inguinal area demonstrating the superficial and deep lymphatic chain. The node of Cloquet lies at the transition between the superficial and deep inguinal nodes. It is located beneath the inguinal ligament in the femoral canal. B. The iliac nodes include those on the common and superficial iliac vessels and the obturator nodes. Obturator nodes should be excised as part of an iliac nodal dissection. (From CM Balch, GW Milton, HM Shaw, S-J Soong [eds]. *Cutaneous Melanoma.* Philadelphia: Lippincott, 1985.)

Location of nodes:
A. External iliac
B. Femoral
C. Common iliac
D. Internal iliac
E. Obturator

Node of Rosenmüller

Node of Cloquet

Wound Closure

The skin edges are examined for viability and trimmed back to healthy skin (usually about 1 cm off each edge). Two closed suction drains are placed through separate stab wounds inferiorly. One is laid medially and the other laterally in the bed of the sartorius. The wound is closed with interrupted 3-0 undyed absorbable sutures and a running 4-0 undyed absorbable monofilament suture.

Postoperative Management

The patient is ambulated the day following surgery and measured for a custom-fit elastic stocking to be used during the day for 6 months. After that period, the stocking may be dis-

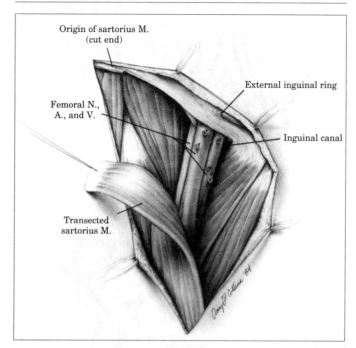

Origin of sartorius M.
(cut end)

External inguinal ring

Femoral N.,
A., and V.

Inguinal canal

Transected
sartorius M.

**Fig. 3-5. Transection of the sartorius muscle at its origin on the anteri-
or superior iliac spine in preparation for transposition over the femoral vessels and nerves. (From CM Balch, GW Milton, HM Shaw, S-J Soong
[eds].** *Cutaneous Melanoma.* **Philadelphia: Lippincott, 1985.)**

continued if no leg swelling occurs. We use a mild diuretic,
such as hydrochlorothiazide, on an individual basis.

Dissection of the Iliac and Obturator Nodes

We perform deep (iliac) dissection for the following indications: (1) known involvement, (2) more than three nodes
grossly involved in the superficial specimen, or (3) frozen section of Cloquet's node reveals metastatic tumor. To gain
access to the deep nodes, we extend the skin incision superiorly. The external oblique muscle is split from a point about
8–10 cm superomedial to the anterior superior iliac spine to
the lateral border of the rectus sheath. The internal oblique
and transversus abdominis muscles are divided, and the
peritoneum is retracted superiorly. An alternative approach
is to split the inguinal ligament just lateral to the femoral
artery. The ureter is exposed as it courses over the iliac
artery. Dissection continues in front of the external iliac
artery separating the external iliac nodes. The inferior epigastric artery and vein are divided if necessary. Dissection of
the lymph nodes continues to the common iliac artery. Nodes
in front of the external iliac vein are dissected to the point at
which the latter proceeds under the internal iliac artery. The

plane of the peritoneum is traced along the wall of the bladder, and the fatty tissues and lymph nodes are dissected off the perivesical fat starting at the internal iliac artery. The superior vesical artery arising from the internal iliac artery toward the bladder may be divided for better exposure if the obturator nodes appear to be involved. Dissection is completed on the medial wall of the external iliac vein, and the nodal chain is further separated from the pelvic fascia until the obturator nerve is seen. Obturator nodes are located in the space between the external iliac vein and the obturator nerve (in an anteroposterior direction) and between the internal iliac artery and the obturator foramen (in a cephalad-caudad direction). The obturator artery and vein usually need not be disturbed. The transversus abdominis, internal oblique, and external oblique muscles may be closed with running sutures. The inguinal ligament, if previously divided, is approximated with interrupted, nonabsorbable sutures to Cooper's ligament medially and to the iliac fascia lateral to the femoral vessels.

Complications

The most common acute postoperative complication is wound infection. Rates range from 5 to 19%. The rate of lymphocele or seroma formation is 3–23%. Leaving suction catheters in place until the drainage decreases to 40–50 ml per day may reduce the incidence of seroma. However, prolonged stay of catheters is associated with a higher rate of infection. Lymphedema is the most serious long-term complication. Three series have now shown a decreased incidence of leg edema after groin dissection as a result of preventive measures including perioperative antibiotics, elastic stockings, leg elevation exercises, and diuretics. Prophylactic measures are important because it is difficult to reverse the progression of edema. Skin flap problems occur with some frequency. Expectant management of ischemic edges often results in full-thickness necrosis and prolonged hospitalization. Therefore if edges are of questionable viability, the patient is returned to the operating room early for flap revision. Clinically detectable deep vein thrombosis is uncommon.

CERVICAL NODE DISSECTION

Metastases to lymph nodes from primary melanomas in the head and neck generally follow a predictable pattern. Melanomas occurring anterior to the pinna of the ear generally metastasize to the parotid, submandibular, submental, upper jugular, and posterior triangle lymph nodes. Lesions occurring inferior to the lateral fissure of the lip will spread to cervical lymph nodes rather than to parotid nodes. Melanomas occurring on the scalp posterior to the pinna of the ear usually spread to occipital, postauricular, posterior triangle, or jugular chain nodes.

Radical neck dissection is generally recommended when nodal metastases are clinically evident. Modified neck dis-

section, sparing the spinal accessory nerve, the sternomas-
toid muscle, and the internal jugular vein, is generally
reserved for patients undergoing elective neck dissection, but
patients with limited metastatic disease are also considered.

Melanomas arising on the scalp or face anterior to the pinna
of the ear and superior to the commissure of the lip are at
risk to metastasize to parotid lymph nodes. This parotid
chain of nodes is contiguous with the cervical nodes. It is
advisable to combine neck dissection with parotid lymph
node dissection when parotid nodes are clinically involved or
at risk.

ADJUVANT THERAPY

No adjuvant therapy for melanoma has been proven to prolong survival. Current therapeutic options include the following.

Radiotherapy

The role of radiotherapy as adjuvant treatment after therapeutic node dissection or as an alternative to ELND in the
regional treatment of patients with intermediate to thick
melanomas has not been clearly defined. Adjuvant radiotherapy, either alone in clinically node-negative patients or
as a surgical adjuvant in pathologically node-positive
patients, has resulted in locoregional control in excess of
85%. Proof of a therapeutic benefit from adjuvant radiotherapy can be obtained only from a prospective randomized
trial. Patients with head and neck primary tumors, with
multiple involved regional nodes, or with extracapsular
extension of regional lymphatic metastases should be considered for adjuvant radiotherapy.

Chemotherapy

No confirmed studies have demonstrated a benefit of adjuvant chemotherapy in melanoma patients at high risk for
relapse. On the contrary, a randomized trial of dacarbazine
(DTIC) given in the adjuvant setting versus no adjuvant
treatment resulted in a statistically significant decrease in
survival in the treatment arm. Adjuvant systemic therapy
should be considered only in the context of a clinical trial.

Biological Therapy

Adjuvant interferon-alpha has been studied in an Eastern
Cooperative Oncology Group randomized trial for melanoma
patients at high risk of recurrence. In that study, a benefit
from adjuvant treatment was suggested by interim analysis;
however, this benefit has not yet achieved statistical significance. In addition, there has been significant treatment-
related toxicity. At present, adjuvant immunotherapy should
be considered only in the context of a clinical trial.

Management of Distant Metastatic Disease

Common sites of distant metastasis in melanoma patients are, in order of decreasing frequency, skin and subcutaneous tissues, lung, liver, and brain. Patients with systemic metastases have poor prognoses. Mean survival is about 6 months. General guidelines for choosing treatment modalities follow, but no treatment for metastatic melanoma has been proven to prolong survival. Experimental treatments are an option for most patients who are diagnosed with distant metastases.

SURGERY

Surgery is a very effective palliative treatment for isolated accessible metastases. Examples of accessible lesions include isolated visceral metastases, particularly brain metastases, and occasionally lung metastases. Some melanoma patients with a solitary pulmonary lesion will have potentially curable primary lung cancer. Gastrointestinal obstruction from metastatic melanoma is usually due to large polypoid lesions that mechanically obstruct the bowel or that act as a lead point for intussusception. These submucosal lesions are generally removed by bowel resection. Liver metastases are associated with such a short survival time (i.e., 2–4 months) that surgical excision is generally not indicated.

Brain metastases from melanoma provide a model for surgical treatment of metastatic disease. Melanoma ranks with small-cell carcinoma of the lung as the most common tumor that metastasizes to the brain. An unusual feature of cerebral metastases is their propensity for hemorrhage, which occurs much more frequently than with other histologic types of metastases. Hemorrhage occurs in 33–50% of patients with melanoma metastases involving the brain. Surgical excision followed by cranial irradiation is the treatment of choice in the case of a solitary, surgically accessible metastasis. Tumor excision is relatively safe; it alleviates symptoms in most patients and prevents further neurologic damage. Although long-term disease-free survival is uncommon, a few patients live more than 5 years after surgery. Radiotherapy is preferred when the lesions are numerous or are located in an area that precludes a safe operation.

RADIOTHERAPY

In the treatment of cutaneous and lymph node metastases with radiation, most authors have observed improved response rates with higher fractional doses. The appropriate recommendation for dose fractionation should be based on considerations of normal tissue tolerance. Multiple or recurrent skin or subcutaneous lesions may be successfully treated by hypofractionated radiotherapy. Symptomatic bony metastases from melanoma also respond to this treatment.

CHEMOTHERAPY

A number of single agents have limited activity against metastatic melanoma, generally inducing partial regression of tumors in 10–20% of patients for a median of 3–5 months. DTIC is the only drug approved for use in melanoma, but antitumor activity has been found with the nitrosoureas (e.g., carmustine), carboplatin, and high-dose cisplatin. Median durations of response have been short, in the range of 3–6 months. If the tumor has no objective response after two or three courses of a particular chemotherapy, it is usually best to discontinue that therapy and evaluate other approaches.

BIOLOGICAL THERAPY

In patients with localized superficial skin metastases and no evidence of bulky disease or visceral metastases, bacille Calmette-Guérin (BCG) can induce regression of most lesions into which it is injected. Interferon also has local activity when injected intradermally or subcutaneously.

The demonstration that interferon-alpha and interleukin-2 (IL-2) are active against melanoma has enabled some new strategies for systemic therapy. Both agents elicit response rates in the range of 10–20%. Although these response rates are not significantly different from those for single-agent chemotherapy, some responses can be dramatic. However, large doses of IL-2 can be highly toxic.

Monoclonal antibody therapy is generally well-tolerated and has shown activity in phase I trials. Monoclonal antibodies have been used to target radiation and potent plant toxins to tumors in patients with metastatic melanoma, and anti-idiotype antibodies have been used to stimulate immune responses.

The use of tumor vaccines is being evaluated in the treatment of advanced disease and as an adjuvant therapy for high-risk patients. These vaccines may contain (1) irradiated tumor cells, usually obtained from the patient; (2) partially or completely purified melanoma antigens; or (3) tumor cell membranes from melanoma cells infected with virus (viral oncolysates). Synthetic vaccines containing genes that encode for tumor antigens or the peptide antigens themselves are also being evaluated, as well as "vaccines" containing genes encoding for immune costimulation signal proteins. Morton has reported encouraging results using a polyvalent melanoma cell vaccine in patients with stage IIIA or IV melanoma. In stage IIIA patients, median survival was 44 months, compared with 29 months in historical controls ($p = .0024$). In stage IV patients, median survival was 23 months, compared with 7.5 months in historical controls ($p = .0001$).

BIOCHEMOTHERAPY

Phase I and II studies have evaluated combinations of IL-2, interferon, and chemotherapy (cisplatin, DTIC, and/or cyclophosphamide). Preliminary results of a series of small studies using combinations of IL-2, interferon-alpha and cisplatin have reported overall response rates of 40%. There is a suggestion that response rates to the combinations may be higher than those for either cytokines alone or for chemotherapy alone. However, toxicity also may be additive.

Follow-Up

Melanoma can have a more variable and unpredictable clinical course than almost any other human cancer. Frequency of follow-up evaluation at M. D. Anderson is as follows: year 1, every 3 months: year 2, every 4 months; years 3–5, every 6 months; and annually thereafter. At each visit the patient undergoes a physical examination, chest radiograph, and liver function studies. Serum lactate dehydrogenase is a useful marker for distant metastases, especially metastasis to the liver. Particular attention should be given to signs or symptoms of central nervous system involvement. Extensive radiographic evaluation of patients with AJCC stage I, II, or III melanoma who are clinically free of disease rarely reveals metastases.

Selected References

Balch CM. The role of elective lymph node dissection in melanoma: Rationale, results and controversies. *J Clin Oncol* 6:163, l988.

Balch CM, Houghton AN, Milton GW, et al. (eds). *Cutaneous Melanoma* (2nd ed). Philadelphia: Lippincott, 1992.

Balch CM, Soong S-J, Murad TM, et al. A multifactorial analysis of melanoma. II. Prognostic factors in patients with stage I (localized) melanoma. *Surgery* 86:343, 1979.

Balch CM, Urist MM, Karakousis CP, et al. Efficacy of 2 cm surgical margins for intermediate-thickness melanomas (1–4 mm): Results of a multi-institutional randomized surgical trial. *Ann Surg* 218:262, 1993.

Cannon-Albright LA, Goldgar DE, Meyer LJ, et al. Assignment of a locus for familial melanoma, MLM, to chromosome 9p 13-p22. *Science* 258:1148, 1992.

Elder DE, Guerry D, VanHorn M, et al. The role of lymph node dissection for clinical stage I malignant melanoma of intermediate thickness (1.5l–3.99 mm). *Cancer* 56:413, l985.

Leinard D, Ewalenko P, Delmotte JJ, et al. High dose recombinant tumor necrosis factor alpha in combination with interferon gamma and melphalan in isolation perfusion of the limbs for melanoma and sarcoma. *J Clin Oncol* 10:52, 1992.

Mansfield PF, Lee JE, Balch CM. Melanoma: Surgical controversies and current practice. *Curr Probl Surg* 31:253, 1994.

McCarthy WH, Shaw HM, Milton GW. Efficacy of elective lymph node dissection in 2,347 patients with clinical stage I malignant melanoma. *Surg Gynecol Obstet* 161:575, l985.

Milton GW, Shaw HM, McCarthy WH, et al. Prophylactic lymph node dissection in clinical stage I cutaneous malignant melanoma: Results of surgical treatment in 1319 patients. *Br J Surg* 69:108, 1982.

Morton DL, Foshag LJ, Hoon DSB, et al. Prolongation of survival in metastatic melanoma after active specific immunotherapy with a new polyvalent melanoma vaccine. *Ann Surg* 216:463, 1992.

Morton DL, Wen DR, Wong JH, et al. Technical details of intraoperative lymphatic mapping for early stage melanoma. *Arch Surg* 127:392, 1992.

Norman J, Cruse CW, Espinoza C, et al. Redefinition of cutaneous lymphatic drainage with the use of lymphoscintigraphy for malignant melanoma. *Am J Surg* 162:432,1991.

Reintgen DS, Cox EB, McCarty KM Jr, et al. Efficacy of elective lymph node dissection in patients with intermediate thickness primary melanoma. *Ann Surg* 198:379, 1983.

Sim FH, Taylor WF, Pritchard DJ, et al. Lymphadenectomy in the management of stage I malignant melanoma: A prospective randomized study. *Mayo Clin Proc* 61:697, l986.

Travis J. Closing in on melanoma susceptability gene(s). *Science* 258:1080, 1992.

Veronesi U, Adamus J, Bandiera DC, et al. Delayed regional lymph node dissection in stage I melanoma of the skin of the lower extremities. *Cancer* 49:2420, l982.

Veronesi U, Adamus J, Bandiera DC, et al. Inefficacy of immediate node dissection in stage I melanoma of the limbs. *N Engl J Me*d 297:627, l977.

Veronesi U, Cascinelli N, Adamus J, et al. Primary cutaneous melanoma 2 mm or less in thickness: Results of a randomized study comparing wide with narrow surgical excision: A preliminary report. *N Engl J Med* 3l8:1159, l988.

Nonmelanoma Skin Cancer

Keith M. Heaton

Epidemiology and Etiology

Basal cell carcinoma (BCC) and squamous cell carcinoma (SCC) of the skin are the most common malignancies in the white population. They account for almost one-third of all cancers in the United States, with more than 600,000 new cases and 2,000 deaths from nonmelanoma skin cancer reported in 1992. These figures most likely underestimate the true prevalence of BCC and SCC because most cases are diagnosed and treated in an outpatient setting and therefore are not recorded in a tumor registry.

Exposure to sunlight is the principal cause of BCC and SCC, although each can occur in sites protected from the sun, such as the genitals and lower extremities. Other known causes of nonmelanoma skin cancer include exposure to ultraviolet (UV) light, chemical carcinogens such as arsenic and hydrocarbons, human papillomavirus, ionizing radiation, cigarette smoking, and chronic irritation or ulceration (e.g., decubitus ulcers). In addition, patients who are immunocompromised have a much higher incidence of skin cancer.

Differential Diagnosis

A variety of benign skin lesions are either precursor lesions of malignant tumors or are difficult to distinguish from malignant tumors.

Keratoacanthoma is a benign tumor that usually presents in elderly people as a single, raised 1- to 2-cm lesion with a characteristic horn-filled crater. Although there is a characteristic phase of rapid growth, spontaneous involution occurs within a few months and is usually complete by 6 months. This lesion can be difficult to distinguish from SCC and therefore requires a biopsy that includes a segment of adjoining normal skin to confirm the diagnosis.

Actinic keratosis also may be confused with early SCC. This benign tumor most commonly presents as multiple lesions on sun-exposed areas in middle-aged individuals with fair complexions, although single lesions can occur. Actinic keratosis is characterized by hyperkeratosis and is usually less than 1 cm in diameter. Cryotherapy or topical fluorouracil are the standard treatments. Persistent lesions require excisional biopsy because the incidence of SCC arising from actinic keratoses approaches 20%.

Bowen's disease represents a benign lesion that has malignant potential. It is frequently solitary and manifests as a slowly enlarging erythematous patch of skin with a sharp but irregular outline. Crusting is commonly noted in the center. Bowen's disease is thought to result from prolonged sun exposure. Histologically, the lesion is an intraepithelial SCC. Complete excision is required because the incidence of SCC developing in patients with Bowen's disease is as high as 11%. Lesions that occur in unexposed areas are frequently due to arsenic ingestion and are associated with an increased incidence of visceral cancer.

There is no known precursor lesion for BCC.

Squamous Cell Carcinoma

Approximately 80% of UV light–induced SCCs develop on the arms, head, and neck. Patients with SCC often have actinic keratoses. SCC associated with exposure to ionizing radiation occurs at sites affected by chronic radiation dermatitis. SCC arises from basal keratinocytes of the skin and typically presents as a firm nodule on an erythematous base with elevated borders and indistinct margins. Central ulceration or crusting may be present. Histologically, SCC is characterized by irregular nests of epidermal cells invading the dermis in varying degrees. Grading is based on the degree of cell differentiation. The greater the differentiation, the less the invasive tendency and the better the prognosis. The more poorly differentiated neoplasms show no evidence of keratinization and exhibit marked cellular atypia making them difficult to distinguish from anaplastic melanoma, lymphoma, or mesenchymal tumors.

SCC may metastasize to regional lymph nodes and eventually to distant sites, including bone, brain, and lungs. The rate of metastases with SCC varies according to prognostic factors such as anatomic site, depth of invasion, and degree of differentiation. For example, SCC arising from actinic keratosis has a low propensity to metastasize (0.5%), whereas SCC arising from a chronic sinus tract or from a previously irradiated area metastasizes much more frequently (20–30%). The overall rate of metastasis for SCC of the skin is 2%.

Basal Cell Carcinoma

BCC is a malignant neoplasm that arises from the basal cell layers of the epidermis and adnexal structures. Ninety-five percent occur in patients older than 40 years. BCC develops on hair-bearing skin, most commonly on sun-exposed areas, and approximately 85% of lesions are found on the head and neck. Pruritis and bleeding are common symptoms, and patients frequently complain of a bleeding sore that heals partially and then ulcerates again.

Histologically, most BCCs are well differentiated. Tumors consist of palisading basal cells with uniform, elongated nuclei and very little cytoplasm.

There are five common forms of BCC:

1. *Noduloulcerative* BCC is characterized by a waxy, nodular lesion with an ulcerated center.

2. *Pigmented* BCC is similar in gross appearance to noduloulcerative BCC but has pigmentation. This lesion can be difficult to distinguish from seborrheic keratosis and nodular melanoma.

3. *Sclerosing or morphea-form* BCC appears as a single, flat, indurated, off-white, ill-defined macule. Histologic sections show a dense, fibrous connective tissue stroma in which small groups and narrow strands of basaloid cells are embedded. It is very similar to the microscopic appearance of metastatic breast carcinoma and desmoplastic epithelioma.

4. *Superficial* BCC occurs commonly on the trunk as an ill-defined, red, scaly macule.

5. *Fibroepithelial* BCC also usually occurs on the trunk and manifests as a flesh-colored papule without surrounding inflammatory changes.

The natural history of BCC depends on the histologic subtype. Fibroepithelial and superficial BCC remain stable and grow slowly. The noduloulcerative and pigmented types also grow slowly but invade locally by peripheral and deep extension. This invasion can, in rare instances, lead to destruction of vital organs and eventually death. Sclerosing BCC is biologically more aggressive and difficult to treat because of indistinct margins and deep infiltration.

Metastases from BCC are very rare (0.0028% in one large study). Lesions at increased risk for metastasis are typically located on the head or neck, are large and locally invasive, and persist despite repeated surgery and radiotherapy. Most metastases are found in the regional lymph nodes, but distant organs may be involved.

Kaposi's Sarcoma

Kaposi's sarcoma (KS), a neoplasm of vascular endothelial cells, is characterized by the presence of bluish-red nodules, edema, and hemosiderin deposition. Prior to 1981, about 100 new cases of this disease were diagnosed in the United States each year. The incidence has since risen dramatically, particularly in immunosuppressed or human immunodeficiency virus (HIV)–positive patients. Prior to 1981 and the HIV disease epidemic, KS most commonly occurred on the feet of men of Jewish or Italian descent in the sixth to eighth decade of life. Typical KS patients today are immunocompromised. These people develop a much more virulent, systemic form of the disease, with occasional lymph node and/or gastrointestinal involvement.

Sebaceous Carcinoma

Sebaceous carcinoma accounts for only 0.2–4.6% of all cutaneous neoplasms. It usually presents as a slow-growing, hard, yellow nodule arising from the sebaceous glands of the face and eyelids. Apocrine and eccrine sweat gland carcinomas are even rarer, with fewer than 100 cases reported annually.

Syndromes Associated with Skin Cancers

Xeroderma pigmentosum is a rare (1 in 250,000 persons) autosomal-recessive disease characterized by severe sun sensitivity, photophobia, cutaneous pigmentary changes, advanced sun damage, and the development of malignant cutaneous neoplasms, especially BCC, SCC, and melanoma.

Sebaceous nevus of Jadassohn usually manifests as a single, oval, alopecic, orange-yellow plaque on the scalp of a child. At puberty, the lesion becomes verrucous. In adult life, both benign and malignant skin tumors (particularly BCC) may develop.

Basal cell nevus syndrome is a genetic form of BCC inherited by an autosomal-dominant gene. The lesions appear on the skin between puberty and 35 years and can range in number from a few to several hundred. Most lesions remain quiescent, but some may become locally aggressive.

Biopsy Techniques

There are four principal biopsy techniques used for cutaneous malignancies. A *shave biopsy* is obtained by slicing a superficial portion of the tumor with a scalpel. A *punch biopsy* obtains a deeper specimen by introducing a sharp, cylindrical instrument into the reticular dermis or subcutaneous tissue. An *incisional biopsy* removes only a portion of the tumor, while the entire lesion is removed with an *excisional biopsy*. To facilitate accurate diagnosis, the technique selected should be the one that yields the optimal pathologic specimen. For example, the diagnosis of SCC can be missed with a shave biopsy. Therefore a deep punch biopsy, incisional biopsy, or excisional biopsy is indicated when SCC is suspected. These more definitive techniques are also indicated in suspected cases of pigmented or sclerosing BCC or to confirm the diagnosis of benign keratoacanthoma. Shave biopsy may be used in cases of noduloulcerative or superficial BCC.

Staging

The current American Joint Committee on Cancer (AJCC) staging system for BCC and SCC of the skin is shown in Table 4-1.

Table 4-1. TNM staging for squamous cell carcinoma and basal cell carcinoma of the skin

Primary tumor (T)

Tx	Not assessable
Tis	Carcinoma in situ
T0	No primary tumor present
T1	Tumor ≤2 cm, strictly superficial, or
T2	Tumor >2 cm but <5 cm or with minimal dermal infiltration
T3	Tumor >5 cm or with deep infiltration of dermis
T4	Tumor involving other structures such as muscle, bone, or

Nodal involvement (N)

Nx	Not assessable
N0	No evidence of regional lymph node
N1	Evidence of mobile ipsilateral regional lymph nodes
N2	Evidence of contralateral mobile lymph nodes
N3	Fixed regional lymph nodes

Distant metastasis (M)

Mx	Not assessable
M0	No known distant metastasis
M1	Distant metastasis present

Staging

Stage I	Any T	N0	M0
Stage II	Any T	N1–3	M0
Stage III	Any T	Any N	M1

Source: Adapted from AK Patterson, RG Geronemu. Cancers of the Skin. In VT DeVita Jr, S Hellman, SA Rosenberg (eds): *Cancer: Principles and Practice of Oncology* (3rd ed). Philadelphia: Lippincott, 1989.

Treatment

Once the histologic diagnosis has been made, numerous factors must be considered in determining the appropriate therapy. These factors include the histopathologic type, location, and size of the tumor; the age and general medical condition of the patient; patient preference; and cost. Commonly used treatments for nonmelanoma skin cancers are excisional surgery, Mohs' surgery, cryosurgery, curettage and electrodesiccation, and radiotherapy.

SURGICAL EXCISION

Excisional surgery is effective for all types of nonmelanoma skin cancer and is a mainstay of therapy. Complete excision of a tumor has the advantage of allowing evaluation of the tumor margins. Most excisions are performed in an elliptical fashion along Langer's cleavage lines (the lines of skin tension) to achieve a good cosmetic result. Elliptical excisions are easily performed on the trunk, extremities, cheeks, forehead, chin, and scalp; however, special consideration must be given to excision of lesions from the lip, eyelids, alar rim of the nose, and ears. In these locations, a wedge-shaped excision may be preferable to minimize distortion. There is no uniform recommendation regarding the size of surgical margins, but many surgeons use margins of 3–5 mm for small, well-defined lesions and margins of at least 1 cm for large lesions or more aggressive subtypes. Simple primary closure, a local flap, a skin graft, or healing by second intention can be used to repair the defect.

For a neoplasm with the potential to metastasize, clinical evaluation of the regional lymph nodes is mandatory. However, lymph node dissection should be performed only if there is clinically palpable lymphadenopathy and a biopsy of an enlarged node has demonstrated metastatic disease.

MOHS' MICROGRAPHIC SURGERY

Mohs' surgery is a specialized technique in which serial horizontal sections of excised tissue are systematically mapped and microscopically evaluated by frozen-section examination. Because margins are checked thoroughly at the time of surgery, this technique is a major improvement in the treatment of difficult and recurrent skin cancers, allowing complete removal of tumor with minimal loss of normal tissue. However, Mohs' surgery is both time-consuming and expensive. The choices for repair after Mohs' surgery are similar to those with excisional surgery.

CRYOSURGERY

Cryosurgery uses liquid nitrogen delivered by a spray apparatus or a cryoprobe under local anesthesia. It is effective in the treatment of premalignant tumors. However, the local failure rate is high even for experienced cryosurgeons. Favorable anatomic sites for cryosurgery include the eyelids, ears, face, neck, and trunk. Particular care must be taken when treating tumors of the nasolabial fold, inner canthi of the eyes, and periauricular areas. These sites usually require a wider margin of freezing to help prevent recurrence because there is often deep infiltration. Cryosurgery should not be the first-choice therapy for malignant tumors.

CURETTAGE AND ELECTRODESICCATION

Dermatologists commonly use curettage and electrodesiccation to treat BCC and superficial SCC. A curette is first used to debulk and delineate the tumor from the surrounding normal skin based on differences in tissue consistency. The remaining lesion is then electrodesiccated or obliterated with a carbon dioxide laser. Usually two or three office visits are required to completely remove the tumor, depending on its size. This method is appropriate for small superficial or noduloulcerative BCCs and for SCCs with clearly defined borders. It should not be used for tumors larger than 2 cm. Because of wound contracture, distortion is especially likely to occur around the eyes and mouth. Curettage and electrodesiccation is particularly useful for lower extremity tumors or when optimal cosmetic results are not essential.

RADIOTHERAPY

Prior to initiation of radiotherapy, a biopsy should always be performed to confirm the diagnosis and document the type of neoplasm. Radiotherapy is most appropriate for primary SCC and BCC, although recurrences (of tumors previously treated by other means) can also be treated. However, treatment is costly and the cure rate is low. Radiotherapy is particularly advantageous in elderly or debilitated patients and in patients at high risk for surgical complications.

CHEMOTHERAPY

Topical fluorouracil may be used to treat premalignant lesions. Available as creams and solutions, fluorouracil is applied twice daily for 4–6 weeks. Treatment causes oozing, crusting, and ulceration of the lesion, with healing taking 3–6 weeks after treatment stops. The recurrence rate after treatment with topical fluorouracil may be higher than with other therapies.

Intralesional interferon-alpha is currently being evaluated as a treatment for noduloulcerative and superficial BCC and for SCC. Although it offers good cosmetic results, studies have found recurrence rates to be higher and cure rates lower than with other treatment modalities. The use of interferon is classified as investigational at this time.

PHOTODYNAMIC THERAPY

Photodynamic therapy, another investigational treatment, involves the intravenous administration of a systemic photosensitizer followed by nonionizing radiation to preferentially destroy neoplastic tissue. The photosensitizer is cleared from most organs by 48–72 hours but is retained by the tumor, skin, and reticuloendothelial system. Exposure to light at 630 nm produces oxygen free radicals and selectively kills the tumor cells. Preliminary results show success rates of 85–100% for BCC. Patients must be shielded from sunlight for the duration of therapy.

Screening and Prevention

The key to preventing nonmelanoma skin cancer is reducing one's exposure to sunlight. People of all ages should protect their skin from sun exposure by staying out of the sun, particularly during the middle of the day, by wearing protective clothing, and by applying sunscreens with a sun protection factor of 15 or higher to all exposed areas. Although most chemical sunscreens (p-aminobenzoic acid [PABA], benzophenones, cinnamates, salicylates, and anthranilates) absorb and filter out UVB radiation, only the benzophenones and anthranilates absorb UVA radiation.

Because there are no completely satisfactory topical sunscreens, other strategies have been attempted. However, chemoprophylaxis with beta-carotene or isotretinoin has failed to show any significant reduction in the risk of developing of nonmelanoma skin cancer.

The rising incidence of skin cancers underscores the need for effective measures to control these cancers. Because of its ease, screening for skin cancer is theoretically promising, but there are few data demonstrating its effectiveness. Nevertheless, monthly at-home examination using full-length and hand-held mirrors of all areas of the body is useful for detecting skin changes. Any change in an existing lesion or the appearance of a new lesion should be brought to the attention of a physician.

Selected References

Arnold HL, Odom RB, James WD (eds). *Andrew's Diseases of the Skin* (8th ed). Philadelphia: Saunders, 1990.

Patterson AK, Geronemu RG. Cancers of the Skin. In VT DeVita, Jr, S Hellman, SA Rosenberg (eds), *Cancer: Principles and Practice of Oncology* (3rd ed). Philadelphia, Lippincott, 1989.

Koh HK, Geller AC, Miller DR, et al. Can screening for melanoma and skin cancer save lives? *Dermatol Clin* 9:795, 1991.

Kuflik EG, Gage AA. The five-year cure rate achieved by cryosurgery for skin cancer. *J Am Acad Dermatol* 24:1002, 1991.

Miller PK, Roenigk RK, Brodland DG, et al. Cutaneous micrographic surgery: Mohs procedure. *Mayo Clin Proc* 67:971, 1992.

O'Donoghue MN. Sunscreen: One weapon against melanoma. *Dermatol Clin* 9:789, 1991.

Preston DS, Stern RS. Nonmelanoma cancers of the skin. *N Engl J Med* 327:1649, 1992.

Robinson JK. Advances in the treatment of nonmelanoma skin cancer. *Dermatol Clin* 9:757, 1991.

Silverman CK, Kopf AW, Grin JM, et al. Recurrence rates of treated basal cell carcinomas. *J Dermatol Surg* 17:713, 1991.

Urbach F. Incidence of nonmelanoma skin cancer. *Dermatol Clin* 9:751, 1991.

Wick MR. Kaposi's sarcoma unrelated to the acquired immunodeficiency syndrome. *Curr Opin Oncol* 3:377, 1991.

Bone and Soft-Tissue Sarcoma

Sarkis H. Meterissian and Kenneth K. Tanabe

Soft-Tissue Sarcomas

EPIDEMIOLOGY AND RISK FACTORS

Approximately 6,000 persons are diagnosed in the United States each year as having soft-tissue sarcomas, rare tumors that account for less than 1% of all newly diagnosed adult cancers in the United States annually. More common in children, soft-tissue sarcomas represent 7% of all malignancies diagnosed in the pediatric population. Because of the ubiquity of connective tissue, soft-tissue sarcomas are found throughout the body, including the extremities, head and neck, abdominal wall, and retroperitoneum. Approximately 50% of sarcomas occur in the extremities, 15% in the trunk, and 15% in the retroperitoneum. Lower extremity lesions are 3.5 times more common than upper extremity lesions. The thigh is the most common area affected by this tumor. The incidence of sarcomas is equivalent in men and women.

Risk factors for soft-tissue sarcoma include the following:

1. *Environmental factors.* Exposure to herbicides has been linked in some studies to an increased risk for the development of soft-tissue sarcoma. Exposure to asbestos has been associated with the development of mesotheliomas.

2. *Previous radiation exposure.* Rarely, sarcomas may develop in areas exposed to radiotherapy, such as the chest wall of women who have received radiotherapy for breast cancer. The risk of postradiotherapy sarcomas increases with increasing dosage. The interval between irradiation and the development of sarcoma is usually at least 10 years. Sarcomas occurring after radiation exposure are most commonly malignant fibrous histiocytomas.

3. *Chronic lymphedema.* Chronic lymphedema such as that experienced after axillary dissection has been associated with lymphangiosarcoma (Stewart-Treves syndrome).

4. *Genetic predisposition.* Specific inherited genetic alterations have been associated with an increased risk of bone and soft-tissue sarcomas. For example, patients with Gardner's syndrome (familial polyposis) have a higher than normal incidence of desmoids; patients with germ line mutations in the tumor suppressor gene *P53* (Li-Fraumeni syndrome) have a high incidence of sarcomas; and patients with von Recklinghausen's disease who have abnormalities in the neurofibromatosis type 1 gene (NF1) tend to develop neurofibrosarcomas.

5. *Oncogene changes.* Germ line defects in *P53* have been identified in families studied who are affected by Li-Fraumeni syndrome, suggesting that inactivation of *P53* by

Table 5-1. The relative incidence of the most common histologic types of soft-tissue sarcoma treated at M. D. Anderson Cancer Center, 1963–1977

Histologic classification	Incidence (%)
Malignant fibrous histiocytoma	20
Neurofibrosarcoma	20
Fibrosarcoma	14
Liposarcoma	14
Synovial sarcoma	8
Unclassified sarcoma	6
Rhabdomyosarcoma	6
Leiomyosarcoma	5
Epithelioid sarcoma	2
Angiosarcoma	1
Other	4

Source: Adapted from RD Lindberg, RG Martin, MM Romsdahl, et al. Conservative surgery and postoperative radiotherapy in 300 adults with soft-tissue sarcomas. *Cancer* 47:2391, 1981.

mutation may play an etiologic role in the development of soft-tissue sarcomas. Amplification of the *MDM2* gene, whose protein product binds to the *P53* protein, has been detected in several sarcoma specimens. Future studies will undoubtedly uncover more information on the genetic alterations that result in sarcoma formation.

PATHOLOGY

Sarcoma is Greek for "fish flesh," referring to the tumor's tendency to feel fleshy when palpated, unlike the more common scirrhous variants of many carcinomas. Mesodermal cells give rise to the connective tissues distributed throughout the body, including pericardium, pleura, blood vessel endothelium, smooth and striated muscle, bone, cartilage, and synovium, and are the cells from which nearly all sarcomas originate. Consequently, sarcomas develop in a wide variety of anatomic sites. Although schwannomas (peripheral nerve sheath tumors) arise from Schwann's cells, which are derived from neuroectoderm rather than mesodermal cells, schwannomas are still commonly considered sarcomas.

Several histologic types of sarcomas have been characterized. Their relative frequencies (Table 5-1) differ among institutions, depending on referral patterns, study exclusion criteria, and the time period examined. For example, malignant fibrous histiocytoma was rarely reported before 1972; however, since that time it has gained increasing recognition and is now the most common histologic diagnosis in many published series.

Approximately 15% of all soft-tissue sarcomas occur in the retroperitoneum. Of tumors that occur in the retroperitoneum, approximately 80% are malignant, with liposarcoma, fibrosarcoma, leiomyosarcoma, and malignant fibrous histiocytoma accounting for the vast majority of histologic types identified. It is not uncommon for a patient's tumor to be classified differently by different pathologists. The concordance rate among competent pathologists in assigning a sarcoma to a histologic subtype is approximately 65%. Few pathologists have the opportunity to study many of these rare tumors during their careers, and this lack of experience may contribute to the relatively low concordance rate. However, when different histologic types are grouped together according to histologic grade, it becomes apparent that tumors of different histologic type but of common histologic grade behave similarly with respect to distant metastasis and effect on patient survival.

There are several different sarcoma grading schemes in use. Knowledge of the histologic grade is critical in the formulation of treatment plans. The criteria used to determine grade include differentiation, cellularity, amount of stroma, vascularity, degree of necrosis, and mitoses per high-power field. Metastases are uncommon in patients with low-grade sarcomas, in contrast to patients with intermediate- or high-grade sarcomas. Only three histologic types of sarcoma metastasize to regional lymph nodes: Epithelioid sarcomas metastasize to regional nodes in approximately 20% of cases, with rhabdomyosarcomas and malignant fibrous histiocytomas metastasizing to regional nodes significantly less frequently (10% and 5%, respectively).

STAGING

The American Joint Committee for Cancer Staging (AJCC) system for staging soft-tissue sarcomas relies on histologic grade, tumor size, nodal status, and the presence or absence of distant metastases (Table 5-2). An alternate system for extremity soft-tissue sarcoma staging has been proposed by Enneking and colleagues and relies on histologic grade (low versus high), anatomic location (intracompartmental versus extracompartmental), and the presence or absence of metastases. In this staging scheme, anatomic location may be a pseudonym for tumor size because large tumors are generally not confined to a single compartment.

In nearly all published reports, histologic grade is a statistically significant prognostic factor for disease-free and overall survival. Tumor size at presentation is also an important determinant of outcome. Tumors larger than 5 cm have a higher incidence of both distant metastasis and local recurrence and are associated with a worse overall survival rate than tumors that are smaller than 5 cm at presentation. Local recurrence is an independent adverse prognostic factor in many published series.

CLINICAL PRESENTATION

Most extremity soft-tissue sarcomas present as an asymptomatic mass, and therefore the size at presentation usually

Table 5-2. The AJCC staging system for sarcoma of soft tissues

Histologic grade of malignancy (G)

GX	Grade cannot be assessed
G1	Well differentiated
G2	Moderately differentiated
G3	Poorly differentiated
G4	Undifferentiated

Primary tumor (T)

TX	Primary tumor cannot be assessed
T0	No evidence of primary tumor
T1	Tumor 5 cm or smaller in greatest dimension
T2	Tumor larger than 5 cm in greatest dimension

Regional lymph nodes

NX	Regional lymph nodes cannot be assessed
N0	No regional lymph node metastases
N1	Regional lymph node metastases

Distant metastases (M)

MX	Presence of distant metastases cannot be assessed
M0	No distant metastases
M1	Distant metastases

Stage grouping

Stage IA	G1	T1	N0	M0
Stage IB	G1	T2	N0	M0
Stage IIA	G2	T1	N0	M0
Stage IIB	G2	T2	N0	M0
Stage IIIA	G3,4	T1	N0	M0
Stage IIIB	G3,4	T2	N0	M0
Stage IVA	Any G	Any T	N1	M0
Stage IVB	Any G	Any T	Any N	M1

Source: Adapted from OH Beahrs, DE Henson, RVP Hutter, et al (eds). *Manual for Staging of Cancer* (4th ed). Philadelphia: Lippincott, 1992.

depends on the anatomic site of the tumor. For example, while a 2- to 3-cm tumor may become readily apparent on the back of the hand, a tumor in the thigh may grow to 10–15 cm in diameter before it becomes apparent. Frequently a traumatic event to the affected area will call attention to the preexisting lesion. Some patients present with pain; however, there appear to be no signs or symptoms that reliably distinguish between benign and malignant soft-tissue tumors. Small lesions that by clinical history have been unchanged for several years may be closely observed without biopsy. However, a biopsy should be performed for all other tumors.

Retroperitoneal soft-tissue sarcomas nearly always present as asymptomatic masses and generally grow to large sizes (median approximately 15 cm) because of the abdomen's ability to accommodate slow-growing tumors with few symptoms. Patients may present with neurologic symptoms from compression of lumbar or pelvic nerves. On occasion, patients may present with obstructive gastrointestinal symptoms related to displacement or direct tumor involvement of an intestinal organ.

EXTREMITY SOFT-TISSUE SARCOMAS

Biopsy

Appropriate biopsy of an extremity lesion suspected of being a soft-tissue sarcoma requires avoidance of several potential pitfalls. Core needle biopsies and fine-needle aspirations have been demonstrated to be accurate diagnostic tools at large centers with extensive experience in the management of these tumors. However, tissue samples larger than those provided by needle biopsy may be necessary to obtain sections of viable tissue adequate for determination of grade and histologic type.

Excisional biopsy is indicated for lesions smaller than 3 cm. Soft-tissue tumors larger than 3 cm in diameter should be assessed by incisional biospy, regardless of whether malignancy is suspected. This technique provides adequate tissue for analysis without disturbing the tissue planes that surround the tumor, and it leaves the bulk of the tumor intact to aid in performing a subsequent wide local excision. The biopsy incision should be oriented so that a subsequent wide local excision can easily encompass the biopsy site and scar. Biopsy incisions should generally be oriented along the long axis of an extremity or parallel to the dominant underlying muscle group on the trunk. An improperly oriented biopsy incision may result in a much larger surgical defect than would otherwise be necessary to appropriately excise the biopsy cavity. This, in turn, may result in significantly larger postoperative radiotherapy fields to encompass all tissues at risk.

The need for adequate hemostasis after a biopsy cannot be overemphasized. Extravasation of blood allows dissemination of tumor cells along the planes of blood extravasation and therefore increases the volume of tissue requiring treatment by radiotherapy or surgical excision.

Work-Up

After establishing a diagnosis of an extremity soft-tissue sarcoma, it is important to assess the extent of local disease and search for distant metastases. Magnetic resonance imaging (MRI) provides a more accurate delineation of muscle groups affected by the primary tumor than does computed tomography (CT). MRI also provides sagittal and coronal views and better distinction between bone and tumor than does CT. However, both techniques provide the information essential for planning a surgical resection. The possibility of bone invasion by tumor should be addressed by either MRI or plain bone radiography. Radionuclide bone scans cannot distinguish between bone invasion by tumor and increased periosteal blood flow in reaction to an adjacent tumor. High-quality cross-sectional images usually obviate the need for arteriography, especially for extremity and trunk tumors. Soft-tissue sarcomas very rarely metastasize to lymph nodes, so lymphangiography is never indicated.

The most common site for the distant spread of extremity sarcomas is the lungs. CT is more sensitive than conventional tomography in the detection of lung, pleural, and mediastinal metastases. However, because it also detects many more lesions that on subsequent evaluation prove to be unrelated benign conditions, CT is less specific than conventional tomography. Searches for bone and brain metastases are rarely indicated, unless symptoms of metastases to these sites are present.

Management of Local Disease

The success of local tumor control depends on several tumor-related and treatment-related prognostic factors. Patients with sarcomas that are recurrent, large (>5 cm), and/or high grade have a higher risk of recurrence. Older patients (>50 years) may have a higher risk of local recurrence than do younger patients. Local control rates based on stage are shown in Table 5-3.

Elective regional lymphadenectomy is rarely indicated in patients with soft-tissue sarcoma and should be considered only in patients with epithelioid sarcomas.

Because the pseudocapsule that forms around a sarcoma always contains malignant cells, shelling a sarcoma out of its pseudocapsule is inadequate treatment and nearly always leads to a local recurrence.

The concept of radical resection with wide surgical margins and entire muscle group excision was a major breakthrough in extremity sarcoma management, with a reduction in the local recurrence rate to 20%. However, although radical resection was a step foward, several problems remained. First, in patients with large lesions, these resections were extremely morbid, often requiring amputation or causing other significant functional and/or cosmetic deficits. Second, many patients who underwent radical resection for large, high-grade lesions developed distant disease despite adequate local control. Finally, some sarcomas arise in areas where anatomic constraints limit the surgical margins obtainable.

Although the need for radical excision may be unavoidable in some instances, the modern approach to extremity soft-tissue sarcoma entails an aggressive effort to achieve limb salvage. Small (<5 cm), low-grade tumors are usually amenable to therapy by wide local excision only, with margins of 2 cm. With larger, higher-grade lesions, adjuvant

Table 5-3. Local control and disease-free survival rates by AJCC stage in 220 patients with soft-tissue sarcomas treated with surgery and radiotherapy at the Massachusetts General Hospital, 1971–1985

| AJCC stage* | Number of patients | 5-year actuarial rates (%) | |
		Local control	Disease-free survival
IA	15	100	100
IB	25	91	96
IIA	32	86	88
IIB	53	85	53
IIIA	31	92	89
IIIB	61	73	44
IVA	3	100	100
Total	220	86	70

*AJCC staging according to 1988 guidelines, which used three categories for histopathologic grade rather than the current four-grade system.
Source: Adapted from HD Suit, HJ Mankin, WC Wood, et al. Treatment of the patient with stage M0 soft tissue sarcoma. *J Clin Oncol* 6:854, 1988.

radiotherapy has been demonstrated to be effective in reducing local recurrence. The addition of radiotherapy to surgery has permitted the increased use of limb-sparing surgery, with local control rates equal to those associated with radical surgery. Radiotherapy may be delivered preoperatively, postoperatively, intraoperatively, or by brachytherapy; no randomized studies have been performed to compare these methods.

At the University of Texas M. D. Anderson Cancer Center radiotherapy is preferentially used preoperatively rather than postoperatively. The radiotherapy fields can be smaller preoperatively because they do not need to encompass all tissue areas and planes exposed during surgical resection. Additionally, radiotherapy doses of 50 Gy given preoperatively yield results comparable to those with higher doses given postoperatively because of relative tissue hypoxia in surgical wounds.

More recently, the use of brachytherapy techniques has resulted in tumor control that is comparable to that achieved with external beam radiotherapy. An additional benefit of brachytherapy is that only 5 days of treatment are required rather than 5–6 weeks needed for external beam radiotherapy. Moreover, there is no delay in resection as with preoperative radiotherapy, which requires 1 week of healing for each 10 Gy of radiation delivered. The frequency of wound complications with brachytherapy is similiar to that seen with postoperative radiotherapy (approximately 10%), as compared with the 30% frequency seen with preoperative irradiation. Finally, because there is less radiation scatter, brachytherapy is the radiotherapy technique of choice for sarcomas near joints, immature epiphyses, or gonads.

Ongoing prospective trials may better define the indications of the various radiotherapeutic approaches. The overall 5-year survival rates are dependent on stage at presentation and are shown in Table 5-3.

Adjuvant Chemotherapy

The role of adjuvant chemotherapy in the treatment of extremity soft-tissue sarcoma remains controversial. Because of the high incidence of distant metastases with high-grade lesions, several prospective studies have been initiated in an attempt to improve outcome. However, prospective randomized adjuvant chemotherapy trials have failed to demonstrate convincingly an improvement in disease-free survival and overall survival for treated patients. Most regimens use combinations of drugs, with doxorubicin and ifosfamide being the most active. Clinical response rates have been 40–50% at best, and the regimens used have been associated with significant toxicities.

Because of the poor response and severe side effects associated with adjuvant chemotherapy, it is used in the neoadjuvant (preoperative) setting at M. D. Anderson. Patients with high-grade lesions who respond with primary tumor shrinkage after two or three courses of multiagent chemotherapy are continued on this treatment regimen after tumor resection. Patients whose tumors do not respond are offered other systemic treatments, thereby avoiding the toxicity of a chemotherapy regimen to which they have demonstrated insensitivity. In a retrospective review of this approach at M. D. Anderson, marked improvement in overall, disease-free, and distant disease-free survival rates was seen in patients who responded to neoadjuvant therapy.

Management of Local Recurrence

It remains unclear whether a local recurrence contributes to distant metastases and diminished survival. Although patients with local recurrences have a worse overall survival rate than those who maintain local disease control, a local recurrence may be a marker rather than a source of distant metastases. Microscopically positive surgical margins increase the risk for local recurrence but do not adversely influence overall survival. Studies have shown that patients with isolated local recurrences may be successfully retreated with additional surgery and adjuvant radiotherapy. In a retrospective analysis of 39 patients with locally recurrent soft-tissue sarcomas, Singer, et al., found that of the 21 patients with an isolated local recurrence, 14 (67%) were successfully retreated by an aggressive re-excision. An isolated local recurrence should be aggressively treated with a negative-margin re-resection (amputation if necessary), with the addition of radiotherapy. Patients previously treated with external beam radiotherapy can still receive radiotherapy by either a brachytherapy or intraoperative radiotherapy technique.

Management of Distant Disease

Distant metastases are the most common cause of death from soft-tissue sarcomas, and the majority of treatment failures at distant sites occur within 2 years. The incidence of metastases is 40% in patients with intermediate- and high-grade extremity sarcomas, compared with only 5% in patients with low-grade sarcomas. Within each histologic grade, the incidence of metastases increases with increasing primary tumor size. The most common site of metastases is the lungs, and 50% of first recurrences are isolated lung metastases.

In the absence of extrapulmonary metastases, lung metastases should be resected if the patient is medically fit to withstand a thoracotomy and the lesions are amenable to resection. A complete resection can result in a 15–30% 5-year survival rate. Disease-free interval and number of metastases have an impact on prognosis. Patients with a disease-free interval of more than 12 months and fewer than four lung nodules have a better prognosis after lung metastases resection. With the advent of thoracoscopic techniques, an aggressive approach to isolated pulmonary metastases should be encouraged.

General Recommendations

General recommendations for management of extremity soft-tissue sarcomas are as follows:

1. Soft-tissue tumors (benign or malignant) smaller than 3 cm should be evaluated by excisional biopsy with 1- to 2-cm margins.

2. Larger soft-tissue tumors should be evaluated by incisional biopsy.

3. Wide local excision with 2-cm margins is adequate therapy for low-grade lesions smaller than 5 cm.

4. Radiotherapy plays a critical role in the management of larger lesions.

5. Patients with high-grade sarcomas should be offered adjuvant chemotherapy.

6. An aggressive surgical approach should be taken in the management of patients with an isolated local recurrence or isolated resectable distant metastases.

RETROPERITONEAL SARCOMAS

Although significant advances in the understanding of extremity soft-tissue sarcomas have resulted in improved treatments and outcomes, similar progress has not been achieved in the understanding and treatment of retroperitoneal soft-tissue sarcomas.

Patients with retroperitoneal soft-tissue sarcomas generally have a worse prognosis than those with extremity sarcomas.

Retroperitoneal soft-tissue sarcomas grow to larger sizes before they become clinically apparent, and they often involve important vital structures that preclude surgical resection. Furthermore, the surgical margins that can be obtained around these sarcomas are often inadequate because of anatomic constraints.

Biopsy

In patients with retroperitoneal tumors, it is important to distinguish a sarcoma from lymphoma or a germ-cell tumor. Therefore, unlike extremity lesions, CT-directed fine-needle aspiration is indicated. If fine-needle aspiration is nondiagnostic, a CT-directed core needle biopsy can be performed. These techniques will spare most patients an open laparotomy for diagnosis.

Work-Up

The single most informative study in the work-up of a retroperitoneal sarcoma is a CT scan, which can identify the mass and adjacent organs that may be involved as well as the presence of liver metastases. Because retroperitoneal soft-tissue sarcomas may metastasize to the lungs, a thoracic CT scan is indicated. MRI will reveal the same information as well as provide coronal and sagittal views and better delineation of the retroperitoneal mass from vessels and bone. Angiography is indicated when CT or MRI suggests the presence of visceral artery encasement. Bilateral renal function must be assessed preoperatively because nephrectomy is frequently required (33%).

Management of Local Disease

The best chance for long-term survival in patients with retroperitoneal sarcoma is offered by a resection with tumor-free margins. Patients with clear radiographic evidence of unresectability should be operated on only for specific symptoms amenable to surgical treatment, such as intestinal obstruction or bleeding. Patients with partially resected tumors have the same overall survival rate as patients who undergo laparotomy with only a biopsy for unresectable disease. However, patients with well-differentiated liposarcomas may benefit symptomatically from repeated debulking.

The first step of an operation for a retroperitoneal sarcoma is determination of resectability based on the absence of liver metastases, sarcomatosis, and tumor invasion of unresectable structures. An organ or mesentery attached to a retroperitoneal sarcoma may be invaded by tumor and should be resected en bloc with the specimen. The tumor itself should not be violated, and a biopsy is rarely indicated, unless the tumor cannot be distinguished from a lymphoma preoperatively. Only 50% of patients who undergo surgical exploration have completely resectable tumors.

Adjuvant Therapy

In patients whose initial or recurrent tumor is not resectable, it may be possible to downstage the lesion with neoadjuvant chemotherapy and radiotherapy. This approach is used only if surgery would be possible with tumor shrinkage; it is not used adjuvantly after resection. No studies have demonstrated a benefit from adjuvant chemotherapy, external beam radiotherapy, or intraoperative radiotherapy after complete resection of a retroperitoneal sarcoma; these modalities remain investigational. At M. D. Anderson, patients selected for neoadjuvant therapy receive ifosfamide with hypofractionated (short-course) external beam radiotherapy (36 Gy over 10 days). This is done in an attempt to avoid radiation enteritis in long-term survivors. After treatment, patients are restudied radiographically to assess resectability. Intraoperative radiotherapy or brachytherapy can be used, depending on the status of margins on frozen section examinations.

Management of Recurrent Disease

In addition to recurring locally in the tumor bed and metastasizing to the lungs, retroperitoneal leiomyosarcoma and malignant fibrous histiocytoma readily spread to the liver. Also, retroperitoneal sarcomas tend to recur diffusely throughout the peritoneal cavity (sarcomatosis). The approach to resectable recurrent disease after treatment of a retroperitoneal sarcoma is similar to the approach taken after the recurrence of an extremity sarcoma. Isolated liver metastases, if stable over several months, may be amenable to resection.

Follow-Up

Follow-up of patients with extremity and retroperitoneal soft-tissue sarcomas must be extremely stringent in the first 2 years after therapy because approximately 80% of all recurrences become evident during this period. Patients should have a complete history and physical examination every 3 months and a chest radiograph every 6 months for the first 2 years. If the chest radiograph reveals a suspicious nodule, a CT scan of the chest should be obtained for confirmation. A CT scan or, if available, an MRI of the tumor site should be performed every 6 months during the initial 2 years, particularly if the primary tumor was deeply situated and the site is therefore not amenable to simple clinical examination. Thereafter, patients should be seen every 6 months for the next 3 years with a chest radiograph and appropriate imaging of the original tumor site done yearly. After 5 years, patients should be seen and a chest radiograph taken on a yearly basis.

Bone Sarcomas

EPIDEMIOLOGY

Malignant tumors arising from the skeletal system are rare, representing only 0.2% of primary cancers. Osteosarcoma and Ewing's sarcoma are the two most common bone tumors. They occur mainly during childhood and adolescence. Chondrosarcoma is the most common bone sarcoma that develops after skeletal maturity.

Osteosarcoma most commonly involves the distal femur, proximal tibia, or humerus. Rarely are the bones of the hands or feet involved. The most common sites of involvement by Ewing's sarcoma are the femur, pelvis, tibia, and fibula. Ewing's sarcoma, unlike osteosarcoma, may involve the flat bones and the axial skeleton. Chondrosarcoma occurs most commonly in the pelvis, proximal femur, and shoulder girdle.

STAGING

As with soft-tissue sarcomas, histologic grade is a crucial component of staging bone sarcomas. The staging system proposed by Enneking is shown in Table 5-4.

DIAGNOSIS

Plain radiography in conjunction with a thorough history and physical examination is essential to make an accurate diagnosis. Malignant bone tumors have irregular, poorly defined borders. In addition, there is evidence of bone destruction and periosteal reaction. Soft-tissue extension is a common finding. Plain radiographs may differentiate Ewing's sarcoma from osteosarcoma based on the characteristic diaphyseal involvement, "moth-eaten" appearance, and classic "onion skin" appearance of the periosteum in Ewing's sarcoma.

Once a malignant bone tumor is suspected, bone scintigraphy, MRI, CT, and angiography are required prior to biopsy to delineate the local tumor extent, vascular displacement, and compartmental localization. The serum alkaline phosphatase level is elevated in approximately 50% of osteosarcoma cases. If elevated at initial presentation, the alkaline phosphatase level is an excellent marker of treatment response and disease recurrence.

BIOPSY

The first step in treatment is a carefully planned and meticulously executed biopsy. If the biopsy incision is poorly placed, the chance for a limb-sparing procedure may be lost. Unlike extremity soft-tissue sarcomas, for which an incisional biopsy is favored, a trephine or core needle biopsy is opti-

Table 5-4. Staging system for sarcoma of bone

Primary tumor (T)			
T1	Intracompartmental lesion		
T2	Extracompartmental lesion		
Tumor grade (G)			
G1	Low grade		
G2	High grade		
Distant metastases (M)			
M0	No distant metastases		
M1	Distant metastases		
Stage grouping			
Stage IA	G1	T1	M0
Stage IB	G1	T2	M0
Stage IIA	G2	T1	M0
Stage IIB	G2	T2	M0
Stage IIIA	G1, 2	T1	M1
Stage IIIB	G1, 2	T2	M1

Source: Adapted from WF Enneking, SS Spanier, MA Goodman. A system for the surgical staging of musculoskeletal sarcoma. *Clin Orthop* 153:106, 1980.

mal for bone sarcomas and is best done under radiographic guidance. Precautions should be taken to avoid contamination of uninvolved soft tissue. Adequate hemostasis is critical.

TREATMENT

Surgery

During the 1950s and 1960s, amputation was the standard surgical approach to bone sarcomas. Currently, treatment involves limb salvage whenever feasible. Management of localized sarcoma requires coordination of staging studies, biopsy, surgery, and adjuvant therapy.

Successful limb-sparing surgery consists of three phases: tumor resection, bone reconstruction, and soft-tissue coverage. The contraindications for limb-sparing surgery include major neurovascular involvement, pathologic fractures, inappropriately placed biopsy incision, and extensive soft-tissue involvement.

Surgical resection is usually the only modality indicated for the management of chondrosarcomas. The indications for primary resection of Ewing's sarcoma are a lesion in an expendable bone, a lesion in the pelvic region (after chemotherapy), a tumor that arises at or below the knee in a child younger than 6 years old, or the expectation that a major uncorrectable functional deformity will result from radiotherapy.

Chemotherapy

Chemotherapy has revolutionized the approach to most bone sarcomas and is considered standard care for osteosarcoma and Ewing's sarcoma. The bleak 15–20% survival rate with surgery alone during the 1960s has improved to 55–80% with the addition of combination chemotherapy to surgical resection. The timing of chemotherapy, the mode of delivery, and the drug combinations continue to be studied in multi-institutional trials. Adjuvant preoperative chemotherapy is an attractive option because of its potential to downstage tumors, thus allowing for the maximal application of limb-sparing surgery.

Radiotherapy

Because osteosarcomas are generally radioresistant, the major role for radiotherapy is in the palliation of large, unresectable tumors. Acceptable palliation can be achieved in up to 75% of patients with large, unresectable primary tumors. Adjuvant external beam radiotherapy may improve 5-year survival rates for osteosarcomas of the maxilla and mandible by enhancing local control.

For most localized Ewing's sarcomas, radiotherapy is the primary mode of therapy. In conjunction with chemotherapy, doses of 50–60 Gy achieve local tumor control in up to 85% of cases without surgery.

RECURRENT DISEASE

Bone tumors disseminate almost exclusively through the bloodstream. Lymphatic metastases are rare and a poor prognostic sign. The lungs are the most common site of distant disease, followed by the bony skeleton. With the use of adjuvant chemotherapy, bony metastases are becoming a more common form of initial distant relapse. It is important to note that patients with Ewing's sarcoma may present with distant disease as long as 15 years after initial diagnosis. Tumor nodules located within the same bone as the initial tumor (skip metastases) are a feature of high-grade lesions. An aggressive approach to recurrent disease, similar to that for soft-tissue sarcomas, should be used.

Selected References

Barkley HT, Martin RG, Romsdahl MM, et al. Treatment of soft tissue sarcomas by preoperative irradiation and conservative surgical resection. *Int J Radiat Oncol Biol Phys* 14:693, 1988.

Brennan MF, Casper ES, Harrison LB, et al. The role of multimodality therapy in soft-tissue sarcoma. *Ann Surg* 214:328, 1991.

Chang AE, Kinsella T, Glatstein E, et al. Adjuvant chemotherapy for patients with high-grade soft-tissue sarcomas of the extremity. *J Clin Oncol* 6:1491, 1988.

Chang AE, Matory YL, Dwyer AJ, et al. Magnetic resonance imaging versus computed tomography in the evaluation of soft tissue tumors of the extremities. *Ann Surg* 205:340, 1987.

Glenn J, Sindelar WF, Kinsella T, et al. Results of multimodality therapy of resectable soft-tissue sarcomas of the retroperitoneum. *Surgery* 97:316, 1985.

Huth JF, Eilber FR. Patterns of metastatic spread following resection of extremity soft-tissue sarcomas and strategies for treatment. *Semin Surg Oncol* 4:20, 1988.

Jaques DP, Coit DG, Hajdu SI, et al. Management of primary and recurrent soft-tissue sarcoma of the retroperitoneum. *Ann Surg* 212:51, 1990.

Lindberg RD, Martin RG, Romsdahl MM, et al. Conservative surgery and postoperative radiotherapy in 300 adults with soft-tissue sarcomas. *Cancer* 47:2391, 1981.

Mazanet R, Antman KH. Adjuvant therapy for sarcomas. *Semin Oncol* 18:603, 1991.

Potter DA, Kinsella T, Glatstein E, et al. High-grade soft tissue sarcomas of the extremities. *Cancer* 58:190, 1986.

Razek A, Perez C, Tefft M, et al. Intergroup Ewing's Sarcoma Study: Local control related to radiation dose, volume and site of primary lesion in Ewing's sarcoma. *Cancer* 46:516, 1980.

Rosenberg SA. Adjuvant chemotherapy of adult patients with soft tissue sarcomas. *Important Adv Oncol* pp 273–94, 1985.

Rosenberg SA, Tepper J, Gladstein E, et al. The treatment of soft-tissue sarcomas of the extremities: Prospective randomized evaluations of (1) limb-sparing surgery plus radiation therapy compared with amputation and (2) the role of adjuvant chemotherapy. *Ann Surg* 196:305, 1982.

Storm FK, Mahvi DM. Diagnosis and management of retroperitoneal soft-tissue sarcoma. *Ann Surg* 214:2, 1991.

Suit HD, Mankin HJ, Wood WC, et al. Treatment of the patient with stage M0 soft tissue sarcoma. *J Clin Oncol* 6:854, 1988.

Verweij A, van Oosterom A, Somers R, et al. Chemotherapy in the multidisciplinary approach to soft tissue sarcomas: EORTC soft tissue and bone sarcoma group studies in perspective. *Ann Oncol* 3(Suppl 2):75, 1992.

Carcinoma of the Head and Neck

John R. Austin

Epidemiology

This chapter focuses on squamous cell carcinomas (SCCs) of the head and neck and on salivary gland tumors; thyroid and parathyroid tumors are discussed in Chapter 15.

Approximately 67,000 cancers of the head and neck are diagnosed in the United States each year. The relative frequencies of primary head and neck tumors by site are 40% in the oral cavity, 25% in the larynx, 15% in the oropharynx, 7% in the major salivary glands, and 13% at other sites. The male to female ratio is 3:1, and the average age at onset is approximately 50 years.

There is an increased incidence of SCC in patients with heavy tobacco and alcohol exposure. Some studies have shown an association between SCC and syphilis, human papillomavirus, exposure to sawdust and metal dust, and neglect of oral hygiene.

Pathology

In early lesions the carcinoma may be intraepithelial, in which case it is termed *carcinoma in situ*. Invasive carcinomas are classified as well differentiated, moderately differentiated, poorly differentiated, or undifferentiated. It is important to distinguish undifferentiated carcinomas from malignant melanoma and lymphoma; immunohistochemical techniques usually allow for correct classification. Head and neck tumors may be either exophytic or infiltrative. Ulceration is common and portends a poor prognosis. Regional metastasis to cervical lymph nodes is common. Distant metastasis occurs late; the most frequent sites are the lungs, liver, and bone.

Clinical Presentation

SCC of the mucous membranes of the head and neck initially appears as a white plaque (leukoplakia), a velvety red area (erythroplakia), or an ulcer. The tumor spreads in area and depth and eventually invades adjacent structures. Symptoms of SCC of the head and neck include a nonhealing ulcer, bleeding, otalgia, unexplained facial pain, and/or a mass in the neck. The presence of such symptoms necessitates a detailed examination that includes both inspection and palpation. Bimanual palpation of the neck, oral cavity, tonsils, and base of the tongue is required in every patient. In addition, the nasal cavity, nasopharynx, oropharynx, hypopharynx, and larynx should be examined; in skillful hands, these examinations can all be done with a mirror, but flexible endoscopy can also provide valuable clinical information. To search for either occult primary tumors or extension of primary disease into the deep cervical structures and to detect nonpalpable lymph nodes, all the above examinations should be supplemented with computed tomography (CT).

Two mistakes commonly made in the evaluation of patients with head and neck tumors can lead to treatment delays. First, an incomplete examination of the upper aerodigestive system can allow one to miss small lesions. It is imperative that patients who present with symptoms suggestive of head and neck cancer be evaluated by a physician experienced in performing a thorough head and neck examination. The second common mistake occurs with patients with a cervical mass, who often experience delays in referral for biopsy while long courses of antibiotic therapy are tried. A patient with persistent adenopathy after a 2-week course of antibiotics should be evaluated with a fine-needle aspiration biopsy.

Staging

Head and neck cancers are staged according to the TNM system of the American Joint Committee on Cancer Staging (AJCC) (Table 6-1). TNM categories are based on physical examination findings and additional information obtained by radiographic studies or endoscopy. The T staging is based on the location of the primary tumor and thus will vary for each site in the head and neck.

Pretreatment Evaluation

After a complete head and neck examination has been performed, a CT scan from the skull base to the clavicle should be obtained. To avoid misinterpretation of postbiopsy edema as a primary carcinoma site, the CT scan should be performed before oral panendoscopy and biopsies. In a patient with a clinically apparent primary tumor, a biopsy specimen can be obtained with a scalpel, punch forceps, or fine needle. The incidence of distant metastatic disease at the time of presentation of the primary tumor is low; therefore a chest radiograph and liver function studies are adequate screening examinations for metastatic disease. An isolated pulmonary nodule seen on chest radiograph in a patient with a known SCC of the head and neck more likely represents a primary lung cancer (second primary) than metastatic disease from the head and neck primary tumor. Therefore a diagnostic biopsy of the lung lesion is necessary before treatment of the head and neck cancer is undertaken.

General Principles of Treatment

Surgery, radiotherapy, or both are the conventional treatment modalities used in the management of head and neck

Table 6-1. AJCC staging system for head and neck cancers

Stage grouping	
Stage I	T1, N0, M0
Stage II	T2, N0, M0
Stage III	T3, N0, M0
	T1-3, N1, M0
Stage IV	T4, N0 or N1, M0
	Any T, N2 or N3, M0
	Any T, any N, M1
Primary tumor (T) dependent on anatomic location	
Regional lymph nodes (N)	
N0	No regional lymph node metastasis
N2a	Metastasis in single ipsilateral lymph node >3 cm but <6 cm
N2b	Metastasis in multiple ipsilateral lymph nodes, none >6 cm
N2c	Metastasis in bilateral or contralateral lymph nodes, none >6 cm
N3	Metastasis in a lymph node >6 cm
Metastatic disease	
M0	No evidence of distant metastasis
M1	Evidence of distant metastasis

Source: Adapted from OH Beahrs, DE Henson, RVP Hutter, et al (eds). *Manual for Staging of Cancer* (4th ed). Philadelphia: Lippincott, 1992.

SCC. In general, chemotherapy and immunotherapy are appropriate only as part of clinical protocols, as palliative measures in patients with incurable disease, or for tumors that persist after conventional therapy.

Surgical resection generally offers the best chance for complete tumor ablation and provides a specimen that can be used to verify the adequacy of excision margins. Morbidity is minimal when the tumor is small and accessible, but significant cosmetic and functional deficits are not unusual after resection of large tumors; disabilities can be minimized with appropriate reconstructive techniques.

Radiotherapy is effective in the treatment of head and neck tumors. The advantage of radiotherapy is that anatomic structures can be preserved while local tumor control is achieved. However, irradiation produces acute mucositis in the head and neck, and over the long term, it produces xerostomia and fibrosis of the skin and soft tissue and can alter pituitary and thyroid function.

Combined surgery and radiotherapy are often used in the management of cancer of the head and neck. Most surgeons prefer to use radiation postoperatively. The main indications for postoperative radiation are high risk of local and regional failure (stage III and IV disease), surgical margins that are not tumor-free, and histopathologic features that suggest unusual tumor aggressiveness (i.e., vessel invasion, perineural invasion, anaplastic appearance, multiple positive nodes, or extracapsular nodal spread).

Neck Dissection

There are three different types of neck dissection that can be performed: radical neck dissection, modified radical neck dissection, or selective neck dissection. The term *radical neck dissection* refers to removal of all ipsilateral cervical lymph nodes in levels I–V (Fig. 6-1). The dissection extends from the inferior border of the mandible to the clavicle, posteriorly to the anterior border of the trapezius muscle, and anteriorly to the lateral border of the sternohyoid muscle. The depth of dissection extends to the fascia overlying the anterior scalene and levator scapulae muscles. The spinal accessory nerve, internal jugular vein, and sternocleidomastoid muscle are removed.

The term *modified radical neck dissection* refers to the excision of all lymph nodes routinely removed in a radical neck dissection, with preservation of the spinal accessory nerve, internal jugular vein, and sternocleidomastoid muscle.

Selective neck dissection is the term reserved for less extensive lymph node dissections. The most common selective dissection is the supraomohyoid neck dissection, in which submental, submandibular, and upper and middle jugular lymph nodes (levels I–III) are removed. Another common selective neck dissection, used to treat patients with posterior scalp melanoma, is the posterolateral neck dissection; in this procedure, the suboccipital, retroauricular, upper jugular, middle jugular, and lower jugular lymph nodes (levels II–V) are removed.

At the University of Texas M. D. Anderson Cancer Center, the neck dissection most commonly performed for a primary cancer of the head and neck is a modified radical neck dissection; it is used both electively and therapeutically. The radical neck dissection is reserved for treatment of disease that has extended into the sternocleidomastoid muscle, jugular vein, or spinal accessory nerve. We believe that a modified radical neck dissection as either a therapeutic or elective procedure produces oncologic cure rates equivalent to those achieved with a radical neck dissection, but with significantly less morbidity.

Carcinoma of the Oral Cavity

In the United States, cancer of the oral cavity develops in about 30,000 people and causes about 10,000 deaths annually. The incidence is twice as high in males as in females. The oral cavity extends from the vermillion border of the lips to the plane between the junction of the hard and soft palate. It

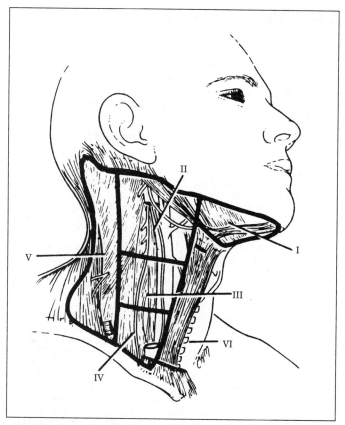

Fig. 6-1. Lymph node groups. Level I, submental and submandibular lymph node groups; level II, upper jugular group; level III, middle jugular group; level IV, lower jugular group; level V, posterior triangle group; level VI, anterior compartment group.

includes the lip, buccal mucosa, gingiva, retromolar trigone, floor of the mouth, hard palate, and anterior two-thirds of the tongue.

The staging system for tumors of the oral cavity is shown in Table 6-2. The treatment for carcinoma of the oral cavity is determined by location and stage of the primary tumor. For small stage T1 and some stage T2 tumors, radiation or surgery will yield similar results. Surgical treatment for stage T1 oral cancer is accomplished by excising the primary tumor with an adequate margin (approximately 1 cm) and repairing the defect either by primary closure, local advancement flaps, or split-thickness skin grafts. Stage T2 disease can be treated in the same way, but a flap closure is almost always necessary for larger defects.

Table 6-2. Staging system for oral cavity tumors

Tis	Carcinoma in situ
T1	Tumor ≤2 cm at greatest dimension
T2	Tumor >2 cm but not 4 cm at greatest dimension
T3	Tumor >4 cm at greatest dimension
T4	Tumor invades adjacent structures (e.g., cortical bone, deep extrinsic muscle of tongue, maxillary sinus, or skin)

Source: Adapted from OH Beahrs, DE Henson, RVP Hutter, et al (eds). *Manual for Staging of Cancer* (4th ed). Philadelphia: Lippincott, 1992.

Radiotherapy as a primary treatment modality for cancers of the oral cavity may involve interstitial radioactive implants, external beam therapy, or both. Small superficial cancers can be treated with interstitial implants. Postoperative adjuvant external beam radiotherapy is effective in improving local control rates for tumors likely to recur (T3 and T4).

Lymph nodes that are clinically involved with tumor are always treated with a neck dissection. However, treatment of the clinically uninvolved neck is still controversial, with three options available: observation, elective neck dissection, or elective irradiation. Most clinicians think that if there is a greater than 20% chance of nodal metastases, treatment of the neck is indicated. At M. D. Anderson Cancer Center, most, if not all, stage T1 and T2 oral cavity carcinomas are treated with primary surgical excision and a supraomohyoid neck dissection. If there is no nodal involvement or if only a single node is involved, without evidence of extracapsular extension, postoperative radiotherapy is not given. If there are multiple positive nodes or extranodal extension, postoperative radiotherapy to the neck is used to lower the incidence of disease recurrence. Radiotherapy for clinically negative cervical nodes is reserved for patients whose primary tumor is to be treated by radiotherapy as well.

The 5-year disease-free survival rate for patients with oral cavity cancers remains about 30–40%, irrespective of specific tumor site; these poor results are related to tumor size and the presence of regional lymph node metastasis and distant metastasis.

LIP

Small lesions of the lip can be cured with either radiation or surgical excision. Most T1 lesions are best treated by surgery alone, with a greater than 90% 5-year survival rate. However, T1 lesions of the commissure are best treated by radiotherapy. Lesions larger than 2 cm should be treated by surgical excision with immediate reconstruction and postoperative radiotherapy. Invasion of the mental nerve is associated with an 80% incidence of node involvement and only a 35% 5-year survival rate.

FLOOR OF THE MOUTH

Small lesions confined to the floor of the mouth can be treated by intraoral excision with tumor-free surgical margins. Floor of the mouth lesions frequently involve adjacent structures, such as the deep muscles of the tongue and mandible. In most cases, a cheek flap with marginal or segmental mandibulectomy is required to obtain adequate margins. Postoperative radiotherapy to the tumor bed is effective in reducing the incidence of local failure.

TONGUE

Carcinoma of the tongue is the most common intraoral malignancy. An intraoral glossectomy can be performed for patients with lesions limited to the anterior or middle third of the oral tongue. Tumor thickness is the most accurate predictor of lymph node involvement. Lesions thinner than 1 cm have a minimal incidence of lymph node involvement. Thicker lesions have a greater than 20% chance of lymph node positivity; therefore a supraomohyoid neck dissection should be included in the treatment of patients with a tongue carcinoma 1 cm or thicker and a clinically uninvolved neck. The lower jugular nodes are typically involved in patients with clinically positive cervical nodes; therefore a complete modified radical neck dissection is required. Tumors of the posterior oral tongue with extension into the base of the tongue are best treated by a transcervical excision combined with an en bloc neck dissection. The surgical defect can be left to heal by primary intention, or a split-thickness skin graft can be used for larger defects; in some instances, the edges of the tongue can be approximated upon itself.

HARD PALATE

Most SCCs of the upper gum and hard palate begin on the gingiva and can be excised with negative margins. Radiotherapy is effective in reducing the incidence of local failure after resection of larger lesions. Large lesions of the palate that have invaded the bone will require a partial maxillectomy. Reconstruction for maxillary defects of the oral cavity are best achieved using a prosthetic dental appliance.

CARCINOMA OF THE LARYNX

The incidence of carcinoma of the larynx in the United States is approximately 13,000 cases per year, with a male to female ratio of 9:1 and with the majority of patients presenting in the sixth decade of life. The major predisposing factors are tobacco and alcohol use; there is also a risk associated with exposure to the human papillomavirus.

The larynx extends superiorly from the epiglottic cartilage and inferiorly to the inferior surface of the cricoid cartilage. It includes the arytenoid cartilages, aryepiglottic folds, false vocal cords, ventricles of the larynx, and true vocal cords. The lymphatics of the larynx are numerous, except over the vocal cords, where the mucosa is thin and tightly adherent to the vocal ligament and lacks lymphatic channels. Above the level of the ventricles, the efferent lymphatics of the superior portion of the larynx extend to the pyriform sinus upward to join the jugular chain. From the inferior larynx, the efferent lymphatics drain into the pretracheal, paratracheal, and deep cervical lymph nodes. The lymphatic drainage of the larynx is usually bilateral, and any laryngeal tumor, except a lesion of the true vocal cords, should be considered a midline cancer with the propensity to metastasize to bilateral neck nodes.

Glottic carcinomas are those that involve the upper surface of the vocal cords and continue down to 1 cm below this plane. Glottic cancers account for 65% of cancers of the larynx. They usually are well differentiated, grow slowly, and metastasize late. A common presenting symptom is hoarseness. Metastasis occurs only after the disease has infiltrated muscle or has spread beyond the limits of the true vocal cords into the paraglottic space or from the anterior commissure into the pretracheal region.

The supraglottis is the region extending upward through the floor of the ventricles to a plane that includes the epiglottis, aryepiglottic folds, arytenoids, and false vocal cords. Supraglottic cancers account for 35% of laryngeal tumors. They are usually aggressive tumors because of both direct extension and lymph node metastasis. The lymphatic channels of the supraglottis drain to the jugulodigastric and middle and inferior internal jugular chains. Supraglottic tumors have a high risk of bilateral nodal involvement.

Subglottic cancers are those that involve the inferior border of the glottis and the area extending to the inferior border of the cricoid cartilage; these cancers are uncommon and account for less than 1% of all laryngeal tumors. They commonly produce extension into the lymph nodes of the prelaryngeal region area, inferior internal jugular chain, and thyroid gland and have a high risk of bilateral cervical metastasis.

The staging system for tumors of the larynx is given in Table 6-3.

PATIENT EVALUATION

The initial presenting symptoms of cancer of the larynx depend on the site and stage of the disease. Glottic tumors tend to produce hoarseness, but this symptom is a late finding with supraglottic cancers. Hence, supraglottic lesions are usually discovered at a much later stage; their earliest symptoms include dysphagia, odynophagia, hemoptysis, or referred otalgia. Often, supraglottic tumors produce a large lesion that can eventually impair motion of the vocal cord.

Early detection of cancers of the larynx requires a thorough examination of the larynx with either a mirror or a flexible

Table 6-3. Staging system for cancers of the larynx

Supraglottis	
T1	Tumor confined to site of origin
T2	Tumor involving adjacent supraglottic sites, without glottic fixation
T3	Tumor limited to the larynx, with fixation and/or extension to the postcricoid medial wall of the pyriform sinus or pre-epiglottic space
T4	Massive tumor extending beyond the larynx to involve the oropharynx, soft tissues of the neck, or destruction of thyroid cartilage
Glottis	
T1	Tumor confined to vocal folds, with normal vocal cord mobility
T2	Tumor extension to supraglottis and/or subglottis with normal or impaired vocal cord mobility
T3	Tumor confined to larynx, with fixation of the vocal cords
T4	Massive tumor, with thyroid cartilage destruction and/or extension beyond the confines of the larynx

Source: Adapted from OH Beahrs, DE Henson, RVP Hutter, et al (eds). *Manual for Staging of Cancer* (4th ed). Philadelphia: Lippincott, 1992.

endoscope. If the tumor is detected early, physical examination reveals either an exophytic or a submucosal lesion. If clinical findings are inconclusive, a direct laryngoscopy and biopsy should be performed. CT is very useful in determining paraglottic, subglottic, pyriform sinus, and extralaryngeal involvement; it is also useful in detecting clinically occult lymph node involvement.

TREATMENT

The goal of treatment for laryngeal carcinoma is to preserve vocal function without compromising the possibility for cure. In general, radiotherapy can satisfy this goal for patients with T1 and T2 lesions. Mucosal stripping of the cord can be effective treatment for patients with premalignant lesions such as carcinoma in situ, but repeated attempts at stripping leave the cord difficult to examine for the development of a malignant lesion. Therefore radiotherapy should be recommended for patients with recurrent premalignant vocal cord lesions.

Surgery

A vertical laryngectomy (hemilaryngectomy) preserves voice function, albeit a hoarse voice, and is used for patients with T1 or T2 vocal cord tumors who are not candidates for radiotherapy (usually due to prior irradiation). Hemilaryngectomy can also be used in select patients with persistent or recurrent disease after radiotherapy.

A supraglottic laryngectomy is used for patients with early (T1 or T2) supraglottic cancers. It is often associated with aspiration and is contraindicated in patients with poor pulmonary function.

Total laryngectomy is the procedure of choice for patients with stage T3 or T4 cancers of the larynx. (This procedure is seldom performed when patients have normal vocal cord mobility.) A wide-field laryngectomy includes the paralaryngeal soft tissue, which extends between the internal jugular veins, and the lymph nodes in levels II–V (see Fig. 6-1). In some instances, portions of the hypopharynx will also need to be removed, in which case a 1-cm mucosal margin is desirable because of the risk of submucosal microscopic disease. An ipsilateral thyroid lobectomy is indicated when the tumor involves the subglottis, pyriform apex, or paratracheal nodes, or when the tumor extends through the thyroid cartilage on the same side as the lesion.

Radiotherapy

Early (stage T1 or T2) glottic and supraglottic cancers respond predictably to external radiation, and tumor control is usually achieved with a 65- to 70-Gy dose. Glottic tumors, which have a low incidence of lymph node involvement, can be treated through small portals that encompass only the larynx. With careful treatment, there is minimal damage to normal tissues, and the patient can retain a normal voice. Supraglottic tumors, because of their higher incidence of lymph node involvement, require larger fields that encompass the lymphatic drainage of the neck. The primary echelon lymph nodes, if clinically uninvolved, should be treated with a 50-Gy dose.

Postoperative radiotherapy to the primary site and/or the regional lymph nodes is indicated for patients who have undergone a total laryngectomy and who have multiple positive lymph nodes, extranodal disease, close or positive surgical margins, T4 disease, or subglottic extension of tumor. Patients who have undergone a tracheotomy to achieve airway control prior to laryngectomy also require postoperative radiotherapy to control disease at the tracheostoma.

The local control rate for T1 and T2 lesions treated by radiotherapy is 71–100% (depending on stage) after 60 Gy. Salvage laryngectomy improves the local control rate to 88–100%. The local control rates for patients with T3 laryngeal carcinomas treated by surgery and radiotherapy is 85%, with a 67% 5-year survival rate. Patients with T4 lesions treated by surgery and radiotherapy can anticipate a 30–50% 5-year survival rate.

Carcinoma of the Oropharynx

Small lesions of the oropharynx are usually curable with radiotherapy alone. Larger lesions most frequently involve the supraglottic larynx and are treated as described above.

Lymph Node Metastasis from an Unknown Primary Tumor

Management of patients who present with an enlarged cervical lymph node and no known primary tumor can be very challenging. The search for the etiology of the adenopathy begins with a history and physical examination that includes the head and neck. The most common etiology of cervical lymph node enlargement aside from inflammatory disease is SCC of the head and neck, followed by lymphoma, and then a variety of solid tumor metastasis including lung cancer, breast cancer, and thyroid cancer.

Should the etiology of the enlarged cervical lymph node still be in doubt after a history and physical examination, a fine-needle aspiration biopsy should be performed. Fine-needle biopsy usually allows a diagnosis of SCC, adenocarcinoma, thyroid carcinoma, or inflammation. Rarely, fine-needle biopsy will not provide a clear diagnosis, and an open lymph node biopsy will be required. The incision for an open biopsy should be oriented in such a fashion that it can later be included in a larger incision for a complete neck dissection.

A diagnosis of inflammation should be followed by a thorough search for a specific cause. The finding of metastatic thyroid carcinoma in a cervical lymph node is sufficient information to proceed with neck exploration and thyroidectomy. Lymphoma can be diagnosed by fine-needle aspiration but cannot be subtyped; therefore an accessible lymph node should be removed. The diagnosis of adenocarcinoma requires an evaluation of the salivary glands if the node is cephalad in the neck. Needle biopsy evidence of adenocarcinoma in inferior neck nodes should prompt an evaluation of the lungs, breasts, pancreas, and colon. The 5-year survival rate for patients with metastatic adenocarcinoma to the cervical lymph nodes is less than 5%.

Metastatic SCC in a cervical node may have originated in many different sites. The location of the node can provide valuable diagnostic information as to the possible origin of the primary tumor. A submental and submandibular nodal metastasis can be expected to have come from a primary tumor of the lip, skin, or floor of the mouth. Subdigastric nodes are usually involved by tumors of the oral cavity, oropharynx, or larynx. Nasopharyngeal carcinoma characteristically metastasizes to the posterior cervical nodes.

Midjugular nodes are involved by tumors of the oral cavity or larynx, and lower jugular nodes are involved by primary tumors of the larynx, postcricoid area, or cervical esophagus.

CT of the head and neck should be performed if fine-needle aspiration biopsy of a cervical node demonstrates metastatic SCC and a primary tumor cannot be identified. If a primary tumor still cannot be found by CT scan, the patient should be prepared for the operating room for an examination under general anesthesia and for possible neck dissection.

An examination under general anesthesia should include an evaluation of the oral cavity, nasopharynx, tonsil, base of the tongue, hypopharynx, esophagus, and larynx. Suspicious areas should be biopsied. In addition, biopsies of normal-appearing nasopharynx, base of the tongue, tonsil, and pyriform sinus should be performed, since these are the most likely sites for small occult tumors.

A patient with a cervical lymph node metastasis and a small tumor of the head and neck that is detected only by an examination under general anesthesia can usually be treated by radiotherapy alone. The cervical lymphatics can be adequately treated with radiotherapy if the involved lymph node is small (<3 cm) based on physical examination and CT scan, although some surgeons advocate a neck dissection in all patients to determine the extent of regional disease. A modified radical neck dissection should be performed if the enlarged lymph node is larger than 3 cm or if residual disease persists after radiotherapy.

When the primary tumor cannot be identified, SCC metastases to cervical lymph nodes are best treated with a modified radical neck dissection. In general, radiotherpy is used to treat the common sites of occult SCC of the head and neck (nasopharynx, tonsil, base of the tongue, and larynx). A complete modified lymph node dissection provides staging information that will guide therapy. If multiple lymph nodes are found to be involved on pathologic evaluation, or if extracapsular extension of lymph node disease is noted, then postoperative radiotherapy to the entire neck would be indicated. Conversely, if only a single node is involved by metastatic SCC, then radiotherapy to the neck can be avoided, along with the complications of neck irradiation.

Five-year survival rates of 50% have been reported for patients with cervical metastases from an unknown primary tumor. After treatment for metastatic carcinoma in the cervical lymph nodes from an unknown primary tumor, close follow-up is mandatory, as the primary site will become evident in 15–20% of patients over 5 years.

Carcinoma of the Major Salivary Glands

Neoplasms of the parotid gland account for 90% of all tumors of the three major salivary glands. About 75% of parotid neoplasms are benign pleomorphic adenomas, and the other 25%

are malignant. Mucoepidermoid carcinoma is the most com-mom parotid malignancy, representing 25% of all such can-cers. Malignant mixed tumor is the second most common parotid malignancy.

Tumors of the submandibular gland are less common but are more frequently malignant. Tumors of the sublingual gland, the third major salivary gland, are extremely rare and are not discussed in this chapter.

The superficial portion of the parotid gland makes up 80% of the structure and lies lateral to the facial nerve. The deeper portion of the gland, referred to as the *deep lobe*, has a retro-mandibular portion, which is related to the ramus of the mandible and extends medially into the loose areolar tissue of the parapharyngeal space. The parotid gland is associated with numerous lymph nodes that lie within the parotid fas-cia and the substance of the gland itself.

The submandibular gland is invested by the superficial layer of the cervical fascia. The medial portion of the gland is inti-mately related to the hypoglossal and lingual nerves, and the marginal mandibular branch of the facial nerve traverses the investing fascia of the superficial portion of the gland. Although the submandibular gland does not contain lymph nodes within its parenchyma, there are lymph nodes within the investing fascia that communicate with the deep jugular chain of lymphatics.

PATIENT EVALUATION

Asymptomatic swelling is the most common initial complaint of patients with salivary gland tumors. Most painful parotid tumors prove to be malignant, but pain is also occasionally associated with rapidly growing benign neoplasms. Swelling of the submandibular gland is often intermittent, painful, and associated with eating. Obstruction of the submandibu-lar duct or inflammation of the gland requires that evalua-tion for a neoplasm be performed. Small malignant tumors of the major salivary glands are often difficult to distinguish from their benign counterparts. Signs that strongly suggest malignancy include rapid tumor growth, pain, involvement or invasion of overlying skin, facial nerve dysfunction, and enlargement of regional lymph nodes.

Fine-needle aspiration, which has a sensitivity greater than 95%, is a useful biopsy technique for distinguishing inflam-matory and neoplastic enlargements of the submandibular gland. The use of fine-needle aspiration for diagnosing parotid lesions is more controversial. Most parotid neo-plasms will require surgical removal; therefore unless the result of a needle aspiration would significantly affect the decision of whether to perform surgery, a needle aspiration is not indicated. The role of CT in the evaluation of parotid tumors is limited to patients with symptoms suspicious of malignancy. A CT scan can identify tumor extension and is useful in differentiating between a deep lobe parotid neoplasm and other parapharyngeal space tumors. A patient with an asymptomatic mass in the parotid gland can be treated appropriately by a superficial parotidectomy without a tissue diagnosis or CT scan.

TREATMENT

Surgery is the treatment of choice for salivary gland neoplasms. Any mass arising in the preauricular area or the angle of the mandible should be presumed to have arisen from the parotid gland. The minimal operation that should be performed is a superficial parotidectomy.

During superficial parotidectomy, every effort should be made to preserve facial nerve function unless the tumor has adhered to or directly invaded the nerve. If the facial nerve must be sacrificed, it should be immediately reconstructed with either a nerve graft or a cranial nerve XII–VII anastomosis. Neither is contraindicated in patients who will be receiving postoperative radiotherapy. Neck dissection is indicated when nodal metastases are detected either before or during surgery.

For lesions of the submandibular gland, adequate surgical excision includes removal of the submandibular gland and the associated investing fascia and lymph nodes. Malignant lesions require that the surgeon be prepared to perform a supraomohyoid neck dissection to remove all of the regional nodes. In some instances, resection of part or all of the mandible, floor of the mouth, and lingual and hypoglossal nerves will be necessary.

Postoperative radiotherapy is indicated for patients with the following histologic tumor types: high-grade mucoepidermoid carcinoma, adenocarcinoma, malignant mixed tumor, SCC, or adenoid cystic carcinoma. Radiotherapy is also beneficial for patients with perineural invasion, positive nodes, or skin involvement. Patients with low-grade mucoepidermoid carcinoma or acinic cell carcinoma usually do not require postoperative radiotherapy.

Patients with benign mixed tumors completely resected by superficial parotidectomy can anticipate a local recurrence rate of less than 5%. The 5-year survival rates for patients with malignant salivary gland tumors ranges from 95% for low-grade mucoepidermoid carcinoma, to 75% for adenoid cystic carcinoma, to 50% for high-grade mucoepidermoid carcinoma and malignant mixed tumors.

Surveillance

Following curative treatment of head and neck cancers, patients must be closely followed for the development of local as well as distant recurrences. Physical examination performed by someone skilled in examination of the head and neck is the most important part of the postoperative follow-up. At M. D. Anderson, we follow patients every 3 months for the first 2 years postoperatively, followed by every 6 months for the next 3 years, and then yearly thereafter. A chest radiograph and liver function studies are performed yearly, as distant metastatic disease is much less common than local recurrence.

Selected References

Byers RM. The Role of a Modified Neck Dissection. In C Jacobs (ed), *Cancers of the Head and Neck*. Boston: Martinus Nijhoff, 1987.

Byers RM, Wolf PF, Ballantyne AJ. Rationale for elective modified neck dissection. *Head Neck* 10:160, 1988.

Crissman JD, Gluckman J, Whiteley J, et al. Squamous cell carcinoma of the floor of mouth. *Head Neck* 3:2, 1980.

Eiband JD, Elias GE, Suter CM, et al. Prognostic factors in squamous cell carcinoma of the larynx. *Am J Surg* 158:314, 1989.

Frankenthaler RA, Luna MA, Lee SS, et al. Prognostic variables in parotid gland cancer. *Arch Otolaryngol Head Neck Surg* 117:1251, 1991.

Lefebvre JL, Degueant C, Castelain B, et al. Interstitial brachytherapy and early tongue squamous cell carcinoma management. *Head Neck* 12:232, 1990.

Mendenhall WM, Million RR, Sharkey DE, et al. Stage T3 squamous cell carcinoma of the glottic larynx treated with surgery and/or radiation therapy. *Int J Radiat Oncol Biol Phys* 10:357, 1984.

Mendenhall WM, Parsons JT, Stringer SP, et al. T1-T2 vocal cord carcinoma: A basis for comparing the results of irradiation and surgery. *Head Neck Surg* 10:373, 1988.

Rice DM, Spiro RH (eds). *Current Concepts in Head and Neck Cancer*. Atlanta: American Cancer Society, 1989.

Robbins KT, Medina JE, Wolfe GT, et al. Standardizing neck dissection terminology. Official report of the Academy's Committee for Head and Neck Surgery and Oncology. *Arch Otolaryngol Head Neck Surg* 117:601, 1991.

Wang RC, Goepfert H, Barber A, et al. Squamous Cell Carcinoma, Metastatic to the Neck from an Unknown Primary Site. In DL Larson, AJ Ballantyne, OM Guillamondegui (eds), *Cancer in the Neck*. New York: Macmillan, 1986.

Weber RS, Byers RM, Petit B, et al. Submandibular gland tumors. *Arch Otolaryngol Head Neck Surg* 116:1055, 1990.

Weber RS, Callender DL. Laryngeal conservation. *Semin Radiat Oncol* 2:149, 1992.

Thoracic Carcinoma

Bruce Toporoff and Paul T. Morris

Esophageal Carcinoma

Carcinoma of the esophagus will account for an estimated 11,300 new cancer cases and over 10,200 deaths in the United States in 1994. Patients at risk for the development of esophageal cancer are men 55–65 years of age with a long-standing history of tobacco abuse and heavy alcohol intake. The 5-year survival rate for patients with esophageal carcinoma is 6–9% and has changed little over the past several decades.

PATHOLOGY

There are two histologic types of esophageal carcinoma: squamous cell carcinoma (SCC) and adenocarcinoma. SCC is associated with race (more common among African-Americans), male gender, cigarette smoking, alcohol abuse, and poor socioeconomic status. The incidence of adenocarcinoma of the esophagus is increasing in comparison to SCC and is higher in middle-aged men. Approximately 15% of all esophageal cancers occur in the upper third of the esophagus, 50% in the middle third, and 35% in the lower third. Adenocarcinoma only occurs in the distal third of the esophagus, usually in association with severely dysplastic columnar epithelium within the esophagus (Barrett's esophagus) or from proximal gastric carcinoma extending into the distal esophagus.

N-nitrosamines are associated with an increased risk for development of esophageal SCC. The carcinogenic effects of N-nitrosamines are enhanced by alcohol, tobacco, and mycotoxins.

Achalasia predisposes patients to SCC. Even if achalasia is successfully treated medically, the increased risk for the development of carcinoma persists.

Barrett's esophagus is associated with gastroesophageal reflux. Twenty percent of patients undergoing esophagoscopy for esophagitis have Barrett's esophagus. Barrett's esophagus is noted in 59–86% of all patients who develop adenocarcinoma. Mutations in the tumor suppressor gene *P53* are common in patients with both Barrett's esophagus and adenocarcinoma and may be causal.

Caustic burns to the esophagus predispose patients to the development of SCC, which is characteristically seen 40–50 years after injury.

The Paterson-Kelley syndrome consists of dysphagia from an esophageal web, iron deficiency anemia, and glossitis. This condition is premalignant, and approximately 10% of individuals will develop SCC of the esophagus or hypopharynx.

There is a high incidence of *Helicobacter pylori* infection in patients at risk for neoplasms of the gastroesophageal junction. In one series, over 15% of patients with Barrett's esophagus were noted to be infected with *H. pylori*. The role of *H. pylori* infection in the subsequent development of esophageal carcinoma remains to be described.

CLINICAL PRESENTATION

The initial symptoms of esophageal carcinoma in 90% of patients are dysphagia and weight loss. Dysphagia occurs when the diameter of the esophagus is narrowed to less than 13 mm. Occasionally, the onset of dysphagia is sudden, but most patients complain of a vague difficulty in swallowing for 3–6 months prior to presentation. Odynophagia (painful swallowing) is seen in about one-half of the patients. Regurgitation of undigested food, retrosternal or epigastric pain, or aspiration pneumonia may be present. More advanced lesions may present with hematemesis, melena, tracheoesophageal fistula, hemoptysis, or problems from nerve involvement. Erosion of an esophageal carcinoma into the aorta may result in exsanguinating hemorrhage. Palpable supraclavicular or cervical lymph nodes should be biopsied to exclude metastases. Metastasis to the bones may produce a paraneoplastic syndrome from hypercalcemia.

DIAGNOSIS

The current diagnostic evaluation of esophageal carcinoma includes a chest radiograph, a barium swallow, and computed tomographic (CT) scans of the chest and abdomen, including the liver and adrenals. CT scans of the chest may accurately identify tracheal or aortic invasion by tumor. All patients need esophagoscopy for histologic diagnosis of the tumor and evaluation of intramural metastases. In patients with complaints of bone pain, a plain film of the bone and a bone scan should be obtained. Bronchoscopy is mandatory for patients with middle or upper third tumors. Both bone scans and bronchoscopy may identify metastases not evident on CT scan. Pulmonary function testing is performed to assess the ability to tolerate surgery. Endoscopic ultrasound may be useful to define both tumor and nodal stage.

STAGING

The TNM staging system for the cervical and thoracic esophagus is outlined in Table 7-1. The stage groupings can also be found in Table 7-1.

TREATMENT

Preoperative Preparation

Patients with esophageal carcinoma can demonstrate nutritional depletion, dehydration, and anemia that will require

Table 7-1. TNM staging for esophageal cancer

Primary tumor (T)

Tx	Primary tumor cannot be assessed
T0	No evidence of primary tumor
Tis	Carcinoma in situ
T1	Tumor invades lamina propria or submucosa
T2	Tumor invades muscularis propria
T3	Tumor invades adventitia
T4	Tumor invades adjacent structures

Regional lymph nodes (N)

Nx	Regional nodes cannot be assessed
N0	No regional node metastasis
N1	Regional node metastasis

Distant metastasis (M)

Mx	Presence of distant metastasis cannot be assessed
M0	No distant metastases
M1	Distant metastasis

Stage grouping

Stage 0	Tis	N0	M0
Stage I	T1	N0	M0
Stage IIA	T2	N0	M0
	T3	N0	M0
Stage IIB	T1	N1	M0
	T2	N1	M0
Stage III	T3	N1	M0
	T4	Any N	M0
Stage IV	Any T	Any N	M1

correction preoperatively. Pulmonary function due to tobacco abuse and hepatic function due to ethanol abuse are frequently compromised in patients with esophageal carcinoma.

Surgery

Surgery is the only curative treatment modality for esophageal carcinoma. Five-year survival rates of 70% are reported for stage I disease. Advanced-stage disease is rarely cured by surgery, but resection, when possible, provides optimal palliation of the dysphagia associated with progressive esophageal carcinoma. In patients with locally advanced disease, chemotherapy or chemotherapy plus radiotherapy may help achieve improved local control compared with surgery alone.

The rich submucosal lymphatic plexus of the esophagus results in longitudinal spread of tumors within the esophagus; therefore a total or subtotal esophagectomy is required for complete removal of esophageal carcinomas. Segmental esophageal resection frequently results in microscopic residual tumor at the surgical margin and a high incidence of local recurrence.

Resection of esophageal carcinoma begins with a midline laparotomy incision. The abdomen is thoroughly explored to evaluate for metastases. The two most common sites of metastatic disease in the abdomen are the liver and celiac lymph nodes. If metastatic disease is identified, resection of the tumor should still be performed if possible to provide palliation. If the tumor cannot be resected completely, it may still be beneficial to remove the bulk of the tumor and mark the residual tumor by metal clips to guide radiotherapy.

After the assessment for metastatic disease is completed, the stomach is fully mobilized by performing a Kocher maneuver, dividing the gastrocolic ligament with care to preserve the right gastroepiploic vessels, and dividing the short gastric vessels. The lesser omentum is opened to identify the left gastric artery, which is then ligated at its origin. A pyloromyotomy or pyloroplasty is performed to avoid gastric stasis, which inevitably occurs after division of the vagus nerves during esophageal transection.

The two popular methods of mobilizing the esophagus and its periesophageal lymphatic tissue are the Ivor-Lewis esophagectomy and the transhiatal esophagectomy. In the Ivor-Lewis esophagectomy, the esophagus is resected through a right thoracotomy incision and an intrathoracic esophagogastric anastomosis is performed at the level of the azygous vein. If total thoracic esophagectomy is to be performed, a right thoracotomy is still used for esophageal mobilization, but the gastric conduit is either brought substernally or through the posterior mediastinum, and the esophagogastrostomy is completed in the left neck.

A transhiatal esophagectomy involves resection of the intrathoracic esophagus performed through the esophageal hiatus and the thoracic inlet without an open thoracotomy. The esophagus is dissected bluntly from both the cervical and abdominal incisions. The mid-portion of the esophagus cannot be visualized from the abdominal or cervical incisions and dissection is done blindly. The gastric conduit is placed into the posterior mediastinum and a cervical anastomosis is performed.

The advantage of the transhiatal technique over the Ivor-Lewis technique is the avoidance of a thoracotomy. A major disadvantage of the transhiatal technique includes the inability to perform the operation under direct vision, which can result in an inadequate periesophageal lymphadenectomy or esophageal resection. Another criticism of the transhiatal technique is the possibility of a vascular injury occurring in the chest without exposure of the bleeding site. The transhiatal approach requires a cervical anastomosis, which is associated with a higher anastomotic leak rate compared with intrathoracic anastomoses.

In a series reported by Goldminc et al., the operative morbitity, mortality, and survival rates did not differ when prospectively comparing the transhiatal technique to the Ivor-Lewis technique.

Reconstruction Following Resection

The stomach, colon, and jejunum have all been successfully used as replacement conduits following esophagectomy. The stomach is easily mobilized, has an excellent vascular supply, and is the preferred conduit following esophagectomy. Pyloroplasty or pyloromyotomy is required to avoid gastric stasis secondary to sacrifice of the vagus nerves during esophagectomy. End-to-end stapling devices have been widely used for esophagogastric anastomosis with results comparable to hand-sewn anastomosis.

The colon is the most commonly used alternative to the stomach, usually due to prior gastric surgery. Either the right or left colon can be used, although the segment of the left and transverse colon supplied by the left colic artery is generally longer. In addition, an intact marginal artery is present more often for the left colon. The colonic arterial anatomy should be evaluated by arteriography, and the colonic mucosa should be evaluated by colonoscopy to be certain no colonic pathology is present.

Free jejunal graft interposition has been used successfully for conduit replacement following resection for carcinoma of the upper cervical esophagus or hypopharynx that does not extend past the thoracic inlet. Once the esophagus is resected, the proximal and distal anastomoses are completed to stabilize the graft. The mesenteric vessels are usually anastamosed to the external carotid artery and the internal jugular vein. Up to 15–20 cm of jejunum may be used as a free graft.

Results of Surgical Resection

The operative mortality rate reported for an Ivor-Lewis esophagectomy is less than 5%, with postoperative complication rates ranging from 10 to 27%. Transhiatal esophagectomy is associated with perioperative mortality rates similar to those of the Ivor-Lewis esophagectomy. Local recurrence rates after transhiatal resection may be slightly higher when compared with the rates reported for the Ivor-Lewis technique. However, survival appears to be unrelated to the operative technique used; instead, stage at presentation is the most important determinant. Five-year survival rates range from 68 to 85% for stage I and II patients and 15 to 28% for stage III patients.

Operative Palliation for Unresectable Tumors

Bypass of an obstructing unresectable esophageal tumor has been advocated as an effective means of palliation. Bypass is usually accomplished with a substernally placed stomach. The esophagus and tumor are excluded from the gastrointestinal tract by suturing or stapling proximally and distally to the tumor. Dysphagia can be relieved in more than 90% of the patients with this procedure. Unfortunately, the operative mortality rate for this procedure is greater than 20%, reflecting the poor condition of patients with unresectable obstructing esophageal tumors. At the University of Texas

M. D. Anderson Cancer Center, we have experienced a high complication rate from this procedure and reserve a palliative by-pass for the rare patient in overall good medical condition who has an unresectable obstructing tumor.

Tracheal-esophageal fistula is another complication of advanced esophageal carcinoma that requires operative palliation. Cervical esophagostomy and gastrostomy can offer effective palliation.

Nonoperative Palliation of Unresectable Tumors

Several effective local therapies are available to relieve the progressive dysphagia that characterizes late disease. Dilatation of the obstructing lesion is the most frequently applied initial palliative therapy. Dilatation is safe and effective, but may require multiple, frequent applications as the disease progresses.

Endoscopic laser therapy or electrocoagulation is another effective method of treating dysphagia, with 80–100% success rates reported.

If either of the above treatments fails, dilatations become too frequent, or an esophagopulmonary fistula forms, an endoprosthesis can be placed. Good results are reported in most patients; however, ulceration, obstruction, dislocation, and aspiration have all been reported in association with this device.

Adjuvant Therapy

Alternative therapeutic modalities for esophageal carcinoma have been developed to address the issue of palliation for patients who cannot benefit from surgical resection, the best form of therapy. Two of these therapies, chemotherapy and radiotherapy, have also been used in an adjuvant setting in an attempt to improve on the poor survival data from surgical resection alone. All of these alternative therapies focus on palliation, which in this patient population means relief of dysphagia with associated malnutrition and pain.

When used alone, radiotherapy results in 5-year survival rates of 0–10%. The results of two phase III prospective studies have shown that chemoradiation is superior to radiation therapy alone. Therefore, at the present time, radiation therapy alone is reserved for palliation in patients whom chemotherapy is contraindicated.

Preoperative radiotherapy alone has not been proven to increase resectability. When used postoperatively, radiotherapy has been shown to decrease local recurrence, but no improvement in survival has been noted. Another form of radiotherapy, endoluminal iridium radiation, has been used in some centers for local tumor control.

Several general principles apply to the evaluation of chemotherapy as treatment for esophageal carcinoma. Most single-agent studies involve SCC, while most recent multiagent studies involve SCC, adenocarcinoma, or both. SCCs are more responsive to chemotherapy compared with adenocarcinomas, and multiagent chemotherapy is more effective than single-agent therapy for SCC. The most common single agents used for the treatment of esophageal carcinoma include 5-fluorouracil, cisplatin, mitomycin C, and methotrexate, which have produced response rates of 0–42%. The most common multiagent regimen, 5-fluorouracil and cisplatin, has produced response rates of 30–70%; these response rates are short in duration and associated with no significant improvement in survival.

The postoperative use of single or multiple chemotherapeutic agents with or without radiotherapy has unfortunately not proven beneficial in terms of improved survival. Preoperative chemotherapy trials were initiated to theoretically downstage tumors to facilitate their resection and improve survival. The results of an Intergroup trial to address this issue is pending. When preoperative chemotherapy was combined with radiotherapy, some complete pathologic responses were seen. However, this did not translate into a survival benefit. In summary, the role of radiotherapy, chemotherapy, or both modalities in either the neoadjuvant or adjuvant settings has not been clearly established.

Lung Cancer

Lung cancer accounts for over 125,000 deaths annually in the United States—25% of all cancer deaths and 5% of all deaths in this country. Lung cancer has replaced breast cancer as the leading cause of cancer death in women. The overall 5-year survival rate for lung cancer patients is approximately 15%, due to the advanced stage at presentation in the majority of cases. However, with early diagnosis and aggressive surgical therapy, 5-year survival rates can approach 60% for early-stage disease.

PATHOLOGY

Squamous Cell Carcinoma

SCC represents 35% of lung cancers and arises mainly in the mainstem, lobar, or segmental bronchi. It is therefore centrally located and prone to cavitation. Superior sulcus tumors are invariably squamous cancers and have a propensity for local invasion into bone, the brachial plexus, and the cervical sympathetic plexus, producing Horner's syndrome. SCCs can secrete a parathormone-like substance causing hypercalcemia.

Adenocarcinoma

Studies have shown that adenocarcinoma of the lung occurs with a frequency equal to that of SCC. Adenocarcinomas are most often peripheral lesions and are thought to be less frequently related to tobacco abuse. Primary lung adenocarcinoma should always be considered in the differential diagnosis of a solid peripheral nodule on chest radiograph. Bronchoalveolar carcinoma is relatively uncommon and accounts for about 5–10% of all primary lung carcinomas. This cell type is the most likely to arise from a scar in the pulmonary parenchyma.

Large-Cell Carcinoma

Large-cell carcinomas are undifferentiated tumors that cannot easily be characterized. They comprise about 10% of all lung cancers. They are poorly differentiated and are associated with early metastases to the mediastinum and brain. Immunohistochemical studies have noted that approximately one-half of these tumors are actually poorly differentiated adenocarcinomas. As many as 30% of these tumors are neuroendocrine in origin and are actually small-cell carcinomas.

Small-Cell Carcinoma

Small-cell carcinoma represents about 20–25% of primary lung carcinomas. Studies indicate that the vast majority of these cells exhibit neuroendocrine characteristics (APUD cells). Over 70% of patients have metastases outside the involved hemithorax at the time of diagnosis. A small but significant portion of these tumors are associated with hypersecretion of hormones such as adrenocorticotropic hormone (ACTH) causing Cushing's syndrome. Other syndromes seen in association with small-cell carcinoma are the syndrome of inappropriate antidiuretic hormone secretion (SIADH) and carcinoid syndrome.

Mesothelioma

Mesothelioma, a rare tumor of the pleura, is strongly associated with exposure to asbetos. Asbestos exposure is not essential to make the diagnosis of mesothelioma since 50% of patients diagnosed with mesothelioma have had no known asbestos exposure. Since the pleura is of mesodermal origin, mesotheliomas are usually classified as soft-tissue sarcomas. Extrapleural pneumonectomy and radical radiotherapy techniques have been used to treat mesothelioma with little success. Response rates for combination chemotherapy have been less than 20%.

Carcinoid

Carcinoids are less aggressive, well-differentiated neuroendocrine tumors that were historically called bronchial adenomas. Carcinoids constitute about 5% of all lung cancers and usually occur in patients in their fourth decade of life. Carcinoids can be successfully treated with sleeve resection of the bronchus because their malignant potential is low.

Metastatic Lung Lesions

Thirty percent of cancer patients die with pulmonary metastases. These lesions are most often peripheral, are detected by chest radiograph, and are asymptomatic 85% of the time. A subgroup of patients representing 10–20% of all patients with pulmonary metastases have disease confined to the lung. Resection of metastases by wedge resection with at least a l-cm tumor-free margin can result in long-term survival benefit. The best results occur for removal of small (less than 3 cm) solitary lesions, but long-term survival for patients with multiple resected metastases can be achieved. Tumors amenable to pulmonary resection of metastatic disease are listed in Table 7-2.

DIAGNOSIS

Signs and symptoms associated with lung carcinoma usually are indicators of advanced disease. Symptoms may be related to growth of the tumor in the airway, causing cough and hemoptysis, or airway obstruction causing stridor or pneumonitis. Peripheral growth of tumors can cause pleuritic chest wall pain. Tumor cavitation can become secondarily infected and result in a lung abscess. Signs or symptoms associated with lung carcinoma should lead to evaluation with chest radiographs.

Anteroposterior and lateral chest radiographs are the initial diagnostic study required to evaluate patients with suspected lung carcinoma. Also, many patients will have a solitary pulmonary nodule (SPN) identified by routine chest radiographs during evaluation of other complaints, which will require additional evaluation. Approximately 150,000 SPNs are diagnosed in the United States each year. Half prove to be either primary or metastatic malignancies. Nonsmoking patients younger than 35 years of age and without a history of prior malignancy may be safely observed with serial chest films. Otherwise, patients should be aggressively evaluated, so that the opportunity to treat and cure an early-stage malignancy is not missed.

Routine chest radiographs cannot accurately provide sufficient staging information for patients suspected of having lung cancer. Chest CT with intravenous contrast is the procedure of choice for noninvasive imaging of the mediastinum. Chest CT includes the thoracic cavity and continues into the abdomen to include the liver and adrenals, the two most common sites of intra-abdominal metastases.

Interpretation of chest CT includes assessment of lymph node metastasis. Nodes less than 1 cm have a low probability of malignancy, nodes 1.0–1.5 cm have a moderate malignant potential, and nodes greater than l.5 cm have a high probability of being malignant. These are inexact guidelines of radiographic interpretation, and one should realize that many lymph nodes less than 1 cm harbor metastatic lung cancer. Some investigators report that 25% of all positive

Table 7-2. Survival rate following resection of metastases of tumors

Tumor	Survival rate (5-year actuarial)
Osteogenic sarcoma	36–66%
Head and neck cancer	41–44%
Soft-tissue sarcoma	26–33%
Melanoma	12–33%
Colorectal carcinoma	9–30%
Breast cancer	12–27%

nodes are less than 1 cm. Conversely, not all nodes greater than 1.5 cm are malignant, especially in the presence of pneumonitis or cavitation.

Lesions noted on chest radiographs and CT can be evaluated and diagnosed cytologically by CT-directed fine-needle aspiration biopsy. The sensitivity of this test is greater than 90% when a malignant lesion is present. A 10–20% risk of pneumothorax is associated with this procedure. A 10% false-negative rate for diagnosing malignant lesions has been reported, most commonly due to the fact that peripheral adenocarcinomas can cytologically be confused with chronic inflammatory conditions. Benign lesions are less reliably diagnosed with the fine-needle aspiration biopsy technique. CT-directed core needle biopsy techniques are gaining wider use and should allow for a better rate of accurate diagnosis for benign lesions.

Thoracoscopic wedge resection using video-assisted thoracic surgery (VATS) is a highly accurate technique for providing diagnostic information. Sensitivity and specificity rates of 100% have been reported for VATS' ability to diagnose benign and malignant lesions. VATS is well tolerated by nearly all patients, with a complication rate of 5% reported.

The role of mediastinoscopy in the evaluation of lung cancer patients is controversial. Positive mediastinal nodes are associated with a poor prognosis; therefore, if involved mediastinal nodes can be demonstrated by mediastinoscopy, diagnostic thoracotomy can be avoided. Some centers routinely perform mediastinoscopy on all patients prior to thoracotomy, because 10–15% of patients will have metastasis to mediastinal nodes despite a negative chest CT. Other centers rely solely on chest CT and accept that a few patients will have a thoracotomy with metastatic disease in the mediastinal nodes. Patients who undergo complete resection of the primary tumor and are found to have mediastinal nodes involved with tumor have a less than 20% 5-year survival.

All patients with mediastinal nodes larger than 1 cm on chest radiograph should be evaluated with mediastinoscopy. Since the prognosis for patients with mediastinal nodal involvement is so poor, alternative treatment strategies should include preoperative chemotherapy and radiotherapy.

Bronchoscopy should always be performed prior to thoraco-tomy. Bronchoscopy allows the surgeon to obtain histologic confirmation of malignancy prior to thoracotomy. In addition the relationship of the tumor to the carina and lobar bronchi can be evaluated, so that the surgeon can be prepared to per-form the appropriate margin-negative resection.

STAGING

The American Joint Committee on Cancer (AJCC) staging for lung cancer is included in Table 7-3.

TREATMENT

Surgical resection is the mainstay of treatment for lung car-cinoma. Patients who have stage I or II tumors based on CT scans, mediastinoscopy, or both should always be considered for surgical resection. Patients with more advanced locore-gional disease should be evaluated for alternative therapies, with the goal of downstaging their disease to allow for even-tual resection. Patients with metastatic disease should not be considered for surgical resection. Patients with a malig-nant pleural effusion documented by cytologic studies of their fluid do not benefit from surgical resection; however, the radiographic diagnosis of pleural effusion is not a con-traindication to lung resection, provided the effusion does not contain malignant cells. Table 7-4 summarizes survival after surgical resection for lung carcinoma based on the stage of disease.

Preoperative Evaluation

Patients being evaluated for lung resections commonly have diminished pulmonary reserve secondary to tobacco abuse. All studies agree that patients with chronic lung disease have a higher incidence of postoperative morbidity and mor-tality following thoracic surgery. Simple spirometry can identify patients at increased risk for complications following lung resection. In general, the minimum acceptable postre-section FEV_1 is 0.8 L. Another method that reliably predicts whether pulmonary reserve is sufficient for a patient to tol-erate a resection is the percentage of the predicted normal FEV_1. Patients having less than 35% of the predicted FEV_1 are at high risk for resection. Arterial blood gas analysis is frequently performed in conjunction with spirometry. Even mild elevations in PCO_2 are indications of pulmonary dys-function, and hypercarbic patients are rarely acceptable can-didates for pulmonary resection. Patients with decreased PO_2 are clearly high risk; however, if a significant amount of atelectasis or shunting is associated with the tumor, the PO_2 may actually improve after resection. A PO_2 less than 50 without evidence of significant atelectasis is usually a con-traindication for resection.

Table 7-3. AJCC-UICC staging system for lung carcinoma TNM system

Primary tumor (T)

TX	Tumor proven by cytologic assessment of secretions but cannot be visualized roentgenographically
T0	No evidence of primary tumor
Tis	Carcinoma in situ
T1	Tumor ≤3 cm
T2	Tumor >3 cm, or tumor of any size that invades visceral pleura, has associated atelectasis or obstructive pneumonitis extending to the hilum, or extends to within 2 cm distal to the carina in a lobar bronchus
T3	Tumor of any size within 2 cm of the carina or with direct extension into the chest wall, diaphragm, mediastinal pleura, or pericardium
T4	Tumor of any size with invasion of the mediastinum, heart, great vessels, trachea, esophagus, vertebral body, or associated malignant pleural effusion

Nodal involvement (N)

N0	No nodal involvement
N1	Peribronchial and/or ipsilateral hilar nodes
N2	Mediastinal or subcarinal nodes
N3	Scalene or supraclavicular nodes or contralateral nodes

Distant metastasis (M)

M0	No distant metastasis
M1	Distant metastasis

Stage grouping

Stage 0	Carcinoma in situ
Stage I	T1 or T2, N0, M0
Stage II	T1 or T2, N1
Stage IIIA	T1 or T2, N2, T3, N0, N1, or N2
Stage IIIB	Any T, N3, T4, any N
Stage IV	Any T, any N, M1

Table 7-4. Survival of surgically treated patients with lung cancer

Stage	Number of patients	5-year survival (%)
T1 N0 M0	591	69
T2 N0 M0	1,012	59
T1 N1 M0	19	54
T3 N0 M0	221	44
T2 N1 M0	176	40
T3 N1 M0	71	18

Source: Adapted from CF Mountain. A new international staging system for lung cancer. *Chest* 89(Suppl):225S, 1986.

When evaluating patients with an FEV_1 less than 2 L pre-operatively, it often becomes imperative to assess the contribution of each lobe of the lung to the total lung capacity. If no obvious shunting is occurring in the lungs, the relative contribution of each lobe can be estimated by figuring that each lobe is responsible for 20% of the total pulmonary function. Patients who have significant atelectasis, pneumonitis, or cavitation should have ventilation/perfusion ($\dot{V}/\dot{Q}$) scans to more accurately define the relative contribution of each lobe to the total lung capacity. The postoperative FEV_1 can be accurately predicted after the data from spirometry and $\dot{V}/\dot{Q}$ scans are combined and operability can thus be assessed. Preoperative training with an incentive spirometer, initiation of bronchodilator therapy for patients whose pulmonary function improves on bronchodilators, weight reduction if appropriate, good nutrition, and the cessation of smoking for at least 2 weeks prior to surgery are helpful adjuncts that can minimize complications for patients with marginal pulmonary reserve.

Surgery

The posterolateral thoracotomy is the incision of choice for the majority of lung resections. The incision is frequently made through the fifth or sixth intercostal space. Approaches that spare the serratus anterior muscle and occasionally the latissimus dorsi muscle can be used to significantly diminish the degree of postoperative discomfort associated with thoracotomy.

Pneumonectomy

Pneumonectomy, once the most frequent resection for lung cancer, now accounts for only 20% of all pulmonary resections. Pneumonectomy is required when the tumor invades the proximal mainstem bronchus or pulmonary arteries, making lung-conserving techniques impossible. The major disadvantage of pneumonectomy is that it removes a large volume of functional lung, which may lead to chronic respiratory failure and the later development of pulmonary hypertension. Intrapericardial dissection is often required during a pneumonectomy to obtain vascular margins on the pulmonary vessels, especially when the tumor involves the pericardium.

Lobectomy, the most frequently performed resection for lung cancer, allows sparing of functional lung while still providing adequate margins and resection of N1 lymph nodes. Complete mediastinal lymph node dissection using frozen sections should always be performed at the time of lobectomy or pneumonectomy. If hilar N1 or N2 disease is confirmed by frozen sections, the surgeon should perform a radical lymph node dissection to accurately stage and potentially cure the patient. Patients who are N0 do not need radical lymphadenectomy.

Lower-lobe tumors drain to the posterior mediastinum; the pleura should be opened from the inferior pulmonary ligament to the subcarinal area and all lymph nodes removed en bloc. If the hilar N1 nodes are positive in a right lower-lobe tumor, it is necessary to resect the right middle lobe for complete resection. When a right upper lobectomy is being performed, it is important to remember that the venous drainage from the right middle lobe drains to the superior pulmonary vein and must be preserved.

Right upper-lobe tumors drain to the inferior mediastinal lymph nodes, which can be resected en bloc with the lobe. The subcarinal area should also be dissected for right upper-lobe tumors, because these tumors frequently spread to the subcarinal area.

During lymph node dissection for left upper-lobe tumors, care must be taken to avoid injury to the recurrent laryngeal nerve when excising lymphatic tissue in the aortopulmonary window. Reports of patients treated by left upper lobectomy and lymphadenectomy of the aortopulmonary window demonstrate up to a 40% 5-year survival provided all other N2 nodes are negative. Unfortunately, most left upper-lobe tumors have spread to the inferior or superior mediastinal nodes at the time of diagnosis.

Many lung carcinomas spread along the bronchial lymphatics, submucosa, and mucosa. When performing a lobectomy, it is necessary to ensure complete resection by evaluating the bronchial margin by frozen section examination prior to closing the chest. If a resection margin is positive, attempts should be made to convert it to a negative one, which may result in performance of a pneumonectomy or sleeve lobectomy.

Sleeve lobectomy is a lung parenchyma-sparing technique used for right upper-lobe tumors involving the right mainstem bronchus. The right mainstem bronchus is resected proximal and distal to the origin of the right upper-lobe bronchus. The cut end of the proximal right mainstem bronchus is anastomosed to the bronchus intermedius. This technique was first used with bronchial adenomas but has now been shown to be a reasonable parenchyma-sparing procedure for patients who cannot tolerate pneumonectomy. The right middle and lower lobes can be spared and the tumor can be completely resected. The survival rates appear to be similar to those for lobectomy and pneumonectomy, provided that a complete nodal excision is performed during the resection.

Segmentectomy is another parenchyma-sparing operation typically used for resection of peripherally placed lesions. The technique should be limited to N0 patients, and the surgeon should always sample the N1 nodes of the tumor to be sure they are uninvolved. Patients who will benefit most from this technique are those with compromised pulmonary function and who may not be able to tolerate a lobectomy.

Wedge resection is the technique of choice for known metastatic lesions (i.e., breast cancer, colon cancer, or sarcoma). This technique can also be used as a parenchyma-sparing procedure. The local recurrence rate has been shown to be about 10% higher at 5 years when wedge resection was compared with lobectomy in a prospective randomized study for N0 patients with lung cancer. The results, however, did justify the use of this technique for patients with compromised pulmonary function. Wedge resection can be performed via a standard thoracotomy incision or using a VATS technique.

Five-year survival rates as high as 50% have been reported for tumors that involve the parietal pleura without lymph node metastases. When N2 disease is associated with a T3 tumor, the prognosis is very poor, and if N2 disease is recognized preoperatively, chemotherapy and radiotherapy should be used as the initial treatment modality. If the tumor involves the intercostal muscles and ribs, en bloc chest wall resection should be done with at least a 2-cm margin of normal tissue. Frozen section confirmation of the margins on the chest wall is recommended.

Posterior chest wall defects that are covered by the scapula and small posterior defects do not require reconstruction. Defects that are on the anterior chest wall or that involve more than two intercostal spaces should be reconstructed using Marlex mesh. Methylmethacrylate can also be added to provide additional chest wall strength.

Treatment for Superior Sulcus Tumors

Superior sulcus tumors originate in the apex of the lungs and were described by Pancoast in 1932. These lesions tend to be locally aggressive, involve adjacent structures very early in their growth, and cause the manifestations of Pancoast syndrome, constant pain in the distribution of the C8, Tl, or T2 nerve roots associated with Horner's syndrome. Because of the early presence of symptoms, the tumor frequently presents before metastasizing to the regional lymph nodes or outside the thorax.

Long-term survival with superior sulcus tumors is directly related to complete resection. Attempts to achieve local control with surgical resection alone have been disappointing, with less than 10% of patients being completely resected. Preoperative radiotherapy can downsize superior sulcus tumors and be followed by a margin-negative surgical resection in 25% of patients. A 50% 5-year survival rate can be expected for patients treated with preoperative radiotherapy and complete resection.

Adjuvant Therapy

Data collected by the Lung Cancer Study Group (LCSG) show that 60–70% of stage I patients will survive 5 years without adjuvant therapy. Reports suggest that stage I SCCs have a better prognosis than adenocarcinomas.

Stage II and III patients were prospectively studied by the LCSG, comparing postoperative radiotherapy (RT) with surgery alone. With RT, the local recurrence rate was reduced significantly from 35% to 3%, but there was no survival benefit, as 5-year survival rates remained less than 10%.

In patients with advanced disease, chemotherapy with *cis*-platinum–based regimens have been effective with response rates of 25–45%. Postoperative chemotherapy has demonstrated a significant prolongation in disease-free survival for patients with completely resected stage II and III adenocarcinoma and large-cell carcinoma of the lung. In the adjuvant setting, *cis*-platinum–based regimens in combination with RT have been shown to have a survival benefit over RT alone in patients with completely resected stage III lung cancer.

Current studies are focusing on the use of preoperative (neoadjuvant) chemotherapy. In one trial, patients with biopsy-proven N2 disease were given preoperative *cis*-platinum and etoposide (VP-16) along with RT to a dose of 45 Gy. Patients responding to the preoperative therapy or with stable disease underwent surgical resection. If resection was complete with negative nodes, no further therapy was given. If the disease was unresectable or incomplete or if the mediastinal nodes were positive, two more cycles of chemotherapy and an additional 15 Gy of RT were given. Seventy-three percent of the patients were completely resected. Twenty-one percent of patients had no evidence of tumor in the resected specimen, and 38% had only a microscopic focus of disease. The preliminary 2-year survival rate for stage IIIA and IIIB patients was 30%, which is double the expected survival.

Small-Cell Carcinoma

Small-cell carcinoma grows more rapidly than non–small-cell lung cancers and is usually widely disseminated at the time of diagnosis. Small-cell tumors are very sensitive to chemotherapy, and over two-thirds of patients will achieve a partial response after systemic treatment. Chemotherapy can induce a complete response in 25–50% of patients with limited disease, but responses are not durable and the 5-year survival rate is less than 10%.

Chemotherapeutic regimens for small-cell carcinoma most commonly include cyclophosphamide, *cis*-platinum, etoposide (VP-16), doxorubicin, and vincristine. RT is effective in achieving local control of the primary tumor in most patients and is frequently included as part of the treatment for small-cell carcinoma.

Patients diagnosed with small-cell carcinoma need a metastatic work-up including mediastinoscopy, bone marrow biopsy, and CT scans of the liver and brain. Brain metastases are noted in 80% of patients with small-cell carcinoma during the course of their disease. Patients without CT evidence of brain metastases who achieve a good response from systemic therapy are usually treated with prophylactic brain irradiation to minimize the chances of suffering the morbidity of metastases to the brain.

There is a role for surgical resection of small-cell lung carcinoma. Solitary pulmonary nodules are occasionally removed and are shown to be unsuspected small-cell carcinoma on frozen section. Patients with such nodules should have complete surgical resection with intraoperative staging of the mediastinum. Chemotherapy should be started before the patient is discharged from the hospital, and prophylactic cranial irradiation should be given.

Patients diagnosed with small-cell lung carcinoma based on a fine-needle aspiration biopsy of a peripheral solitary pulmonary nodule and a negative extensive metastatic evaluation should be treated surgically. These patients will do well with lobectomy. Five-year survival is at least 50% when postoperative chemotherapy is given for T1N0 and T2N0 small-cell tumors. If intraoperative staging reveals N1 disease that is completely resected, patients can do well after postoperative chemotherapy, with survival rates greater than 50% at 5 years.

Mediastinoscopy should always be performed prior to thoracotomy for a patient with a diagnosis of small-cell carcinoma even if the metastatic work-up is negative. If the mediastinoscopy is positive, there is no benefit to surgery over chemotherapy and RT. Even if mediastinoscopy is negative, the 5-year survival for a primary centrally located small-cell tumor is 20% with chemotherapy and RT alone. Surgery has not been demonstrated to improve this survival rate.

SURVEILLANCE

Follow-up of patients treated for lung carcinoma includes history and physical examination, chest radiographs, and liver function studies every 3 months for the first 2 years. Patients are evaluated twice a year from years 2–5 postresection, and yearly thereafter. If local recurrence occurs, re-resection is usually not attempted and patients are treated with RT. Solitary pulmonary nodules detected on surveillance may represent a second primary tumor. Resection using parenchyma-sparing procedures may be necessary. Visceral metastatic disease is usually treated with chemotherapy. Metastasis in the brain, a common site of recurrence for lung carcinoma, can be treated with RT. Lung carcinoma is the most frequent carcinoma that metastasizes to the small bowel, causing obstruction. Resection of the involved portion of intestine can provide significant palliative benefit.

Mediastinal Tumors

Mediastinal tumors are located within the chest, above the diaphragm, between the parietal pleura, posterior to the

Table 7-5. The frequency of mediastinal tumors and the mediastinal compartment where they are usually located

Tumor	Frequency (%)	Compartment
Neurogenic tumors	21	Posterior
Cysts (pericardial, bronchogenic, enteric)	20	Anterosuperior and middle
Thymomas	19	Anterosuperior
Germ cell neoplasms	13	Anterosuperior
Mesenchymal tumors	7	Anterosuperior
Endocrine (thyroid, parathyroid, and carcinoid)	6	Anterosuperior

sternum, anterior to the spinal column, and below the thoracic outlet. The mediastinum is further subdivided into compartments, which is clinically relevant because specific histologic types of tumors have a predilection to occur in a particular mediastinal compartment (Table 7-5).

CLINICAL PRESENTATION

One-half of mediastinal tumors are asymptomatic, 90% of which prove to be benign on histologic examination. The most common symptoms related to mediastinal tumors include pain, cough, and dyspnea. Signs and symptoms usually attributed to malignant lesions are pain, superior vena cava syndrome, recurrent laryngeal nerve paralysis, and Horner's syndrome. The symptoms of myasthenia gravis in association with a thymoma may be present in up to 50% of patients. Symptoms of excess hormone production are noted in patients with thyroid, parathyroid, germ cell, and neurogenic tumors.

DIAGNOSIS

A routine chest radiograph is the initial basis of the diagnostic evaluation for a mediastinal tumor. Posteroanterior and lateral chest radiographs demonstrate a mass in 97% of patients with proven mediastinal tumors. The aortopulmonary window and subcarinal region are portions of the mediastinum not well visualized on routine chest radiographs.

Chest CT is the imaging modality of choice to evaluate a suspected mediastinal tumor. Aside from the ability of CT to localize a tumor to its mediastinal compartment, which has diagnostic significance (see Table 7-5), CT can be used to examine the relationship of the tumor to critical structures such as the great vessels, esophagus, and bones of the chest.

Other studies that are used to diagnose mediastinal tumors include an iodine-131 thyroid scan, which will demonstrate a large goiter extending into the superior mediastinum.

Esophagoscopy or barium swallow may be required to evaluate esophageal lesions. Tumor serum markers such as alpha-fetoprotein or human chorionic gonadotropin are helpful to establish the diagnosis of a germ cell tumor, especially in a young male. Urinary catecholamine levels should be evaluated for patients suspected of harboring a pheochromocytoma or other neurogenic tumor.

Mediastinal lesions can be diagnosed histologically by fine-needle aspiration biopsy under fluoroscopic or CT guidance. Mediastinoscopy and anterior mediastinotomy are particularly useful procedures to biopsy enlarged mediastinal lymph nodes caused by sarcoidosis or lymphoma. If lymphoma is suspected, a portion of an excised node should be kept sterile for the required studies to subtype the lymphoma.

NEUROGENIC TUMORS

Neurogenic tumors, the most common mediastinal tumors, are typically located in the posterior compartment. Neurilemomas represent one-half of mediastinal neurogenic tumors, ganglioneuromas and neuroblastomas one-third, and neurofibromas 10%. Paragangliomas are extremely rare and can be hormonally active. Thoracotomy is frequently required to provide a definitive diagnosis. Before surgery is performed on a patient with a posterior mediastinal tumor, urinary catecholamine levels need to be evaluated. Patients with catecholamine-producing tumors need to undergo alpha-adrenergic blockade preoperatively (see Chapter 14) to avoid catastrophic intraoperative complications.

THYMOMA

Thymoma is the most common anterosuperior mediastinal tumor and the second most common neoplasm of the mediastinum as a whole. Myasthenia gravis is noted in 10–50% of thymoma patients, while about 15% of myasthenia gravis patients have an associated thymoma. About one-half of thymomas are well encapsulated and amenable to complete surgical resection. Twenty percent invade the mediastinal fat but can be completely resected without removal of adjacent structures. The remainder of thymomas are locally invasive into mediastinal structures. The recurrence rate for noninvasive thymomas that are completely resected is less than 2%. Other patients should be treated with postoperative RT. Systemic metastases are uncommon but when present are treated with doxorubicin and *cis*-platinum–containing regimens.

Selected References

Akiyama H, Hiyama M, Hashimoto C. Resection and reconstruction for carcinoma of the thoracic oesophagus. *Br J Surg* 63:206, 1976.

Goldminc M, Madden G, Lefrise E, Mevnier B, et al. Oesophagectomy by a transhiatal approach or thoracotomy: A prospective randomized trial. *Br J Surg* 80:367, 1993.

Grillo HC, Austen WG, Wilkens EW. *Current Therapy in Cardiothoracic Surgery*. Philadelphia; B.C. Decker, 1989.

Mountain CF. A new international staging system for lung cancer. *Chest* 89(Suppl):225S, 1986.

Orringer MB. Transhiatal Blunt Esophagectomy Without Thoracotomy. In *Modern Technics in Surgery. Cardiac Thoracic Surgery*. Mt. Kisco, NY: Futura, 1983. Pp 0–61.

Pancoast HK. Superior sulcus tumor: Tumor characterized by pain, Horner's syndrome, destruction of bone and atrophy of hand muscles. *JAMA* 99:1391, 1932.

Postlethwait RW. *Surgery of the Esophagus* (2nd ed). New York: Appleton-Century-Crofts, 1986.

Putnam JB, Roth JA. Neoplastic Diseases of the Esophagus. In RH Bell, LF Rikkers, MW Mulholland (eds), *Digestive Tract Surgery: A Text and Atlas*. Philadelphia: Lippincott (in press).

Roth JA, Lichter AS, Putnam JB, Forastiere AA. Cancer of the Esophagus. In RJ McKenna, GP Murphy (eds), *Cancer: Principles and Practice of Oncology* (4th ed). Philadelphia: Lippincott, 1983. Pp 776–817.

Roth JA, Ruckdeschel JC, Weisenburger TH. *Thoracic Oncology*. Philadelphia: Saunders, 1990.

Sabiston DC, Spencer FC. *Surgery of the Chest* (5th ed). Philadelphia: Saunders, 1990.

Gastric Carcinoma

Charles A. Staley

Epidemiology

It is estimated that gastric carcinoma, the eighth most common cause of cancer mortality in the United States, will account for 24,000 new cases and 13,600 deaths in 1994. The incidence of gastric cancer in the United States declined steadily from 1930 to 1980, but from 1980–1990, the incidence has plateaued. The approximate incidence in the United States is 10 per 100,000 people, compared with 780 per 100,000 people in Japan. Survival of patients with gastric cancer remains poor, with the overall 5-year survival rate being 15%.

Risk Factors

Many factors have been associated with an increased risk of gastric cancer. Animal studies have shown that polycyclic hydrocarbons and dimethylnitrosamines can induce malignant gastric tumors. In the United States, male sex, black race, and low socioeconomic class are associated with a higher risk of gastric carcinoma. A specific occupational hazard may exist for metal workers, miners, and rubber workers, and for workers exposed to dust from wood and asbestos. Diets rich in starch and poor in animal protein and vitamins are thought to be a factor in gastric carcinogenesis. An association of carcinoma with blood group A patients was described in 1953, but the relative risk is only 1.2. Familial clusterings, though rare, have been reported.

Helicobacter pylori, a gram-negative microaerophilic bacterium, has been implicated as a possible promoter agent in the development of gastric carcinoma. This association is based on the increased incidence of *H. pylori* infection in China, where there is a high rate of gastric cancer and an increased incidence of infection in patients with gastric cancer in the United States.

Gastric polyps are rarely precursors of gastric cancer. Hyperplastic polyps, the polyps most commonly found in the stomach, are benign lesions. Villous adenomas do have malignant potential but represent only 2% of all gastric polyps. Pernicious anemia is associated with a 10% incidence of gastric cancer, a risk that is about 20 times that of the normal population. The risk of developing carcinoma in a chronic gastric ulcer is small, but gastric resections for benign peptic ulcers are associated with an increased risk of subsequent stomach cancer. Even so, there is typically a 15- to 40-year lag period after the initial surgery before the cancer develops. Atrophic gastritis and intestinal metaplasia have been associated with gastric carcinoma but do not appear to be direct precursor conditions.

Pathology

Ninety-five percent of gastric cancers are adenocarcinomas. Lymphoma, carcinoid, leiomyosarcoma, and squamous cell carcinoma make up the remaining 5%. The stomach is the most common site for lymphoma in the gastrointestinal (GI) tract. In the United States, the morphologic classification of gastric cancer is divided into ulcerative (75%), polypoid (10%), scirrhous (10%), and superficial (5%).

Two histologic types of gastric cancer are recognized: intestinal and diffuse. Each type has distinct clinical and pathologic features. The *intestinal* type is found in regions with a high incidence of gastric cancer and is characterized pathologically by the tendency of malignant cells to form glands. The tumors are usually well differentiated; consist of papillary, glandular, and tubular variants; are associated with metaplasia or chronic gastritis; occur more commonly in older patients; and tend to spread hematologically to distant organs. The *diffuse* type is identified by the lack of organized gland formation, is usually poorly differentiated, and is composed of signet ring cells. This type of tumor is more common in younger patients with no history of gastritis and spreads by transmural extension through lymphatic invasion. The incidence of diffuse tumors is relatively constant among many countries and appears to be increasing overall.

In the past, the majority of gastric cancers were localized in the antrum (60–70%). However, from 1980–1990, there has been an increase in tumors of the cardia, which now account for 33% of all gastric carcinomas. Nine percent of patients have tumor involvement of the entire stomach, known as linitis plastica. In general, gastric tumors are more common on the lesser curve of the stomach than on the greater curve. In the United States, the incidence of synchronous lesions is 2.2%, compared to a 10% incidence in Japanese patients with pernicious anemia.

Clinical Presentation

Gastric carcinoma usually lacks specific symptoms early in the course of the disease. The vague epigastric discomfort and indigestion are usually ignored by the patient. Patients are often treated presumptively for benign disease for 6–12 months without diagnostic studies even being performed. Rapid weight loss, anorexia, and vomiting occur more frequently in advanced disease. The most frequent presenting symptoms of 1,121 patients at Memorial Sloan-Kettering Cancer Center were weight loss, pain, vomiting, and anorexia. The epigastric pain is usually similar to benign ulcer pain, can mimic angina, and many times is relieved by eating food. Dysphagia is usually associated with tumors of the cardia or gastroesophageal junction. Antral tumors may cause symptoms of gastric outlet obstruction. Large tumors that directly invade the transverse colon may present with colonic obstruction. Up to 30% of patients will present with a palpable mass, and about 10% present with one or more signs of metastatic disease. The most common indications of metastasis include a palpable supraclavicular node (Virchow's node), Blumer's rectal shelf, periumbilical node (Sister Mary Joseph), ascites, jaundice, a liver mass, or a pelvic mass. The most common site of hematogenous spread is to the liver. Gastric tumors may be associated with chronic blood loss, detected as occult blood in the stool, but massive upper GI bleeding is rare.

Preoperative Evaluation

The only chance to cure gastric cancer is through early diagnosis. Historically, the barium upper GI x-ray series was the gold standard for the diagnosis of gastric cancer. However, this test has an accuracy of only 70–80% and a false-negative rate of 10–20%. The development of fiberoptic flexible endoscopy was a major advance in the accurate tissue diagnosis of gastric cancer. An accurate diagnosis can be made from 4–6 biopsies and cytologic brushings in greater than 90% of patients.

Once the tissue diagnosis has been made, computed tomography (CT) evaluation allows visualization of the stomach, perigastric area, and distant sites such as the liver, nodal basins, and peritoneum. Overall, CT scans have an accuracy of 90% for liver disease, 60% for nodal disease, and 50% for peritoneal disease. Focal wall thickening may be an important but sometimes misleading CT finding. Early small tumors, peritoneal disease, and invasion of adjacent organs are often missed by CT. In Cook and colleagues' report on 37 patients who underwent laparotomy after preoperative CT scans, 61% of the patients were understaged by CT, most frequently because of missed nodal, liver, or peritoneal disease. In addition, not all adenopathy seen on CT scan represents metastasis. CT evaluation of regional lymph nodes has a sensitivity of 67% and a specificity of 61%. Komaki, et al., found that massive adenopathy represented metastatic disease in 96% of cases but that a single enlarged node was metastatic only 48% of the time. Yet most authors agree that nodes larger than 6 mm are suspicious for cancer.

In view of the deficiencies of CT, endoscopic ultrasound (EUS) has become the gold standard for preoperative staging of gastric cancer. EUS is more accurate than CT in staging the depth of primary tumor invasion (T) and regional lymph nodes metastases (N). EUS is not helpful in evaluating distant metastatic disease.

Elevated levels of carcinoembryonic antigen (CEA) are seen in only 30% of patients with gastric carcinoma. Because the CEA level is usually normal in early cancer, it is not a useful screening marker. Serial determinations of CEA level may be helpful in evaluating tumor recurrence or tumor response to treatment in patients who present with an elevated level.

Table 8-1. TNM staging system for gastric carcinoma

T1	Tumor invades lamina propria or submucosa		
T2	Tumor invades muscularis propria or subserosa		
T3	Tumor penetrates serosa		
T4	Tumor invades adjacent organ structures		
N0	No metastases in lymph nodes		
N1	Metastasis in perigastric lymph node(s) within 3 cm of primary tumor		
N2	Metastasis in perigastric lymph node(s) >3 cm from primary tumor, or in lymph nodes along left gastric, common hepatic, splenic, or celiac arteries		
M0	No evidence of distant metastasis		
M1	Evidence of distant metastasis		
Staging	IA	T1	N0	M0
	IB	T1	N1	M0
		T2	N0	M0
	II	T1	N2	M0
		T2	N1	M0
		T3	N0	M0
	IIIA	T2	N2	M0
		T3	N1	M0
		T4	N0	M0
	IIIB	T3	N2	M0
		T4	N1	M0
	IV	T4	N2	M0
		Any T, N	M1	

Source: Adapted from OH Beahrs, DE Henson, RVP Hutter, et al (eds). *AJCC Manual for Staging of Cancer* (4th ed). Philadelphia: Lippincott, 1992.

The limitations of CT and EUS in evaluating peritoneal disease have led many surgeons to use diagnostic laparoscopy to avoid an unnecessary laparotomy in patients with unsuspected metastatic disease. Kriplani and Kapur reported a series of 40 patients thought to have resectable gastric tumors preoperatively. Laparoscopy identified 16 patients who were unresectable: 5 with distant metastases (12.5%) and 11 (27.5%) with locally advanced unresectable tumors. The overall accuracy of laparoscopy was 91.6%, and there was no morbidity or mortality associated with the procedure. Overall, 40% of the patients were spared a futile laparotomy. In our experience at the University of Texas M. D. Anderson Cancer Center, laparoscopy will change the original stage assignment in 25% of patients. Diagnostic laparoscopy is an important part of the preoperative evaluation, unless a palliative resection for bleeding or obstruction is planned.

Staging

The current American Joint Committee on Cancer (AJCC) staging for gastric cancer is listed in Table 8-1. This system uses depth of penetration of the gastric wall as the guideline for T stage. Nodal involvement is classified as N0-N2 as

Table 8-2. Lymph node groupings according to site of tumor*

	Location of primary tumor			
Group	Entire stomach	Lower third	Middle third	Upper third
N1	1–6	3–6	1, 3–6	1–4
N2	7–11	1, 7–9	2, 7–11	5–11
N3	12–14	2, 10–14	12–14	12–14

*1–14 correspond to the lymph nodes described in Fig. 8-1.
Source: Adapted from KE Behrns, RR Dalton, JA van Heerden, et al. Extended lymph node dissection for gastric cancer. Is it of value? *Surg Clin North Am* 72:433, 1992.

Table 8-3. Japanese classification of gastric resection

R0	Total gastrectomy with incomplete removal of N1 nodes
R1	Total gastrectomy with complete removal of N1 nodes
R2	Total gastrectomy with complete removal of N2 nodes
R3	Total gastrectomy with complete removal of N3 nodes
R4	Total gastrectomy with complete removal of N4 nodes

described in Table 8-2. Nodes in the retropancreatic, para-aortic, hepatoduodenal, and mesenteric areas are considered M1 disease.

The staging system used in Japan for gastric cancer is very different from that in Western countries, making it difficult to compare reports on the disease. The most confusing difference is in the staging classification of the lymph nodes. The Japanese system describes four major nodal groups (N1–N4) that encompass 16 separate locations of nodal tissue (Fig. 8-1). Nodes closest to the primary tumor and within the perigastric tissue of the lesser and greater curvatures constitute the N1 group of nodes. (It is important to note that the specific nodal tissue included in the N1 nodal grouping varies depending on the anatomic location of the tumor.) Lymph nodes along the blood vessels from the celiac axis to the stomach make up the N2 nodal group. N3 nodes are found in the hepatoduodenal ligament, retropancreatic tissue, and celiac axis. N4 nodes are located in the para-aortic tissue (Table 8-2). The N3 and N4 designations in the Japanese system would constitute distant metastatic disease (M1) in the AJCC system.

The Japanese also use a coding system for the extent of lymph node resection. These resections are labeled R0 through R4, as outlined in Table 8-3.

Surgical Treatment

LYMPHADENECTOMY

Radical lymphadenectomy was adopted based on an initial report in 1981 by Kodama, et al., that showed a survival benefit for patients with serosal or regional lymph node involvement who underwent an R2 or R3 lymphadenectomy.

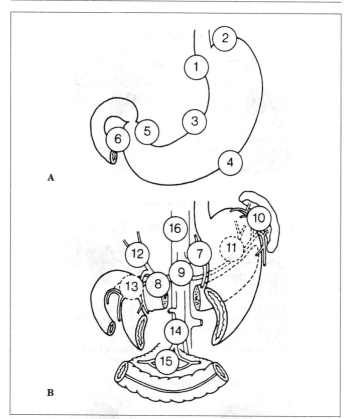

Fig. 8-1. Japanese classification of regional gastric lymph nodes.
A. Perigastric lymph nodes. 1: right pericardial; 2: left pericardial;
3: lesser curvature; 4: greater curvature; 5: suprapyloric; 6: infrapyloric. B. Extraperigastric lymph nodes. 7: left gastric artery; 8: common
hepatic artery; 9: celiac artery; 10: splenic hilus; 11: splenic artery:
12: hepatic pedicle; 13: retropancreatic; 14: mesenteric root; 15: middle
colic artery; 16: para-aortic. (Adapted from Y Kodama, K Sugimachi, K
Soejima, et al. Evaluation of extensive lymph node dissection for carcinoma of the stomach. *World J Surg* 5:242, 1981.)

Patients undergoing radical lymphadenectomy had a 39% 5-
year survival rate compared with 18% with an R1 lymphadenectomy. Figure 8-2 shows the site-specific extent of
dissection for an R1 and R2 lymphadenectomy. Many other
studies from Japan have shown a similarly significant survival benefit for patients undergoing radical lymphadenectomy. Unfortunately, most Western studies have not been able
to repeat the Japanese results, so the role of radical lymphadenectomy in the treatment of gastric cancer remains
controversial.

The reason for the difference in survival between Japanese
and Western studies appears to be multifactorial. Mass

Lower third lesions

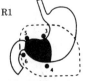

R1

3 Lesser curvature
4 Greater curvature
5 Suprapyloric
6 Infrapyloric

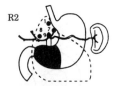

R2

1 R Cardiac
7 L Gastric artery
8 Hepatic
9 Celiac

Middle third lesions

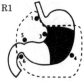

R1

1 R cardiac
3 Lesser curvature
4 Greater curvature
5 Suprapyloric
6 Infrapyloric

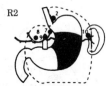

R2

2 L cardiac*
7 L gastric artery
8 Hepatic artery
9 Celiac
10 Splenic hilar
11 Splenic artery

Upper third lesions (includes cardia)

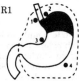

R1

1 R cardiac
2 L cardiac
3 Lesser curvature
4 Greater curvature
   and short gastric

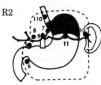

R2

5   Suprapyloric*
6   Infrapyloric*
7   L gastric artery
8   Hepatic artery
9   Celiac
10 Splenic hilar
11 Splenic artery
110 Paraesophageal
    (cardia lesions)

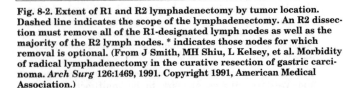

Fig. 8-2. Extent of R1 and R2 lymphadenectomy by tumor location. Dashed line indicates the scope of the lymphadenectomy. An R2 dissection must remove all of the R1-designated lymph nodes as well as the majority of the R2 lymph nodes. * indicates those nodes for which removal is optional. (From J Smith, MH Shiu, L Kelsey, et al. Morbidity of radical lymphadenectomy in the curative resection of gastric carcinoma. *Arch Surg* 126:1469, 1991. Copyright 1991, American Medical Association.)

screening programs in Japan have increased the percentage of early-stage cancers (30% versus 5% in the United States), which could account for part of the difference. It is also postulated that there may be an inherent difference in the biology of gastric cancer in the two countries, with the Japanese having a less aggressive form of tumor. Furthermore, the significant differences in the staging systems between the two countries make it difficult to compare the survival rate stage for stage between studies. In addition, the Japanese nodal dissection and pathologic analysis is much more meticulous and extends out to the quaternary nodes (N4) in many cases. Western series, on the other hand, potentially understage patients because in many cases only perigastric nodes are dissected and the involvement of N2 and M1 nodes is not examined. Another problem with most of the Japanese data is that they compare results of radical lymphadenectomy to historical controls from previous decades rather than conducting prospective randomized trials. A higher percentage of early-stage gastric cancer being diagnosed currently in Japan (as mentioned above) could account, at least in part, for this increased survival over historical controls. Interestingly, one report from Japan was unable to show any benefit for an R3 over R2 dissection.

In studies in the Western literature, Gilbertson reviewed 1,983 patients whose tumors were resected between 1936 and 1963. Patients who underwent an R2 lymphadenectomy had a decreased survival and increased postoperative morbidity when compared to similarly staged patients undergoing an R1 dissection. Similar results have been shown in a prospective study from South Africa. In contrast, Shiu et al. retrospectively reviewed 210 patients with gastric cancer at Memorial Sloan-Kettering Cancer Center and found that a lymphadenectomy that failed to include the lymph nodes at least one echelon beyond the histologically involved nodes was predictive of a poor prognosis. They also showed that there was not a significant difference in morbidity between the R1 and R2 nodal dissections.

Prospective trials are currently underway in an attempt to definitively resolve the controversy over the role of radical lymphadenectomy.

SURGICAL OPTIONS

In the absence of documented metastatic disease, aggressive surgical resection of gastric tumors is justified. The appropriate surgical procedure for a given patient must take into account the location of the lesion and the known pattern of spread.

PROXIMAL TUMORS

The optimal surgical management of proximal gastric tumors is controversial. The options include total gastrectomy and proximal subtotal gastrectomy. In general, proximal tumors are more advanced at presentation and have a poorer long-term prognosis than distal cancers. Consequently, palliative resections are twice as likely to be performed in patients with proximal tumors as in patients with distal cancers. Because of the advanced stage at diagnosis of most tumors of the cardia, some authors argue that any operation is realistically a palliative procedure and therefore one should always perform the simpler proximal subtotal gastrectomy, especially because total gastrectomy does not improve prognosis for patients with stage III and IV disease. However, a survival benefit and lower recurrence rate have been shown for patients with stage I and II disease who undergo a total gastrectomy.

At M. D. Anderson, we perform a total gastrectomy with Roux-en-Y reconstruction for proximal gastric lesions. This procedure has the advantage of avoiding alkaline reflux gastritis associated with proximal subtotal gastrectomy. There is no significant increase in mortality or morbidity with total gastrectomy compared with proximal subtotal gastrectomy.

Mid-Body Tumors

Mid-stomach tumors comprise 15–30% of all gastric cancers. Based on the same arguments that were discussed for proximal tumors, we recommend total gastrectomy for tumors located in the mid-body of the stomach.

Distal Tumors

Distal tumors account for about 35% of all gastric cancers. The standard operation for these lesions is a distal subtotal gastrectomy with or without a regional lymphadenectomy. This procedure entails resection of approximately three-fourths of the stomach, including the majority of the lesser curvature. Studies have shown that there will be no microscopic invasion beyond a distance of 6 cm from the gross tumor. We therefore recommend a 5- to 6-cm resection margin when possible. Even if this distance is achieved, margins must still be checked by frozen-section analysis.

Splenectomy

Splenectomy is not performed unless there is tumor adherence or invasion of the spleen. Routine splenectomy does not influence survival but does increase the morbidity of gastrectomy. If a splenectomy is contemplated due to tumor adherence, Pneumovax (pneumococcal) vaccine should be given preoperatively.

SURGICAL TECHNIQUE

Total Gastrectomy

Once preoperative work-up excludes the presence of distant metastases or an unresectable tumor, the patient should undergo diagnostic laparoscopy. If laparoscopy is negative, an open laparotomy, exploration, and gastrectomy are performed through a midline or bilateral subcostal incision. For a total gastrectomy, the dissection is begun by holding up the omentum and dissecting down the anterior leaf of the transverse mesocolon, thereby separating the omentum from the mesocolon. This plane is developed over the anterior surface of the pancreas. The right gastroepiploic vessels are ligated at their origin, and the subpyloric nodes are dissected with the specimen. The first portion of the duodenum is mobilized and divided 2 cm distal to the pylorus. The lesser omentum is then dissected free at the inferior edge of the liver. The left gastric artery is ligated at its origin. It is important to remember that an aberrant or accessory left hepatic artery may originate from the left gastric artery and reside in the lesser omentum. If an R2 lymphadenectomy is done, the celiac, hepatic artery, and periaortic nodes are dissected along with the specimen. The short gastric vessels are ligated up to the gastroesophageal junction (GEJ). Dissection around the GEJ will free 7–8 cm of distal esophagus, which facilitates transection of the esophagus with adequate proximal margins. After the esophagus is divided, the resection margins are checked by frozen-section examination. If the tumor is adherent to the spleen, pancreas, or mesocolon, the involved organs are removed en bloc.

There are many types of reconstruction, but the most frequently used is a Roux-en-Y anastomosis. If a significant portion of the distal esophagus is resected, a left thoracoabdominal or right Ivor-Lewis approach may be used. Reconstruction with pouches and loops to act as reservoirs has no benefit over a straight Roux-en-Y reconstruction. A feeding jejunostomy tube is placed for postoperative nutritional support.

Subtotal Gastrectomy

A subtotal gastrectomy is approached in the same way as described above for a total gastrectomy except that only about 80% of the distal stomach is resected (Fig. 8-3). A small remnant of stomach remains and is supplied by the short gastric vessels. We prefer to perform a Roux-en-Y reconstruction, but a loop gastrojejunostomy can be done if there is no tension on the anastomosis.

Complications

Postoperative complications are listed in Table 8-4. The most devastating complication of a gastric resection is an anastomotic leak, which is seen in 3–12% of patients. A barium upper GI series is usually obtained on postoperative day 7 to investigate the anastomosis before oral feeding is begun. Because the food reservoir is gone, these patients must change their eating habits to six small meals per day. Many patients are discharged on supplemental jejunostomy feedings until their oral intake is adequate.

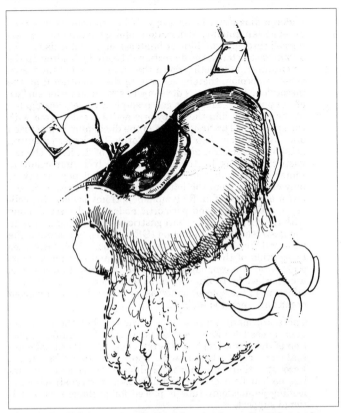

Fig. 8-3. Resection margins of subtotal gastrectomy. Inset shows placement of anastamosis. (From JS MacDonald, G Steele, LL Gunderson. Cancer of the Stomach. In VT DeVita, S Hellman, SA Rosenberg [eds], *Cancer: Principles and Practice of Oncology* [4th ed]. Philadelphia: Lippincott, 1993.)

Early Gastric Cancer

In the early 1960s, the Japanese defined early gastric cancer as carcinoma limited to the mucosa and submucosa regardless of the presence or absence of lymph node metastasis. This pathologic classification is based on the high cure rate in this group of patients. Although the incidence of early gastric cancer has increased in the United States (from approximately 5% to 15% of all gastric cancers), aggressive screening in Japan has resulted in an even greater increase in incidence in that country, from 5% to 30%, during the last 15 years. The mean age of patients at diagnosis in Western studies is 63 (55 in Japanese patients), and most patients present with GI symptoms similar to those of peptic ulcer disease, including epigastric pain and dyspepsia. In contrast

Table 8-4. Complications of gastric resection

Complication	Percentage of patients
Pulmonary	3–55
Infectious	3–22
Anastomotic	3–21
Cardiac	1–10
Renal	1–8
Bleeding	0.3–5
Pulmonary embolus	1–4

to advanced gastric cancer, it is uncommon to see significant weight loss in these patients at the time of diagnosis.

The use of endoscopy and biopsy has been instrumental in the ability to diagnose early gastric cancer. In collected Western series, only 22% of cancers were diagnosed by a barium upper GI study as compared to 80% by endoscopy. The Japanese have classified early gastric cancer pathologically based on its gross endoscopic appearance. They define three basic types of tumors: (1) type I: protruded; (2) type II: superficial; and (3) type III: excavated (Fig. 8-4). By the TNM classification, early gastric cancer would include all T1 tumors with any N stage of disease.

The surgical procedure performed in the patient with early gastric cancer is based on the location, extent of the lesion, and nodal disease. The majority of reports in the Western literature favor subtotal gastrectomy as the procedure of choice for early gastric cancer. Total gastrectomy is reserved for proximal tumors or multifocal disease. This approach has resulted in a 5-year survival rate of approximately 85%, which compares favorably with the Japanese experience of a 5-year survival rate reportedly greater than 90%. The Japanese have been unable to show a survival benefit for radical lymphadenectomy in patients with histologically uninvolved lymph nodes. However, an improved survival rate has been noted in patients with lymph node metastases who undergo a radical lymphadenectomy compared to patients undergoing an R1 dissection. Despite a high potential cure rate, it must be remembered that 10–15% of these early tumors will have positive lymph nodes that may occasionally extend to the N2 nodal basin. Therefore several authors recommend that an extended lymphadenectomy (R2) be performed in these highly curable patients.

Surgical Results

The overall 5-year survival rate for gastric cancer is 10–21% in most Western series, a consequence of the advanced stage of disease at presentation in the majority of patients. There is a slightly better prognosis in patients resected for cure (24–57% 5-year survival rate). This is in contrast to the 50% 5-year survival reported in the Japanese literature. Overall

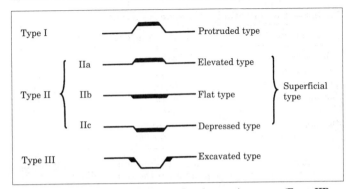

Fig. 8-4. Macroscopic classification of early gastric cancer. (From HR Nava, MA Arredondo. Diagnosis of gastric cancer. *Surg Oncol Clin North Am* **2:371, 1993.)**

5-year survival rates for Japan and the United States are listed by TNM stage in Table 8-5.

In 1989, Cady et al. reviewed their series of 211 gastric cancer patients. Of these, 17% were not explored due to distant metastatic disease or diffuse peritoneal spread identified preoperatively, while 83% underwent a laparotomy. Of those patients undergoing laparotomy, 58% underwent resection; 34% of the procedures were performed for cure and 24% for palliation. These patients were treated before the more widespread availability of diagnostic laparoscopy. The overall 5-year survival rate for all 211 patients was 21%, but those patients who underwent surgical resection had a 5-year survival rate of 36%. This figure increased to 58% for those patients resected with curative intent. The percentage of patients with proximal cancers undergoing curative resection was half that of patients with distal cancers. Fifteen percent of the patients had linitis plastica; these patients had a median survival of 12 months. Resection should be avoided in these patients unless palliation of an obstructing or bleeding tumor is necessary.

Multiple prognostic variables for gastric cancer were reviewed by Shiu et al. in 1989. The five independent variables found to correlate with a poor prognosis were high TNM stage, metastatic involvement of four or more lymph nodes, poorly differentiated tumors, splenectomy, and regional lymphadenectomy not extensive enough relative to the nodal stage. These variables all had a negative impact on survival.

Adjuvant Therapy

POSTOPERATIVE CHEMOTHERAPY

Only a minority of patients who undergo resection for gastric cancer are actually cured, as 70–80% develop recurrences

Table 8-5. Five-year survival rates after gastrectomy (%)

Stage		Japan	United States
N0	T1	80	90
	T2	60	58
	T3	30	50
	T4	5	20
N1		53	20
N2		26	10
N3		10	—
N4		3	—
Overall		50	15

Source: Adapted from Y Noguchi Y, T Imada, A Matsumoto, et al. Radical surgery for gastric cancer: A review of the Japanese experience. *Cancer* 64:2053, 1989.

after gastric resection. Therefore, adjuvant therapy could potentially impact on survival. Two early studies conducted by the Veterans Administration Surgical Adjuvant Group (VASAG) investigated the use of thiotepa and floxuridine (FUDR) following surgical resection. There was no survival benefit seen in either study, and the toxicity of thiotepa was substantial.

Three trials have studied the use of 5-fluorouracil (5-FU) and semustine (methyl-CCNU) as adjuvant therapy. The Gastrointestinal Tumor Study Group (GITSG) evaluated patients who were randomly assigned to receive no additional therapy or 18 months of 5-FU and methyl-CCNU. A survival benefit was noted in patients receiving chemotherapy. However, an Eastern Cooperative Oncology Group (ECOG) trial using the same doses and schedule of chemotherapy failed to demonstrate any survival benefit. A third study by VASAG using the same agents but a different dosing schedule also found no survival benefit. Without a clear benefit in using 5-FU and methyl-CCNU and with a significant risk of treatment-induced acute nonlymphocytic leukemia, many investigators believe that this adjuvant regimen is inappropriate.

A single study from Spain by Estape et al. with a follow-up of 10 years, has shown a survival benefit with the use of adjuvant mitomycin C. The chemotherapy schedule used in this study was 20 mg/m^2 given IV once every 6 weeks for four cycles. Of 37 patients in the control arm, 31 died of recurrent disease, compared to 16 of 33 patients in the treatment group. The most significant advantage was seen in patients with T3, N0, M0 tumors. The major criticism of this study is the relatively small sample size. Other studies have used mitomycin C in combination with 5-FU and either cyclophosphamide or cytosine arabinoside. These studies have been unable to show any survival benefit in the group of patients receiving adjuvant chemotherapy.

More recently, chemotherapy regimens that include doxorubicin have been studied. Several groups have reported no survival benefit in trials with 5-FU, doxorubicin, and mito-mycin C (FAM) in the adjuvant setting.

Two studies have looked at patients randomly assigned to receive no additional therapy or radiotherapy with concurrent 5-FU. Dent studied 142 patients but found no benefit to this combined regimen. A second study by Moertel showed a benefit of chemotherapy plus radiotherapy, but the study results were skewed by 10 patients who were randomized to the experimental arm but refused treatment.

In general, no survival benefit has been reproduced consistently with adjuvant treatment of gastric cancer. There have been two unconfirmed studies, one with 5-FU and methyl-CCNU (GITSG) and the other with mitomycin C alone, that have shown a survival benefit to adjuvant therapy. A current Radiation Therapy Oncology Group trial is randomizing patients to receive either 5-FU, leucovorin, and radiotherapy or observation after gastric resection.

PREOPERATIVE CHEMOTHERAPY

Preoperative, or neoadjuvant, chemotherapy offers the potential to downstage disease and the ability to evaluate tumor sensitivity to a chemotherapeutic regimen. If the tumor responds to the neoadjuvant therapy, treatment can be continued postoperatively. Several trials have evaluated etoposide, cisplatin, and either 5-FU or doxorubicin in the neoadjuvant setting. Response rates have ranged from a clinical response of 21–31% to a complete pathologic response rate of 0–15%. Currently, M. D. Anderson is evaluating a neoadjuvant regimen consisting of 5-FU, cisplatin, and interferon-alpha. Until randomized trials are performed, neoadjuvant therapy should be reserved for a protocol setting.

INTRAOPERATIVE RADIOTHERAPY

Most of the data available on intraoperative radiotherapy (IORT) for gastric cancer is based on the reports of Abe and Takahashi from Japan. Their prospective nonrandomized trial looked at 110 patients who had surgery alone and 84 patients who had surgery plus IORT. The 5-year survival rates were similar in stage I patients; however, a suggestion of a survival benefit was seen in stage II, III, and IV patients receiving IORT. In contrast, a small (less than 40 patients) randomized IORT study done at the National Cancer Institute showed neither a disease-free nor an overall survival benefit with IORT.

Management of Recurrent Disease

The problem of disease recurrence has been analyzed in autopsy, reoperative, and clinical series. Some component of disease failure can be found in up to 80% of patients following gastrectomy. In 1982, Gunderson and Sosin analyzed patterns of failure in a prospective study of 109 patients who had undergone a gastric resection and were then subjected to reoperation at the University of Minnesota. Of the 107 evaluable patients, 86 (80%) had recurrent disease. Locoregional failure alone occurred in only 22 (9%) of the patients, but peritoneal seeding was seen as a component of recurrence in 53.7% of those patients who failed. Isolated distant metastases were uncommon but occurred as some component of failure in 29% of the group.

In 1986, Landry et al. from Massachusetts General Hospital reviewed disease recurrence in 130 patients resected for cure. The overall locoregional failure rate was 38% (49/130): 21 patients (16%) had locoregional failure alone, 28 patients (22%) had locoregional failure and distant metastasis, and 39 patients (30%) had distant metastases alone. Locoregional recurrence increased with the degree of tumor penetration through the gastric wall. The most frequent sites of locoregional recurrence were the gastric remnant at the anastomosis, the gastric bed, or the regional nodes. The overall incidence of distant metastases was 52% (67 patients), and an increased incidence was seen with advancing stage of disease. The overall recurrence rate was 68% (88 patients).

Management of Advanced Disease

PALLIATIVE SURGERY

Because the majority of patients present with advanced disease, only 30% are eligible for curative resection. The procedures available for palliation are resection, bypass, intubation, or laser fulguration. The particular treatment rendered must be individualized for each patient. The symptoms that commonly require palliation are obstruction, bleeding, and intractable pain. Pyloric obstruction can be relieved by a gastroenterostomy or resection. Obstruction of the cardia is best treated by resection, but laser ablation may be used for patients at high operative risk with a reasonable degree of success. The best results with laser ablation are obtained with lesions smaller than 5 cm in diameter. Acute bleeding may be controlled by endoscopy and cautery, angiographic embolization, or resection. Chronic blood loss may be treated with cautery or radiotherapy. Good palliation is obtained with surgery 50% of the time. The operative mortality ranges from 6 to 22%. Mean survival after palliative treatment is 4.2 months and ranges from 0 to 13 months.

CHEMOTHERAPY

The effect of chemotherapy on advanced gastric carcinoma has been disappointing. Several single-agent drug regimens have been tested including 5-FU, doxorubicin, and mitomycin C. The response rates have ranged from 17 to 30%;

however, the responses have generally been brief and have not had a significant impact on survival.

Numerous attempts have been made to develop effective combination chemotherapy using known active agents. The combination of 5-FU, doxorubicin, and mitomycin C (FAM) was studied in the 1980s. Initially, it produced a response rate of 42% and a median response duration of 9 months, but there were no complete responses. Other reports on FAM have shown similar results. Etoposide has been used in combination with doxorubicin and cisplatin (EAP). Although a single report reported a 64% response rate, other investigators have not been able to achieve such high response rates and have documented significant morbidity and mortality due to myelosuppression. As a result, etoposide has been tried in combination with other chemotherapeutic agents including leucovorin and 5-FU, with varying results. This regimen is well tolerated by older, high-risk patients. Mitomycin C has been combined with doxorubicin and 5-FU in clinical trials to produce a regimen termed FAMTX. Response rates have ranged from 33 to 59% with complete response rates and median survival times reported as high as 21% and 9 months, respectively.

In summary, no regimen of combination chemotherapy has been shown to be decisively superior to single-agent therapy. However, many investigators are encouraged by the initial results with FAMTX.

RADIOTHERAPY

There are several isolated case reports of radiotherapy being beneficial when used as palliative treatment for advanced gastic carcinoma. However, no large prospective trial has been able to show any long-term benefit for radiotherapy in advanced disease.

INTRAPERITONEAL HYPERTHERMIC PERFUSION

The use of intraperitoneal (IP) chemotherapy has been investigated for several years, particularly in the treatment of ovarian and colorectal cancers. IP 5-FU was initially shown to decrease peritoneal recurrence in patients with colorectal cancer. Most of the more recent IP therapy for advanced gastric cancer has been reported in the Japanese literature. Koga, et al., reviewed their experience with a combination of hyperthermia and mitomycin C used in an adjuvant setting. The authors showed that this procedure was technically feasible and safe. Patients who underwent perfusion did not have an increased incidence of postoperative complications. Fujimoto, et al., evaluated 59 patients who underwent gastrectomy followed by randomization to no further therapy or IP hyperthermic perfusion therapy. The perfused patients survived longer than the controls (1-year survival rate 80.4% versus 34.2%, respectively). Patients with peritoneal seeding also had a significant survival benefit when perfused with hyperthermic mitomycin C. The findings of this study have yet to be confirmed by other investigators but may indicate that IP hyperthermic perfusion therapy has the potential to extend survival for patients with advanced gastric cancer. This technique is currently under investigation in several centers in the United States.

Figure 8-5 outlines the treatment strategy for gastric adenocarcinoma at the M. D. Anderson Cancer Center.

Surveillance

Patients are examined every 3 months for the first 2 years following resection of a gastric adenocarcinoma. A careful history and physical examination is performed along with a chest radiograph and laboratory studies (complete blood count and liver function tests). Patients should have a CT scan performed 1 year after surgery and yearly thereafter. Those patients who undergo a subtotal gastrectomy should have yearly endoscopy performed as well.

Gastric Lymphoma

In contrast to the decreasing incidence of gastric adenocarcinoma, the incidence of gastric lymphoma is steadily increasing. Gastric lymphoma accounts for two-thirds of GI lymphomas. The average age of patients is 60 years. The most frequent symptoms at the time of presentation are pain (68%), weight loss (28%), bleeding (28%), and fatigue (16%). Obstruction, perforation, and massive bleeding are uncommon.

Before the advent of endoscopy, the diagnosis of gastric lymphoma was usually made at operation. Endoscopy permits a correct tissue diagnosis approximately 80% of the time. The majority of lesions are located in the distal stomach and spread locally by submucosal infiltration. Once the diagnosis has been made, a careful work-up including a physical examination (with special attention to adenopathy), routine laboratory tests along with lactate dehydrogenase and beta$_2$-microglobulin determinations, a bone marrow biopsy, pedal lymphangiogram, chest radiograph, and CT scan of the abdomen should be done to fully stage the extent of disease. Pathologic examination shows most cases to be B cell non-Hodgkin's lymphoma (diffuse histiocytic subtype predominant). The disease is staged using the modified Ann Arbor staging system. Histologic grade and pathologic stage are two variables that independently predict survival.

The treatment of gastric lymphoma varies among institutions, with some centers using surgery alone and others promoting chemotherapy and radiation. Surgery is necessary in some cases to confirm the diagnosis. Surgical resection is curative in many patients with localized disease and can pre-

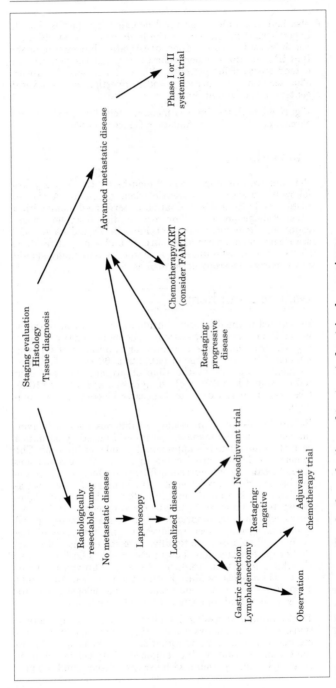

Fig. 8-5. M. D. Anderson outline for the evaluation and treatment of gastric adenocarcinoma.

vent bleeding or perforation in patients receiving radiotherapy or chemotherapy. Moreover, more accurate staging is obtained at surgery. An attempt should always be made to resect the entire lymphoma while leaving uninvolved stomach intact. Several studies have shown adjuvant radiotherapy to be of no benefit.

Many patients with GI lymphoma receive chemotherapy in addition to resection. In fact, cure rates of 70% have been seen in patients with stage IE and IIE gastric lymphoma treated by chemotherapy alone. In contrast, other studies have found no survival benefit with adjuvant chemotherapy. Still other authors believe that patients will benefit from a combination of radiotherapy and chemotherapy without any need for surgery. On the other hand, Talamonti, et al., reported a 5-year survival rate of 82% with surgery alone for stage I and II patients, whereas radiotherapy only produced a 50% 5-year survival rate in similar patients.

At M. D. Anderson, patients with gastric lymphoma are initially treated with a chemotherapeutic regimen based on doxorubicin and cyclophosphamide (Cytoxan). A complete response has been documented in greater than 90% of patients treated by this aggressive protocol. Radiotherapy and surgery are reserved for those patients who do not achieve a complete response to chemotherapy or for patients with recurrent disease.

Selected References

Abe M, Takahashi M. Intraoperative radiotherapy: The Japanese experience. *Int J Radiat Oncol Biol Phys* 7:863, 1981.

Adams YG, Efron G. Trends and controversies in the management of carcinoma of the stomach. *Surg Gynecol Obstet* 169:371, 1989.

Ajani JA, Ota DM, Jessup M, et al. Resectable gastric carcinoma. *Cancer* 68:1501, 1991.

Alexander HR, Grem JL, Pass HI, et al. Neoadjuvant chemotherapy for locally advanced gastric adenocarcinoma. *Oncology* 7:37, 1993.

Behrns KE, Dalton RR, van Heerden JA, et al. Extended lymph node dissection for gastric cancer. *Surg Clin North Am* 72:433, 1992.

Boddie AW, McBride CM, Balch CM. Gastric cancer. *Am J Surg* 157:595, 1989.

Boring CC, Squires TS, Tong T. Cancer statistics, 1993. *Cancer J Clin* 43:7, 1993.

Bozzetti F, Bonfanti G, Bufalino R, et al. Adequacy of margins of resection in gastrectomy for cancer. *Ann Surg* 196:685, 1982.

Brady MS, Rogatko A, Dent LL, et al. Effects of splenectomy on morbidity and survival following curative gastrectomy for carcinoma. *Arch Surg* 126:359, 1991.

Cady B, Rossi RL, Silverman ML, et al. Gastric adenocarcinoma. *Arch Surg* 124:303, 1989.

Cook AO, Levine BA, Sirinek KR. Evaluation of gastric adeno-carcinoma: Abdominal computed tomography does not replace celiotomy. *Arch Surg* 121:603, 1986.

Dent D, Werner I, Novis B, et al. Prospective randomized trial of combined oncologic therapy for gastric carcinoma. *Cancer* 64:385, 1979.

Estape J, Grau J, Alcobendas F, et al. Mitomycin C as an adjuvant treatment to resected gastric cancer. A 10-year follow-up. *Ann Surg* 213:219, 1991.

Frazee RC, Roberts J. Gastric lymphoma treatment. *Surg Clin North Am* 72:423, 1992.

Fujimoto S, Shrestha RD, Kokubun M, et al. Positive results of combined therapy of surgery and intraperitoneal hyperthermic perfusion for far-advanced gastric cancer. *Ann Surg* 212:592, 1990.

Gilbertson VA. Results of treatment of stomach cancer: An appraisal of efforts for more extensive surgery and a report of 1,983 cases. *Cancer* 23:1405, 1969.

Gouzi JL, Huguier M, Fagniez PL, et al. Total versus subtotal gastrectomy for adenocarcinoma of the gastric antrum. *Ann Surg* 209:162, 1989.

Gunderson LL, Sosin H. Adenocarcinoma of the stomach: Areas of failure in a re-operation series clinicopathologic correlation and implications for adjuvant therapy. *Int J Radiat Oncol Biol Phys* 8:1, 1982.

Kelson D. Adjuvant therapy of upper gastrointestinal tract cancers. *Semin Oncol* 18:543, 1991.

Kodama Y, Sugimuchi K, Soejima K, et al, Evaluation of extensive lymph node dissection for carcinoma of the stomach. *World J Surg* 5:241, 1981.

Koga S, Hamazoe R, Maeta M, et al. Prophylactic therapy for peritoneal recurrence of gastric cancer by continuous hyperthermic peritoneal perfusion with mitomycin C. *Cancer* 61:232, 1988.

Komaki S, Toyoshima S. CT's capability in advanced gastric cancer. *Gastrointest Radiol* 8:307, 1983.

Kriplani AK, Kapur BML. Laparoscopy for pre-operative staging and assessment of operability in gastric carcinoma. *Gastrointest Endosc* 37:441, 1991.

Landry J, Tepper JE, Wood WC, et al. Patterns of failure following curative resection of gastric carcinoma. *Int J Radiat Oncol Biol Phys* 19:1357, 1990.

Lawrence M, Shiu MH. Early gastric cancer. *Ann Surg* 213:327, 1991.

Lightdale CJ. Endoscopic ultrasonography in the diagnosis, staging, and follow-up of esophageal and gastric cancer. *Endoscopy* 24(Suppl 1): 297, 1992.

MacDonald JS. Gastric cancer: Chemotherapy of advanced disease. *Hematol Oncol* 10:37, 1992.

MacDonald JS, Steele G, Gunderson LL. Cancer of the Stomach. In VT DeVita, S Hellman, SA Rosenberg (eds), *Cancer: Principles and Practice of Oncologyy* (3rd ed). Philadelphia: Lippincott, 1989.

Moertel C, Childs D, O'Fallon J. Combined 5-FU and radiation therapy as a surgical adjuvant for poor prognosis gastric carcinoma. *J Clin Oncol* 2:1249, 1984.

Ota DM, Mansfield PF, Ajani JA. Operative and adjuvant treatment strategies for gastric carcinoma. *Cancer Bull* 44:286, 1992.

Shiu MH, Moore E, Sanders M, et al. Influence of the extent of resection in survival after curative treatment of gastric carcinoma: A retrospective multivariate analysis. *Arch Surg* 122:1347, 1987.

Shiu MH, Perrotti M, Brennen MF. Adenocarcinoma of the stomach: A multivariate analysis of clinical, pathologic, and treatment factors. *Hepatogastroenterology* 36:7, 1989.

Smith JW, Brennen MF. Surgical treatment of gastric cancer. *Surg Clin North Am* 72:381, 1992.

Smith JW, Shiu MH, Kelsey L, et al. Morbidity of radical lymphadenectomy in the curative resection of gastric carcinoma. *Arch Surg* 126:1469, 1991.

Stipa S, Di Giorgio AD, Ferri M. Surgical treatment of adenocarcinoma of the cardia. *Surgery* 111:386, 1992.

Talamonti MS, Dawes LG, Joehl RJ, et al. Gastrointestinal lymphoma. A case for primary surgical resection. *Arch Surg* 125:972, 1990.

Thirlby RC. Gastrointestinal lymphoma: A surgical perspective. *Oncology* 7:29, 1993.

Small-Bowel Malignancies and Carcinoid Tumors

James C. Cusack, Jr., and Douglas S. Tyler

Epidemiology

Malignancies of the small intestine are rare, with only 3,600 new cases anticipated in the United States in 1994. The small intestine represents 75% of the length and 90% of the surface area of the alimentary tract, accounting for only 1% of gastrointestinal (GI) neoplasms. The incidence of this rare malignancy is 0.7–1.6 per 100,000 population, with a slight male predominance. Mean age at presentation is 57 years. Associated conditions include familial polyposis, Gardner's syndrome, Peutz-Jeghers syndrome, and Crohn's disease. In addition, immunosuppressed patients (e.g., immunoglobulin [Ig] A deficiency) are thought to be at increased risk of developing small-bowel malignancies. As many as 25% of affected patients have synchronous malignancies, including neoplasms of the colon, endometrium, breast, and prostate.

The peak incidence of carcinoid tumors is in the sixth and seventh decades of life, although these tumors have been reported in patients as young as 10 years. The sites of origin of carcinoid tumors are shown in Table 9-1. Approximately 85% of carcinoid tumors are found in the GI tract, with the appendix being the most common site. Nonintestinal sites include the lungs, pancreas, biliary tract, thymus, and ovary. Ileal carcinoids are the most likely to metastasize, even when small, in contrast to appendiceal carcinoids, which rarely metastasize.

Risk Factors

Several distinctive characteristics of the small intestine may explain its relative sparing from malignancy. Benzopyrene hydroxylase, an enzyme that converts benzopyrene to a less carcinogenic compound, is found in large amounts in the mucosa of the small intestine. In contrast, anaerobic bacteria, which convert bile salts into potential carcinogens, are generally lacking in the small intestine. Unlike the stomach or colon, the small intestine is protected from the tumorigenic effects of an acidic environment and from the irritating effects of solid GI contents. In addition, the rapid transit of liquid succus entericus through the small bowel is thought to reduce its tumorigenicity by minimizing the contact time between potential enteric carcinogens and the mucosa. Secretory IgA, also found in large quantities in the small intestine, safeguards against oncogenic viruses.

GI dysfunction may predispose the small intestine mucosa to tumorigenesis. Stasis secondary to partial obstruction or

Table 9-1. Site of origin of carcinoid tumors

Tumor site	Percentage of cases
Stomach	2.8
Duodenum	2.9
Jejunoileum	25.5
Appendix	36.2
Colon	6.0
Rectum	16.4
Bronchus	9.9
Ovary	0.5
Miscellaneous	0.2
Unknown primary	3.3

blind loop syndrome leads to bacterial overgrowth and has been implicated in the development of small-intestine malignancies.

Clinical Presentation

SMALL-BOWEL MALIGNANCY

Seventy-five percent of patients with malignant lesions of the small bowel will develop GI symptoms compared with only 50% of patients with benign tumors. Sixty-five percent will present with intermittent abdominal pain that is dull and crampy and radiates to the back, 50% with anorexia and weight loss, and 25% with signs and symptoms of bowel obstruction. Only 10% of patients with small-bowel malignancies will develop bowel perforation. A palpable abdominal mass is present in 25% of patients.

The nonspecificity of symptoms, when present, frequently results in a 6- to 8-month delay in diagnosis. The correct diagnosis is established preoperatively in only 50% of cases. Late detection and inaccurate diagnosis contribute not only to the advanced stage of disease at the time of surgery but also to a 50% rate of metastasis at presentation and thus to the overall poor prognosis for patients with malignant tumors of the small intestine.

CARCINOID TUMORS

The presentation of carcinoids varies depending not only on their physical characteristics and site of origin but also on whether they are producing substances that are hormonally active. In general, most carcinoids are small, indolent tumors that remain asymptomatic and undetected while the patient is alive. Carcinoid tumors are categorized either pathologically by microscopic features or according to their embryologic site of origin. The embryologic classification of carcinoids is more commonly used and is outlined in Table 9-2.

Table 9-2. Characteristics of carcinoid tumors based on their embryologic site of origin

Characteristics	Foregut	Midgut	Hindgut
Location	Bronchus Stomach Pancreas	Jejunum Ileum Appendix	Colon Rectum
Histology	Trabecular	Nodular, solid Nests of cells	Trabecular
Secretion:			
Tumor 5-HT	Low	High	None
Urinary 5-HIAA	High	High	Normal
Carcinoid syndrome	Yes	Yes	No
Other endocrine secretions	Frequent	Frequent	No

5-HT = 5-hydroxytryptamine; 5-HIAA = 5-hydroxyindoleacetic acid.

This classification system subdivides carcinoids into those of the foregut (stomach, pancreas, and lungs), midgut (small bowel and appendix), or hindgut (colon and rectum). Foregut carcinoids are more commonly associated with an atypical presentation due to secretion of peptide hormone products other than serotonin, such as gastrin, adrenocorticotropic hormone, or growth hormone. Gastric carcinoids, when symptomatic, cause abdominal pain or bleeding. Patients with bronchial carcinoids may present with hemoptysis, wheezing, or postobstructive pneumonitis. Midgut carcinoids produce symptoms of hormone excess only when bulky or metastatic. The vast majority of appendiceal carcinoids are found incidentally, but carcinoids rarely may be the cause of appendicitis. Patients with small-bowel carcinoids usually present with symptoms similar to those described for other small-bowel tumors. Not uncommonly, as a small-bowel carcinoid progresses, it induces fibrosis of the mesentery, which may by itself cause intestinal obstruction as well as lead to varying degrees of mesenteric ischemia. Hindgut carcinoids tend to be clinically silent tumors that rarely produce serotonin even in the presence of metastatic disease. Patients with hindgut tumors most commonly present with bleeding but on occasion also have abdominal pain.

The hormonal manifestations of carcinoid tumors —"carcinoid syndrome"— are seen in only 10% of patients and occur when the secretory products of these tumors gain direct access to the systemic circulation and avoid metabolism in the liver. This situation occurs in the following situations: (1) when hepatic metastases are present; (2) when there is extensive retroperitoneal disease with venous drainage directly into the paravertebral veins; and (3) when the primary carcinoid tumor is outside the GI tract, such as with bronchial, ovarian, or testicular tumors. Ninety percent of the cases of carcinoid syndrome are seen in patients with midgut tumors.

Table 9-3. Clinical symptoms of carcinoid syndrome and tumor products suspected of causing them

Symptom	Tumor product
Flushing	Bradykinin
	Hydroxytryptophan
	Prostaglandins
Telangiectasia	VIP
	Serotonin
	Prostaglandins
	Bradykinin
Bronchospasm	Bradykinin
	Histamine
	Prostaglandins
Endocardial fibrosis	Serotonin
Glucose intolerance	Serotonin
Arthropathy	Serotonin
Hypotension	Serotonin

VIP = vasoactive intestinal polypeptide.

The main symptoms of carcinoid syndrome are watery diarrhea, flushing, sweating, wheezing, dyspnea, abdominal pain, hypotension, and/or right heart failure due to tricuspid regurgitation or pulmonic stenosis caused by endocardial fibrosis. The flush is often dramatic and is an intense purplish color on the upper body and arms. Facial edema is often present. Repeated attacks can lead to the development of telangiectasias and permanent skin discoloration. The flush can be precipitated by consuming alcohol, blue cheese, chocolate, red wine, and exercise. The mediators of these symptoms are shown in Table 9-3.

A life-threatening form of carcinoid syndrome, called *carcinoid crisis*, is usually precipitated by a specific event such as anesthesia, surgery, or chemotherapy. The manifestations include an intense flush, diarrhea, tachycardia, hypertension or hypotension, bronchospasm, and alteration of mental status. The symptoms have a tendancy to be refractory to fluid resuscitation and administration of vasopressors.

Diagnostic Work-Up

SMALL-BOWEL MALIGNANCIES

A high index of suspicion is essential to the early diagnosis and treatment of small-intestine malignancies. The patient presenting with nonspecific abdominal symptoms should undergo a complete history, physical examination, and screening for occult fecal blood. Laboratory work-up should include a complete blood count, measurement of serum electrolytes, and liver function tests. Further laboratory testing, including measurement of urinary 5-hydroxyindoleacetic acid (5-HIAA), should be directed by clinical suspicion.

Retrospective reviews report that 50–60% of small-intestine neoplasms are detected using conventional radiographic techniques, including upper GI series with small-bowel follow-through (UGI/SBFT) and enteroclysis. Hypotonic duodenography, using anticholinergic agents or glucagon to reduce duodenal peristalsis, may enhance diagnostic yield to as high as 86% for more proximally located duodenal malignancies. Upper GI endoscopy, when performed to the ligament of Treitz, was diagnostic in eight of nine patients with duodenal malignancies reviewed by Ouriel and Adams. Because it images only 50% of small-bowel neoplasms, computed tomography (CT) rarely aids in diagnosis, but it may provide important staging information. Angiography demonstrates a tumor blush in specific subtypes of small-bowel malignancies, most notably carcinoid and leiomyosarcoma, but is rarely indicated in the initial diagnostic work-up.

Enteroscopy should be considered when all previous diagnostic studies are negative. Lewis et al. reviewed the experience at Mt. Sinai Medical Center with two endoscopic techniques—push enteroscopy and small-bowel enteroscopy—in 258 patients with obscure GI bleeding. Push enteroscopy uses a pediatric colonoscope that is passed orally and then pushed distally through the small intestine, facilitating intubation of the jejunum 60 cm distal to the ligament of Treitz. This technique established a diagnosis in 50% of patients examined. Small-bowel enteroscopy using a 120-degree, forward-viewing, 2,560-mm, balloon-tipped endoscope that is carried distally by peristalsis permitted intubation of the terminal ileum in 77% of cases within 8 hours.

Most retrospective studies report only moderate success in diagnosing small-bowel neoplasms preoperatively, with large series reporting a correct preoperative diagnosis in only 50% of cases, with the remainder diagnosed at laparotomy. Exploratory laparotomy remains the most sensitive diagnostic modality in evaluating a patient suspected of having a small-bowel neoplasm and should be considered in the diagnostic evaluation of a patient with occult GI bleeding, unexplained weight loss, or vague abdominal pain. Because most tumors will present as large, bulky lesions with lymph node metastasis, laparoscopy is potentially useful for establishing the diagnosis of malignancy when the work-up is otherwise negative and for obtaining adequate tissue samples if a diagnosis of lymphoma is suspected. Early detection and treatment remain the most significant variables in improving outcome from small-bowel malignancy, necessitating the thoughtful and expedient diagnostic work-up of patients presenting with vague abdominal symptoms.

CARCINOIDS

The diagnosis of carcinoid tumor is made using a combination of biochemical tests and imaging studies. Overall, about 50% of patients with carcinoids will have elevated urinary

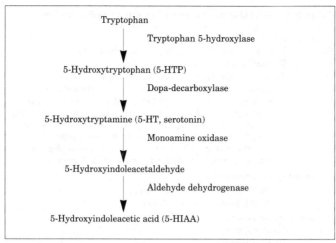

Tryptophan

Tryptophan 5-hydroxylase

5-Hydroxytryptophan (5-HTP)

Dopa-decarboxylase

5-Hydroxytryptamine (5-HT, serotonin)

Monoamine oxidase

5-Hydroxindoleacetaldehyde

Aldehyde dehydrogenase

5-Hydroxindoleacetic acid (5-HIAA)

Fig. 9-1. Biochemical steps in the production of 5-hydroxytryptamine (5-HT, serotonin) and 5-hydroxyindoleacetic acid (5-HIAA).

levels of 5-HIAA, irrespective of whether they have symptoms of carcinoid syndrome. When urinary 5-HIAA levels are nondiagnostic, then a more extensive work-up should be undertaken, consisting of measurement of urinary 5-hydroxytryptamine (5-HT, serotonin) and 5-hydroxytryptophan (5-HPT), plasma 5-HPT, platelet 5-HT, and serum levels of other secretory products such as chromogranin A, neuronspecific enolase, substance P, and neuropeptide K. An overview of serotonin metabolism is shown in Fig. 9-1.

Localization of the tumor also may help confirm the diagnosis. Bronchial carcinoids are best visualized with a chest radiograph or CT scan. Gastric, duodenal, colonic, and rectal carcinoids are usually seen on endoscopy and barium studies. Small-intestine carcinoids are initially evaluated as described for other small-bowel malignancies. Abdominal CT scan is most useful for assessing mesenteric fibrosis, involvement of the retroperitoneum, and the presence of liver metastasis.

Nuclear medicine scans have also been used in localization. Scans using metaiodobenzylguanidine (MIBG) radiolabeled with ^{131}I or [121]I can identify primary or metastatic carcinoid tumors approximately 50% of the time, when MIBG is taken up by the tumor and stored in its neurosecretory granules. Tyr-3-octreotide, a somatostatin analogue, radiolabeled with ^{123}I, has also been used in an attempt to take advantage of the finding that most carcinoids display receptors for somatostatin. Scans with this analogue appear useful in localizing 70–80% of carcinoids but are not widely available.

On occasion, a patient may benefit from angiography or selective venous sampling if other diagnostic maneuvers prove unsuccessful.

Table 9-4. AJCC staging of small-intestine malignancies

Primary tumor (T)

T1	Tumor invades lamina propria or submucosa
T2	Tumor invades muscularis propria
T3	Tumor invades through the muscularis propria into the subserosa or into the nonperitonealized perimuscular tissue (mesentery or retroperitoneum) with extension ≤2 cm
T4	Tumor perforates the visceral peritoneum or directly invades other organs or structures (includes other loops of the small intestine, mesentery, or retroperitoneum >2 cm, and the abdominal wall by way of the serosa; for the duodenum only, includes invasion of the pancreas)

Regional lymph nodes (N)

N0	No regional lymph node metastasis
N1	Regional lymph node metastasis

Distant metastasis (M)

M0	No distant
M1	Distant metastasis

Staging

Stage I	T1-2	N0	M0
Stage II	T3-4	N0	M0
Stage III	Any T	N1	M0
Stage IV	Any T	Any N	M1

Source: Adapted from OH Beahrs, DE Henson, RVP Hutter, et al (eds). *AJCC Manual for Staging of Cancer* (4th ed). Philadelphia: Lippincott, 1992.

Table 9-5. Distribution of primary malignant neoplasms in the small intestine by subsite of cancer and histologic type as a percentage of total (N = 1,413)

Subsite specified	Adenocarcinoma	Carcinoid	Lymphoma	Sarcoma
Duodenum	21.9	1.3	0.8	1.8
Jejunum	14.7	2.5	5.1	5.0
Ileum	8.7	25.5	8.9	3.6
Total	45.3	29.3	14.8	10.4

Source: Adapted from NCI SEER Registries 1973–82. In NS Weiss, C Yang. Incidence of histologic types of cancer of the small intestine. *J Natl Cancer Inst* 78:653, 1987.

Staging

Only recently has the American Joint Committee on Cancer (AJCC) published a staging system for small-bowel malignancies (Table 9-4).

Malignant Neoplasms

The distribution of small-bowel malignancies, reported by Weiss and Yang in a review of nine population-based cancer registries participating in the National Cancer Institute's

Surveillance, Epidemiology, and End Results (SEER) Program, is shown in Table 9-5. Information on tumor biology, modes of lymphatic spread, and patterns of recurrence for small-bowel malignancies is limited.

The most common histologic types of malignant tumors of the small intestine are adenocarcinoma (45.3%), carcinoid (29.3%), lymphoma (14.8%), and sarcoma (10.4%). Adenocarcinoma is the most common malignancy in the proximal small intestine, whereas carcinoid is the most common malignancy in the ileum. Sarcoma and lymphoma may develop throughout the small intestine but are more prevalent in the distal small bowel.

ADENOCARCINOMA

Pathology

Adenocarcinoma of the small intestine occurs most commonly in the duodenum, with 65% of these neoplasms clustered in the periampullary region. These tumors infiltrate into the muscularis propria and may extend through the serosa and into adjacent tissues. Ulceration is common, causing occult GI bleeding and chronic anemia. Obstruction may develop from progressive growth of apple core lesions or large intraluminal polypoid masses and manifests itself as gastric outlet obstruction in cases of duodenal lesions or severe cramping pain in cases of more distally located lesions. Adenocarcinoma of the small bowel follows a pattern of tumor progression similar to that of colon cancer, with similar survival rates when compared stage for stage. Seventy to eighty percent of small-bowel lesions are resectable at the time of diagnosis, with a 5-year survival rate of 20–30% reported for patients undergoing resection. Approximately 35% of patients will have metastasis to regional lymph nodes at the time of diagnosis, with an additional 20% having distant metastasis. Mural penetration, nodal involvement, distant metastasis, and perineural invasion correlate with a poor prognosis.

Treatment

Wide excision of the malignancy and surrounding zones of contiguous spread is performed to provide complete tumor clearance for lesions located in the jejunum and ileum. Treatment strategies ranging from pancreaticoduodenectomy to local excision have been proposed for the management of duodenal adenocarcinoma. Pancreaticoduodenectomy has been touted as a superior operation for duodenal adenocarcinoma because of its more radical clearance of the tumor bed and regional lymph nodes. In fact, some authors, including Lai et al. continue to recommend pancreaticoduodenectomy for all primary duodenal adenocarcinomas. However, segmental resection for adenocarcinoma of the duodenum satisfies the principles of en bloc resection, without the morbidity of a pancreaticoduodenectomy, and should be considered when technically feasible.

Unlike pancreatic cancer, which diffusely infiltrates into the surrounding soft tissues, adenocarcinoma of the duodenum extends into adjacent tissues as a more localized process. Therefore, tumor-free resection margins, critical to a curative extirpation, may be accomplished without necessarily resecting a generous portion of the surrounding soft tissues and adjacent organs; however, the tumor-free status of resection margins must be confirmed on frozen-section evaluation of the resected specimen.

In a comparison of pancreaticoduodenectomy to segmental resection for management of duodenal adenocarcinoma at the University of Texas M. D. Anderson Cancer Center, Barnes et al. found no significant difference in survival rates but did find a difference in 5-year local control rates—76% versus 49% for pancreaticoduodenectomy and segmental resection, respectively. Several other reviews, including those of Lowell et al., Joestling et al., and vanOoijen and Kals-beck, which compared survival following pancreaticoduodenectomy or segmental resection for lesions in the third and fourth portion of the duodenum, have demonstrated no significant difference in 5-year survival. In these studies, a more limited resection, with less associated morbidity and mortality, provided a survival benefit equal to that of a more extensive resection.

At M. D. Anderson, a Whipple pancreaticoduodenectomy is performed for lesions involving the proximal duodenum to the right of the superior mesenteric artery (SMA). A segmental resection is performed for duodenal lesions to the left of the SMA. Local excision is considered for small lesions on the antimesenteric wall of the second portion of the duodenum.

Experimental Therapy

Electron beam intraoperative radiotherapy (EB-IORT) and external beam radiotherapy have been administered at M. D. Anderson in a limited number of cases of microscopic involvement of resection margins or unresectable disease. However, adenocarcinoma of the small intestine is generally considered to be radioresistant. Chemotherapy, based on 5-fluorouracil (5-FU) and nitrosoureas, has been recommended in both the adjuvant setting and cases of unresectable disease, yet most retrospective studies have failed to demonstrate a significant response to chemotherapy. Because most centers have only limited experience treating adenocarcinoma of the small intestine, the efficacy of chemotherapy needs further study, and patients should continue to be enrolled in prospective randomized trials.

CARCINOID

Pathology

Carcinoids are known mainly for their ability to secrete serotonin and are the most common endocrine tumors of the GI

Table 9-6. Biologically active substances that can be secreted by carcinoid tumors

Amines
5-HT
5-HIAA
5-HTP
Histamine
Dopamine

Tachykinins
Kallikrein
Substance P
Neuropeptide K

Others
Prostaglandins
Pancreatic polypeptide
Chromogranins
Neurotensin
HCGa
HCGb

5-HT = 5-hydroxytryptamine; 5-HIAA = 5-hydroxyindoleacetic acid;
5-HTP = 5-hydroxytryptophan; HCG = human chorionic gonadotropin.

system. They arise from enterochromaffin cells, which are located predominantly in the GI tract and mainstem bronchi. In addition to serotonin, these tumors can secrete a number of biologically active substances (Table 9-6), including amines, tachykinins, peptides, and prostaglandins.

Carcinoids occur most commonly in the terminal 60 cm of the ileum as tan, yellow, or gray-brown intramural or submucosal nodules. The presence of multiple synchronous nodules in 30% of patients mandates careful inspection of the entire small intestine in these patients.

Primary carcinoid tumors are indolent, slow-growing lesions that become symptomatic late in the course of the disease. Rarely ulcerative, these tumors infiltrate the muscularis propria and may extend through the serosa to involve the mesentery or retroperitoneum and to produce a characteristically intense desmoplastic reaction.

Metastatic disease, present in 90% of symptomatic patients, correlates not only with the depth of invasion but also with the size of the primary lesion. There is a 2% incidence of lymph node metastasis for lesions smaller than 1 cm in diameter, a 50% incidence for lesions 1–2 cm, and an 80% incidence for lesions larger than 2 cm. Distant sites of metastases include the liver and, to a lesser degree, the lungs and bone.

Treatment of Localized Disease

Surgical extirpation is the definitive treatment for localized primary carcinoid tumors. The extent of resection is determined by the size of the primary lesion and is based on the likelihood of mesenteric lymph node involvement. The incidence of metastasis depends on the location of the tumor, its depth of invasion, and its size.

Appendiceal carcinoids smaller than 1 cm rarely metastasize and are adequately treated by appendectomy alone unless the base of the appendix is involved, in which case a partial cecectomy may be necessary. Because the incidence of metastasis increases with size, treatment of appendiceal carcinoids between 1 and 2 cm is more controversial. In general, most authors recommend appendectomy alone for lesions smaller than 1.5 cm and right hemicolectomy for the lesions larger than 1.5 cm or for any lesion with invasion of the mesoappendix, blood vessels, or regional lymph nodes.

In contrast to appendiceal carcinoids, carcinoids of the small bowel are more likely to metastasize even when smaller than 1 cm. As a result, most surgeons recommend a wide en bloc resection that includes the adjacent mesentery and lymph nodes. Such a resection may be difficult at times if fibrosis and foreshortening of the mesentery are present. Although some surgeons advocate local excision for small midgut carcinoids, up to 70% of these tumors will metastasize to the lymph nodes. Therefore a wide resection not only may cure many of these patients but also should provide better local disease control. Because of the slow-growing nature of these tumors, wide excision is advocated even when distant metastases are present. In addition, approximately 40% of patients with midgut carcinoids have a second GI malignancy. Therefore the entire bowel and colon should be evaluated prior to any planned surgical intervention.

Treatment of Advanced Disease

The role of surgery for unresectable and metastatic disease is not clearly defined, but it appears that surgery may potentially benefit patients. When metastatic disease is present, it is necessary to establish whether the patient has symptoms of carcinoid syndrome and whether curative resection is possible. If there are no contraindications to surgery, then an attempt at complete extirpation should be made because it may lead to prolonged disease-free survival as well as provide symptomatic relief. Patients with metastatic carcinoid should all begin receiving octreotide therapy preoperatively to prevent a carcinoid crisis from occurring (see below). The duration of effective relief from these palliative procedures is generally less than 12 months, and no survival benefit has been consistently demonstrated.

Patients with mildly symptomatic carcinoid syndrome can be treated medically. Diarrhea can usually be controlled with loperamide, diphenoxylate, or the serotonin receptor antagonist cyproheptadine. Flushing can frequently be controlled with either adrenergic blocking agents such as clonidine or phenoxybenzamine, or a combination of type 1 and 2 histamine receptor antagonists. Albuterol (a beta-adrenergic blocking agent) and aminophylline are effective in relieving bronchospasm and wheezing.

For patients whose symptoms cannot be controlled with these conservative measures or who develop a carcinoid crisis, the somatostatin analogue octreotide has shown tremendous promise. A trial from the Mayo Clinic found that flushing and diarrhea could be controlled in the vast majority of patients with as little as 150 mg of octreotide administered subcutaneously three times per day. The duration of the responses was on the average over 1 year. Interestingly, a number of studies have now shown that octreotide is also able to slow tumor growth significantly in over 50% of patients and cause tumor regression for variable periods in another 10–20% of individuals.

Because such good results can be obtained with octreotide, interferon, and/or hepatic artery chemoembolization (see below), surgical debulking procedures, which used to be recommended for patients with symptomatic carcinoid syndrome and liver metastasis, are rarely required. Patients with unresectable disease, if asymptomatic, should just be monitored. Local complications related to the tumor can be addressed if and when they develop. Our current indications for surgical intervention in unresectable and widely metastatic disease include complications of bulky carcinoid tumors such as obstruction and perforation. In addition, surgical debulking is considered for severe intractable symptoms unresponsive to medical treatment, if a dominant mass or liver metastasis can be identified.

Despite the advanced stage of disease at presentation and the limited effectiveness of currently available therapies, the natural history of carcinoids affords affected patients a better prognosis compared with other malignancies of the small bowel. The 5-year survival rate for localized disease approaches 100% after complete resection. Resection of metastatic disease is associated with a 68% 5-year survival rate, while unresectable disease has a 38% 5-year survival rate.

Experimental Therapy

A number of chemotherapeutic agents have been tried in patients with carcinoid tumors. Results of chemotherapy trials with such agents as doxorubicin, dacarbazine, and streptozotocin, either alone or in combination, have been disappointing. Most chemotherapy trials show response rates of less than 30%, with the duration of these responses being only a few months. The role of chemotherapy is still investigational, but for patients with advanced disease that cannot be controlled with standard measures, monitored clinical trials should be recommended.

One biological agent, interferon, in both the alpha-2a and alpha-2b forms, has shown some promising results in diminishing urinary levels of 5-HIAA as well as symptoms of carcinoid syndrome. The majority of patients in most studies had either a partial regression or stabilization of their disease for a prolonged period. Unfortunately, objective responses with reduction of tumor size occurred in only about 15% of patients.

In some centers, hepatic artery chemoembolization has been used with some success to diminish the size of liver metastases and decrease levels of biologically active mediators of carcinoid syndrome.

While external beam radiation has not proven effective in treating carcinoid tumors, targeted radiation in the form of radioactive iodine coupled to either MIBG or octreotide are two therapeutic strategies that may hold some promise for the future.

SARCOMA

Pathology

Sarcomas of the small intestine are typically slow-growing lesions; they occur more frequently in the jejunem and ileum than in the duodenum. Sharing a similar growth pattern to other GI sarcomas, these malignancies invade locally into adjacent tissues, with metastasis occurring predominantly via the hematogenous route to the liver, lungs, and bones. The most common clinical presentations are pain (65%), abdominal mass (50%), and bleeding. More than 75% of tumors exceed 5 cm in diameter at diagnosis, with extramural extension, rather than intramural or intraluminal extension, representing the typical growth pattern. For this reason, obstruction is rarely a manifestation of this disease process.

CT of these lesions typically demonstrates a heterogeneous mass with focal areas of necrosis where the tumor has outgrown its nutrient blood supply and formed localized abscesses.

Leiomyosarcoma accounts for 75% of small-intestine sarcomas; fibrosarcoma, liposarcoma, and angiosarcoma are seen less frequently. In summary, sarcoma represents only 10% of small-bowel malignancies, yet the variety of different subtypes encompasses a broad range of biological behavior—the scope of which exceeds this review.

Treatment

Surgical resection is the primary treatment modality for sarcoma of the small bowel. Because sarcoma infrequently metastasizes to regional mesenteric lymph nodes, unlike adenocarcinoma and carcinoid, an extensive mesenteric lymphadenectomy is unnecessary and will not improve survival. En bloc resection of the lesion with tumor-free margins is recommended for a potentially curative resection; however, at the time of diagnosis, 50% of lesions are unresectable and most exceed 5 cm in diameter. Local resection should be considered in the presence of widely metastatic disease for control of bleeding and relief of obstruction.

Experimental Therapy

While there is no clearly defined benefit from chemotherapy or radiotherapy used in the adjuvant setting, combined chemotherapy and radiotherapy may be considered for unresectable sarcomas in an attempt to downstage the disease and possibly make an unresectable lesion resectable. Chemotherapy is used in the treatment of recurrent or metastatic disease. Currently at M. D. Anderson, we use the adriamycin-based multiagent regimen of mesna, doxorubicin, ifosfamide, and dacarbazine (MAID) with PIXY321 (Immunex, Seattle, WA), a granulocyte macrophage–colony-stimulating factor/interleukin-3 fusion protein. Response rates to various chemotherapy regimens range from 10 to 40%, yet improvement in survival has been minimal.

Sarcoma of the small bowel is typically radioresistant; however, EB-IORT has been used for palliation with some success. External beam irradiation has also demonstrated moderate effectiveness in the palliation of pain related to unresectable disease.

LYMPHOMA

Pathology

The distribution of lymphoma in the small intestine parallels the distribution of lymphoid follicles in the small intestine, with the lymphoid-rich ileum representing the most common location of small-bowel lymphoma. Lymphoma arises from the lymphoid aggregates in the submucosa; infiltration of the mucosa can result in ulceration and bleeding. The tumor may also extend to the serosa and adjacent tissues, producing a large obstructing mass associated with cramping abdominal pain. Perforation occurs in as many as 25% of patients. Lymphoma may arise as a primary neoplasm or as a component of systemic disease with GI involvement. As with sarcoma, bulky disease is a characteristic of lymphoma, with approximately 70% of tumors larger than 5 cm in diameter.

Primary tumors are staged according to the Kiel classification (see Chapter 16) as low-, intermediate-, or high-grade, with high-grade lesions being diagnosed most frequently. Prognostic factors include tumor grade, extent of tumor penetration, nodal involvement, peritoneal disease, and distant metastasis. The 5-year survival rate ranges from 20 to 33%.

Treatment

Extended surgical resection of the primary lesion and accompanying regional mesenteric lymph nodes is the mainstay of treatment for lymphoma of the small bowel. Because of the extensive submucosal infiltration of lymphoma, frozen section should be performed to microscopically confirm tumor-free margins. Lymph node metastases are frequent, necessitating an en bloc resection of the adjoining mesentery. Resection alone provides adequate therapy for low-grade lymphomas, while resection combined with adjuvant chemotherapy is indicated for intermediate- and high-grade lymphomas. The first-line chemotherapy regimen currently used at M. D. Anderson is cyclophosphamide, doxorubicin, vincristine, and prednisone (CHOP).

Experimental Therapy

Chemoradiation has been used at some institutions for nodal metastasis, positive resection margins, and the presence of unresectable disease. However, a survival benefit from such treatment regimens has not been demonstrated. The use of radiotherapy alone has been associated with significant tumor necrosis, bleeding, and bowel perforation but may be considered in elderly patients unable to tolerate the toxicity of chemotherapy.

METASTATIC MALIGNANCIES

Pathology

Metastases are the most common form of malignancy in the small intestine and develop as a result of hematogenous or lymphatic spread from a primary tumor to the mucosa or submucosal lymphatics of the small intestine. The primary tumors that most commonly metastasize to the small bowel include ovarian, colon, lung, and melanoma. Metastatic melanoma is unique in that once localized in the small bowel, the metastatic focus may further disseminate to involve the small-bowel mesentery and draining lymph nodes. In general, however, small-bowel metastases remain localized to the bowel wall, and they may produce small-bowel obstruction or perforation.

Although the typical presentation of metastatic lesions is obstruction or perforation, the more common cause of obstruction and perforation in patients who have previously undergone resection of a GI primary tumor is related to the initial procedure—that is, either recurrence of the primary tumor or adhesions resulting from the initial exploration.

Segmental bowel resection is the primary treatment for small-bowel metastases. Except for melanoma metastases, which may function as a source of further lymphatic dissemination, a regional lymphadenectomy is not performed for metastatic tumors of the small intestine.

PALLIATION

At the time of diagnosis, most small-bowel malignancies are locally advanced, with significant bulky disease and/or metastases. When the advanced stage of disease precludes surgical resection, enteric bypass should be performed to prevent obstruction. In the event of bleeding from an unresectable small-bowel malignancy, intra-arterial embolization of nutrient arteries may be considered, but the benefits must be weighed against the significant risks of this procedure. Our experience with this technique at M. D. Anderson Cancer Center has been discouraging because of the significant rate of bowel ischemia and perforation associated with embolization of the small-bowel mesentery.

Chemotherapy or combined chemoradiation may offer effective control of locally advanced unresectable disease, particularly in the case of lymphoma, and should be considered among palliative treatment options.

Surveillance

Routine follow-up for patients should include a complete history and physical examination, complete blood count, serum electrolyte determination, and liver function tests performed at regular intervals. A chest radiograph should be obtained every 6 months for the first 3 years after resection, followed by subsequent yearly exams. Assessment of locoregional recurrence in patients who have undergone a right hemicolectomy for ileal malignancy or segmental resection for duodenal malignancy should include endoscopy at 6-month intervals. Assessment for recurrence at other sites may include CT, UGI/SBFT, angiography, or enteroscopy and must be directed by clinical suspicion based on patient history and physical and laboratory findings.

Selected References

Ajani JA, Carrasco H, Samaan NA, et al. Therapeutic options in patients with advanced islet cell and carcinoid tumors. *Reg Cancer Treat* 3:235, 1990.

Ashley SW, Wells SA. Tumors of the small intestine. *Semin Oncol* 15:116, 1988.

Barnes G, Romero L, Hess KR, et al. Primary adenocarcinoma of the duodenum: Management and survival in 67 patients. *Ann Surg Oncol* 1:73, 1994.

Bomanji J, Mather S, Moyes J, et al. A scintigraphic comparison of iodine-123 metaiodobenzylguanidine and iodine-labeled somatostatin analog (tyr-3-octreotide) in metastatic carcinoid tumors. *J Nucl Med* 33:1121, 1992.

Carrasco CH, Charnsangavej C, Ajani J, et al. The carcinoid syndrome palliation by hepatic artery embolization. *AJR Am J Roentgenol* 147:149, 1986.

Cattell RB, Braasch JW. A technique for the exposure of the third and fourth portions of the duodenum. *Surg Gynecol Obstet* 11:379, 1960.

Crist DW, Sitzman JV, Cameron JL. Improved hospital morbidity, mortality, and survival after the Whipple procedure. *Ann Surg* 206:358, 1987.

Cubilla AL, Fortner J, Fitzgerald PJ. Lymph node involvement in carcinoma of the head of the pancreas area. *Cancer* 41:880, 1978.

Farouk M, Niotis M, Branum GD, et al. Indications for and the techniques of local resection of tumors of the papilla of Vater. *Arch Surg* 126:650, 1991.

Godwin JD II. Carcinoid tumors: An analysis of 2837 cases. *Cancer* 36:560, 1975.

Hanson MW, Feldman JE, Blinder RA, et al. Carcinoid tumors: Iodine-131 MIBG scintigraphy. *Radiology* 172:699, 1989.

Joestling DR, Beart RW, vanHeerden JA, et al. Improving survival in adenocarcinoma of the duodenum. *Am J Surg* 141:228, 1981.

Johnson AM, Harman PK, Hanks JB. Primary small bowel malignancies. *Am Surg* 51:31, 1985.

Kvols LK, Moertel CG, O'Connell MJ, et al. Treatment of the malignant carcinoid syndrome: Evaluation of a long acting somatostatin analogue. *N Engl J Med* 315:663, 1986.

Lamberts SW, Bakker WH, Reubi JC, et al. Somatostatin-receptor imaging in the localization of endocrine tumors. *N Engl J Med* 323:1246, 1990.

Lai EC, Doty JE, Irving C, et al. Primary adenocarcinoma of the duodenum : Analysis of survival. *World J Surg* 12:695, 1988.

Lewis BS, Kornbluth A, Waye JD. Small bowel tumors: Yield of enteroscopy. *Gut* 32:763, 1991.

Lowell JA, Rossi RL, Munson L, et al. Primary adenocarcinoma of third and fourth portions of duodenum. *Arch Surg* 127:557, 1992.

Maglinte DT, O'Connor K, Bessette J, et al. The role of the physician in the late diagnosis of primary malignant tumors of the small intestine. *J Gastroenterol* 86:304, 1991.

Martin RG. Malignant tumors of the small intestine. *Surg Clin North Am* 66:779, 1986.

Moertel CG, Weiland LH, Nagorney DM, et al. Carcinoid tumor of the appendix: Treatment and prognosis. *N Engl J Med* 317:1699, 1987.

Motojima K, Tsukasa T, Kanematsu T, et al. Distinguishing pancreatic cancer from other periampullary carcinomas by analysis of mutations in the Kirsten-ras oncogene. *Ann Surg* 214:657, 1991.

Oberg K, Eriksson B. The role of interferons in the management of carcinoid tumors. *Br J Haematol* 79:74, 1991.

O'Rourke MG, Lancashire RP, Vattoune JR. Lymphoma of the small intestine. *Aust NZ J Surg* 56:351, 1986.

Ouriel K, Adams JT. Adenocarcinoma of the small intestine. *Am J Surg* 147:66, 1984.

Strodel WE, Talpos G, Eckhauser F, et al. Surgical therapy for small-bowel carcinoid tumors. *Arch Surg* 118:391, 1983.

Thompson GB, van Heerden JA, Martin JK Jr, et al. Carcinoid tumors of the gastrointestinal tract: Presentation, management, and prognosis. *Surgery* 98:1054, 1985.

vanOoijen B, Kalsbeck HL. Carcinoma of the duodenum. *Surg Gynecol Obstet* 166:343, 1988.

Vinik AI, Thompson N, Eckhauser F, et al. Clinical features of carcinoid syndrome and the use of somatostatin analogue in its management. *Acta Oncol* 28:389, 1989.

Weiss NS, Yang C. Incidence of histologic types of cancer of the small intestine. *J Natl Can Inst* 78:653, 1987.

Welch JP, Malt RA. Management of carcinoid tumors of the gastrointestinal tract. *Surg Gynecol Obstet* 145:223, 1977.

Willett CG, Warshaw AL, Connery K, et al. Patterns of failure after pancreaticoduodenectomy for ampullary carcinoma. *Surg Gynecol Obstet* 176:33, 1993.

Wilson H, Cheek RC, Sherman RT, Storer EH. Carcinoid tumors. *Curr Probl Surg* Nov 1, 1970.

Cancer of the Colon, Rectum, and Anus

Thelma Hurd and Haim Gutman

Colorectal Cancer

EPIDEMIOLOGY

Colorectal cancer comprises 13% of all cancers and is responsible for 10% of all deaths from cancer. In 1994, 149,000 cases will be diagnosed and 56,000 Americans will die of this disease.

The age-specific incidence of colorectal cancer increases steadily from the second through the eighth decades of life, with a male predominance. At diagnosis, 10% of patients will have in situ disease, one-third will have local disease, and one-third regional disease; 20% of patients will have distant disease.

The overall 5-year survival rate for colorectal cancer is 50%. However, when stratified by local, regional, and distant disease, the survival rates are 90%, 58%, and 5%, respectively. The age-adjusted death rate increased steadily for males and females from 1930 to 1950. Since 1950, the death rate in females has declined slightly, while that of males has remained constant.

RISK FACTORS

Diet

Dietary factors may promote or inhibit carcinogenesis. Consumption of red meat and animal fat, as well as the presence of high fecal levels of cholesterol, correlate with and may be causally related to an increased risk of colorectal carcinoma.

One mechanism of carcinogenesis involves alterations in bile acid metabolism. Fat and high fecal cholesterol levels both increase bile acid production and favor anaerobic bacterial proliferation. As a result, bacterial production of fecapentaenes and 3-ketosteroids increases, which promotes carcinogenesis.

Increased intake of fiber, calcium, and selenium decreases the incidence of colorectal carcinoma. Fiber acts by lowering intraluminal pH and NH_3, inhibiting bile acid dehydroxylation, and enhancing production of butyrate, a differentiating agent that prolongs tumor doubling time and growth rate. Intestinal transit time is also significantly reduced by a diet rich in fiber. This constellation of effects results in a favorable change in the bacterial population of the bowel. Calcium acts to decrease bile acid concentration by forming insoluble salt complexes. Selenium, an important trace element, protects cells from oxidative damage through the action of glutathione peroxidase.

Polyps

Intestinal polyps are found in 6% of the general population. The majority of colon carcinomas arise from polyps—thus the importance of these lesions. Carcinoma develops through a complex series of genetic alterations. Mutations or deletions of chromosomes 5, 12 (*ras*), 18q (*DCC* gene, deleted in colon carcinoma gene), and 17 (*P53*) can be found in normal colonic epithelium, early adenoma, late adenoma, and frank carcinoma. Whether these changes occur simultaneously or sequentially is unknown.

Polyps coexist with colorectal cancer in 60% of patients and are associated with an increased incidence of synchronous and metachronous colonic neoplasms. Patients with a primary cancer and a solitary associated polyp have a lower incidence of synchronous and metachronous lesions when compared to patients with multiple polyps (7.3% and 2.7% versus 14.6% and 12.4%, respectively). The natural history of polyps supports an aggressive approach to their treatment: 24% of patients with polyps left untreated will develop invasive cancer at the site of the polyp within 20 years.

There are three histologic variants of adenomatous polyps. *Tubular adenomas* represent 75% of polyps and are found with equal frequency throughout all segments of the bowel. Less than 5% of tubular adenomas are malignant. *Tubulovillous adenomas* constitute 15% of polyps. They are also equally distributed throughout the bowel, with 20% being malignant. The remaining 10% of polyps are *villous adenomas*, which are usually localized to the rectum; 35–40% of these polyps are malignant. The size of a polyp is correlated with the histology of the lesion and thus the biologic behavior. Larger polyps have a greater degree of villous components, dysplasia, and malignant involvement.

Since only 5% of all polyps harbor invasive carcinoma at the time of presentation, endoscopy has assumed a major role in the diagnosis and treatment of polyps. Endoscopic polypectomy is less invasive than surgery and can provide equivalent control of malignant disease in carefully selected patients without the risk of major surgery and general anesthesia. However, as previously mentioned, a clear understanding of the adenoma to carcinoma sequence is necessary to properly manage colorectal polyps.

Carcinoma in situ (CIS) is localized to the colonic epithelium and does not invade the muscularis mucosa. The lymphatics of the colon are limited to the submucosal layer; therefore CIS can not metastasize to regional lymph nodes. It is unlikely that the natural history of CIS in a sessile polyp is any different than in a pedunculated polyp. Although there are studies that show a higher incidence of recurrent disease and regional lymph node metastases for sessile polyps, this finding is most likely due to the technical difficulty of removing sessile polyps endoscopically with margins free of tumor.

Overall, 9% of polyps harboring invasive carcinoma will metastasize to regional lymph nodes. Four unfavorable pathologic features of malignant colorectal polyps are known to increase the probability that regional lymph nodes will be involved with tumor: (1) poor differentiation, (2) vascular and/or lymphatic invasion, (3) invasion below the submucosa, and (4) positive resection margin. Poorly differentiated lesions (grade 3) are associated with a higher incidence of lymphovascular involvement and recurrent disease when compared with well and moderately differentiated lesions (grades 1 and 2). Vascular invasion is uncommon; when it occurs, it is associated with recurrent disease or lymphatic invasion in about 40% of patients.

Depth of invasion is the single most important prognostic factor for mesenteric lymph node involvement with cancer. Haggitt et al. stratified pedunculated polyps based on the depth of invasion as follows: level 0, above the muscularis mucosa; level 1, invades the muscularis but limited to the head; level 2, neck invasion; level 3, stalk invasion; and level 4, submucosa and muscularis propria involvement. Sessile polyps with evidence of invasive carcinoma are classified as level 4. Level 1 and 2 lesions have a good prognosis in the absence of other unfavorable histologic features. Conversely, 13% and 15% of patients with level 3 and 4 lesions, respectively, will have residual disease or lymphatic involvement or will develop recurrence if only endoscopic polypectomy is performed.

Forty-two percent of patients with close or positive margins will develop recurrent disease or have lymphatic involvement. Negative margins alone do not ensure a good outcome: 74% of patients with negative margins and poor histologic features (vascular invasion, level 4 or grade 3 lesions) had a poor clinical outcome compared with 1.8% of patients who had negative margins and good histologic features.

Although clinical factors such as age, location, number of polyps, and gender are collectively known to be prognostic factors, only age greater than 60 years has been identified as an independent risk factor.

Polypoid carcinomas arise from benign adenomas in which the entire epithelium in the head of the polyp is replaced by cancer. The biologic behavior of these lesions is governed by the depth of invasion and the presence of unfavorable histologic features as described for other colorectal polyps.

Complete endoscopic polypectomy is the treatment of choice for moderately or well-differentiated cancer in the absence of vascular or lymphatic invasion and when clear margins of resection can be obtained. Grade 3 differentiation, venous or lymphatic invasion, and positive resection margins are unfavorable features that mandate surgical resection. Pedunculated polyps or polypoid carcinomas with invasion confined to the head of the polyp, in the absence of other unfavorable features, can be treated by polypectomy alone as long as negative margins are obtained. Stalk invasion with favorable histologic features and clear margins can also be treated with polypectomy alone since less than 1.5% of patients treated in this way will have an adverse outcome. Sessile polyps with invasive carcinoma should be surgically removed since they are by definition level 4 lesions and are associated with a poor outcome in 15% of patients.

Hereditary Polyposis Syndromes

Hereditary polyposis represents a constellation of syndromes rather than a single disease entity. All are characterized by multiple intestinal polyps as well as associated extraintestinal manifestations. Familial adenomatous polyposis (FAP) is the best characterized of the syndromes; 1–2% of patients diagnosed with colon carcinoma will have FAP. The genetic alteration associated with FAP has been determined to be a point mutation in a gene located on the long arm of chromosome 5. It is inherited in an autosomal dominant pattern, with 90% penetrance. Affected individuals develop polyps throughout the gastrointestinal (GI) tract but most commonly in the colon, duodenum, small bowel, and stomach. More than 80% of affected individuals harbor carcinomas by age 40 years. Gardner's syndrome is also inherited in an autosomal dominant pattern and is thought to represent a variant of FAP. It is characterized by colonic and small-bowel adenomas, lipomas, abdominal desmoids, sebaceous cysts, osteomas, and fibromas. Oldfield's syndrome is associated with multiple sebaceous cysts, polyps, and carcinomas. Patients with Turcot syndrome experience intestinal polyposis and associated central nervous system tumors. This syndrome occurs less frequently than the others and has an autosomal recessive pattern of inheritance.

Although the hereditary syndromes are rare, the identification of a genetic alteration in patients with familial polyposis has provided a unique opportunity to investigate the molecular events involved in the pathogenesis of colon cancer.

Hereditary Nonpolyposis Syndromes

Lynch I and II syndromes are nonpolyposis autosomal dominant diseases that occur five times more frequently than familial polyposis. Isolated colonic involvement occurs in the Lynch I syndrome. Colonic, breast, pancreatic, and endometrial tumors characterize the Lynch II syndrome. Patients present with carcinoma at about age 45 years, which is approximately 10 years earlier than patients with sporadic colon tumors. In contrast to the hereditary polyposis syndromes, in hereditary nonpolyposis syndromes, tumors more frequently involve the colon proximal to the splenic flexure. Twenty percent of patients have synchronous or metachronous lesions. The incidence of metachronous lesions rises to 40% after 10 years. Lynch et al. have identified a group of patients in this cohort with an increased incidence of ovarian, renal pelvis, and uterine tumors.

Inflammatory Bowel Disease

Ulcerative colitis carries a 30-fold increased risk of colorectal carcinoma. The incidence rises steadily with increasing duration of disease. After 30 years, the risk of colorectal cancer rises to 35% in this population. Forty to fifty percent of tumors arise in the proximal colon; 10–20% of patients will have multiple synchronous lesions.

Previous Colon Carcinoma

Patients with a history of colon cancer have a threefold increased risk of developing a second primary colon carcinoma; 5–8% of these patients develop metachronous lesions.

SCREENING

Fecal occult blood testing (Hemoccult or Hemoquant) and endoscopy are the most widely used screening tools for colorectal cancer. However, few studies have been able to document a significant impact of these tests on overall survival. Several factors have contributed to this finding. Compliance rates with fecal occult blood testing are reported to vary between 40% and 68%. There is also an inherent error from random sampling of stool and improper specimen handling. The low sensitivity of occult blood screening (<30% rate of cancer detection) is another major criticism.

Although the introduction of flexible sigmoidoscopy has improved patient comfort and decreased risk compared with rigid sigmoidoscopy, the incidence of cancers proximal to the splenic flexure has increased, especially in women, which decreases the sensitivity of the test. Only 10% of tumors are palpable on digital rectal examination, and only 35% are accessible with a rigid scope.

The study of Winawer et al. from Memorial Sloan-Kettering Cancer Center showed a significant reduction in mortality (43%) in people who were screened with fecal occult blood testing and rigid sigmoidoscopy. Other prospective randomized trials have shown that tumors identified in screened populations of patients tend to be earlier stage tumors at the time of diagnosis, as compared with tumors found in control groups of unscreened patients. However, the effect on mortality remains to be analyzed in these particular studies.

Carcinoembryonic antigen (CEA) has no role in screening for primary lesions. The sensitivity ranges from 30 to 80%, depending on the stage of disease. False-positive results occur in benign disease (lung, liver, and bowel) as well as malignancies of the pancreas, breast, ovary, prostate, head and neck, bladder, and kidney. The CEA level is also elevated in smokers. Overall, 60% of tumors will be missed by CEA screening alone.

Based on this information, the National Board of Directors of the American Cancer Society at its June 1992 meeting recommended the following guidelines for screening asymptomatic patients with no family history of colorectal cancer:

1. Sigmoidoscopy, preferably flexible, every 3–5 years for men and women older than 50 years.

2. Digital rectal examination every year for men and women older than 40 years.

3. Fecal occult blood test yearly for men and women older than 50 years.

Patients with inflammatory bowel disease need to have colonoscopy every 6 months. All clinically suspicious areas should be biopsied. Random biopsies should also be performed at 10-cm intervals throughout the entire length of the colon.

Patients with familial polyposis should undergo colonoscopy every 6 months with biopsy and polypectomy as indicated by clinical findings. Sporadic polyposis can be managed with yearly colonoscopy for the first 2 years following the initial identification of polyps. If no lesions are detected on follow-up, then colonoscopy can be performed every 2 years.

PATHOLOGY

Histologically, greater than 90% of colon cancers are adenocarcinomas. On gross appearance there are four morphologic variants of adenocarcinoma. Ulcerative adenocarcinoma is the most common configuration seen and is most characteristic of tumors in the descending and sigmoid colon. Exophytic (also known as polypoid or fungating) tumors are most commonly found in the ascending colon, particularly in the cecum. These tumors tend to project into the bowel lumen, and patients will often present with a right-sided abdominal mass and anemia. Annular (scirrhous) adenocarcinoma tends to grow circumferentially into the wall of the colon resulting in the classic "apple core" lesion seen on barium enema x-ray study. Rarely, a submucosal infiltrative pattern can be seen that is similar to linitis plastica seen with gastric adenocarcinoma.

Other epithelial histologic variants of colon cancer that are occasionally seen include mucinous (colloid) carcinoma, signet-ring cell carcinoma, adenosquamous carcinoma, and undifferentiated carcinoma. Other rare tumors include carcinoids and leiomyosarcomas.

The most commonly used grading system is based on the degree of formation of glandular structures, nuclear pleomorphism, and the number of mitoses. Grade 1 tumors have the most developed glandular structures with the fewest mitoses.

Table 10-1. Modified Astler-Coller classification of the Dukes staging system for colorectal cancer

Stage	Description
A	Lesion not penetrating submucosa
B1	Lesion up to, but not through, serosa
B2	Lesion through serosa, with involvement of adjacent organs
C1	Lesion up to, but not through, serosa; regional lymph node metastasis
C2	Lesion through serosa, with involvement of adjacent organs; regional lymph node metastasis
D	Distant metastatic disease

Table 10-2. TNM staging classification of colorectal cancer

Primary tumor (T)

T1		Invades submucosa
T2		Invades muscularis propria
T3–T4		
	Serosa	
	T3	Invades into subserosa, but not through serosa
	T4	Invades through serosa into free peritoneal cavity or into contiguous organ
	Serosa	
	T3	Invades through muscularis propria
	T4	Invades contiguous organs

Regional lymph nodes (N)

N0	No lymph node metastases
N1	Lymph node metastases in 1–3 nodes
N2	Lymph node metastases in 4 or more nodes
N3	Lymph node metastases in central nodes

Distant metastases (M)

M0	No distant metastases
M1	Distant metastases present

STAGING

The Dukes and TNM staging systems for colorectal carcinoma are presented in Tables 10-1 and 10-2.

CLINICAL PRESENTATION

One-half of patients with colorectal cancer present with bleeding, abdominal pain, change in bowel habits, anorexia, or weight loss. Twenty percent of patients will have obstruction or an abdominal mass; 50% of splenic flexure and 15% of rectal lesions present with obstructions. Obstructing lesions are commonly associated with advanced disease. Two-thirds of patients will have Dukes stage B and C lesions, while one-third will have Dukes stage D lesions.

DIAGNOSIS

Colon Cancer

Clinical evaluation of carcinoma of the colon should include colonoscopy and biopsy, air contrast barium enema (BE), chest radiograph, complete blood count, CEA determination, urinalysis, and liver function tests (LFTs). BE and colonoscopy are complementary tests. The colonoscope allows evaluation of the distal 2–3 cm of the anorectal canal that is obscured by the BE catheter balloon, while the BE facilitates the visualization of the splenic and hepatic flexures, which may be obscured during colonoscopy. In addition, polypectomy or biopsy can be performed during colonoscopy. Air contrast barium enema study and flexible sigmoidoscopy can be substituted if colonoscopy is not available.

The use of abdominopelvic computed tomography (CT) in the preoperative evaluation of patients with colon cancer remains controversial. The extracolonic abdomen should be evaluated with CT in patients with large bulky lesions to detect metastatic involvement of contiguous organs, para-aortic lymph nodes, and the liver. Some authors only recommend CT scan when preoperative LFTs are abnormal. Both lactate dehydrogenase (LDH) and alkaline phosphatase (AP) levels are useful for detecting hepatic involvement. However, abnormal LFTs are present in only approximately 15% of patients with liver metastases. In contrast, the false-positive rate for LFTs is close to 40%. Therefore a significant number of unnecessary CT scans would be performed if all patients with abnormal LFTs underwent CT scan. The preoperative CEA level can also reflect disease extent and prognosis: CEA levels surpassing 20 ng/ml are associated with liver metastasis, and the tumor recurrence rate is higher when the CEA level exceeds 5 ng/ml. Some surgeons believe that preoperative evaluation of the liver is important because 15–20% of liver metastases will be nonpalpable at the time of surgery. However, 10–15% of lesions will be missed by combined preoperative and operative evaluation. Intraoperatve ultrasonography has been shown to be the most accurate method of detecting liver metastasis.

The majority of patients with colon cancer will require an operative procedure even in the presence of liver metastasis; surgery is the best method to prevent the complications of colon tumors, such as obstruction and bleeding. Therefore the only advantage of a preoperative CT is in helping to plan possible treatment options for metastatic disease to the liver. At the University of Texas M. D. Anderson Cancer Center, we do not routinely obtain preoperative CT scans in patients with colon tumors. The decision to perform a preoperative CT is individualized based on the results of physical examination, LFTs, and CEA level.

The role of routine preoperative urinary tract evaluation is controversial. Patients who are symptomatic or have large bulky lesions should have a preoperative intravenous pyelogram or CT scan to evaluate the urinary tract. Up to 40% of these patients will have urinary tract abnormalities.

Rectal Cancer

In addition to the history and physical examination, chest x-ray, complete blood count, LFTs, electrolytes and urinalysis, endorectal ultrasound (EU), proctoscopic examination, and abdominopelvic CT scan should be performed to accurately stage patients with rectal cancer.

EU is the most useful test in determining tumor (T) stage. All layers of the rectal wall can be identified with 69–93% accuracy. Superficial tumors are the most difficult to stage. Peritumoral edema can compress the bowel wall layers, making it almost impossible to distinguish tumor from edema. EU evaluation of depth of bowel wall penetration is superior to that of either CT scanning or magnetic resonance imaging (MRI), which are only 30% accurate. EU is limited by the inability to detect microscopic disease. Lymph nodes are more difficult to assess with EU than is depth of bowel wall penetration. However, accuracy can be improved through measurement of size and degree of reflection of ultrasound waves. Lymph nodes that are greater than 3 mm and hypoechoic are more likely to contain metastatic deposits. In addition, it is possible to perform fine-needle aspiration of suspicious lymph nodes under EU guidance. EU is invaluable when evaluating patients for preoperative adjuvant therapy, but it is unable to accurately assess response to preoperative adjuvant therapy due to the obliteration of tissue planes by edema and fibrosis.

Abdominopelvic CT scanning is important in assessing the presence of distant spread of disease and involvement of adjacent organs. In the management of rectal cancer it is extremely important to accurately assess the local spread of disease and the involvement of adjacent organs. While EU is superior to CT in detecting depth of penetration, CT provides a better assessment of contiguous organ involvement. MRI at this time remains inferior to CT scanning.

MANAGEMENT OF COLON CANCER

The goal of primary surgical treatment of colon carcinoma is to eradicate disease in the colon, the draining nodal basins, and contiguous organs. Careful surgical planning is essential. Patient age, the stage of disease and extent of tumor, and the presence of synchronous colonic tumors are significant factors in determining the optimal surgical approach. Overall medical condition is also important since most perioperative deaths result from cardiovascular or pulmonary complications.

Anatomy

Thorough knowledge of the arterial, venous, and lymphatic anatomy of the colon and rectum is essential to appropriate surgical management (Fig. 10-1). The ascending and proximal transverse colon are embryologically derived from the midgut and receive their arterial blood supply from the superior mesenteric artery via the ileocolic, right, and middle colic arteries. The distal transverse, descending, and sigmoid colon are hindgut derivatives whose arterial blood supply arises from the inferior mesenteric artery (IMA) through the left colic and sigmoid arteries. The rectum, also a hindgut derivative, receives its blood supply to the upper third from the IMA via the superior hemorrhoidal artery. The middle and lower thirds of the rectum are supplied by the middle and inferior hemorrhoidal arteries, which are branches of the hypogastric artery. Collateral blood supply for the colon is provided through the marginal artery of Drummond. The venous drainage of the colon and rectum parallels the arterial supply, with the majority draining directly into the portal system. This provides a direct route for metastatic spread of tumor to the liver. The only minor anatomic variation in the venous drainage compared to the arterial supply is that the inferior mesenteric vein (IMV) joins the splenic vein prior to emptying into the portal system. The rectum has dual venous drainage; the upper rectum drains into the portal system, while the distal one third of the rectum drains into the inferior vena cava via the middle and inferior hemorrhoidal veins.

The lymphatic drainage of the bowel is more complex than the vascular supply. Lymphatics begin in the bowel wall as a plexus beneath the lamina propria and drain into the submucosal and intramuscular lymphatics. The epicolic lymph nodes drain the subserosa and are located in the colon wall. This nodal group runs along the inner bowel margin between the intestinal wall and the arterial arcades. These nodes in turn drain into the paracolic nodes, which follow the routes of the marginal arteries. The epicolic and paracolic nodes represent the majority of the colonic lymph nodes and are the most likely sites of regional metastatic disease. The paracolic nodes drain into the intermediate nodes, which follow the main colic vessels. Finally, the intermediate nodes drain into the principal nodes, which begin at the origins of the superior and inferior mesenteric arteries and are contiguous with the para-aortic chain.

The route of lymphatic flow parallels the arterial and venous distribution of the colon. The right colon will drain to the superior mesenteric nodes through the intermediate nodes or to the portal system via the lymphatics of the superior mesenteric vein. The left colon's lymphatic drainage follows the marginal artery to the left colic intermediate nodes and finally to the inferior mesenteric nodes. The lymphatic drainage of the upper third of the rectum follows the IMV, while the lower two-thirds drain into the hypogastric nodes,

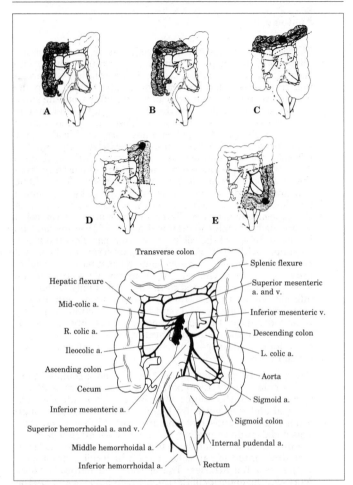

Fig. 10-1. Anatomy of colonic blood supply along with a pictorial description of the various anatomic resections used for colon carcinoma. A. Right hemicolectomy. B. Extended right hemicolectomy. C. Transverse colectomy. D. Left hemicolectomy. E. Low anterior resection. (From PH Sugarbaker, J MacDonald, L Gunderson. Colorectal Cancer. In VT DeVita, S Hellman, SA Rosenberg [eds], *Cancer: Principles and Practice of Oncology* [3rd ed]. Philadelphia: Lippincott, 1984.)

which, in turn, drain into the para-aortic nodes. The lower third of the rectum can also drain along the pudendal vessels to the inguinal nodes.

Surgical Options

At laparotomy, the primary tumor and its lymphatic, venous, and arterial supply are extirpated. Contiguously involved organs should be removed en bloc since attempts to "shave" the tumor off or divide the "adhesions" decreases survival by as much as 90%.

Exploratory laparotomy for colorectal tumors should be performed through an incision large enough to enable a complete and thorough search for metastases and assessment of the extent of the tumor. The liver should be carefully palpated and intraoperative hepatic ultrasound performed if suspicious lesions are noted and the technology is available. The ureters, duodenum, superior and inferior mesenteric vessels, and marginal artery of Drummond should be identified to avoid injury.

The various surgical options, as well as their indications and major morbidities, are briefly discussed below.

A. *Right hemicolectomy:* Removal of the distal 5–8 cm of the ileum, right colon, hepatic flexure, and transverse colon just proximal to the middle colic artery. This procedure is indicated for cecal, ascending colonic, and hepatic flexure lesions. Major morbidities include ureteral injury, duodenal injury, and bile acid deficiency (rarely seen and only with extensive resection of the terminal ileum).

B. *Right radical hemicolectomy*: Removal of the transverse colon (including resection of the middle colic artery at its origin) in addition to the structures removed in the right hemicolectomy. Indications for the procedure are hepatic flexure or transverse colon lesions. Morbidities include anastomotic dehiscence and diarrhea in addition to the complications associated with right hemicolectomy.

C. *Transverse colectomy*: Segmental resection of the transverse colon. This procedure is indicated for mid–transverse colon lesions. The major morbidity is anastomotic dehiscence. At M. D. Anderson this procedure is rarely performed due to the difficulty in achieving a tension-free anastomosis with adequate blood supply (as the marginal artery of Drummond is sacrificed). We prefer to perform an extended right radical hemicolectomy with an ileosigmoid anastomosis.

D. *Left hemicolectomy*: Removal of the transverse colon distal to the right branch of the middle colic artery and the descending colon up to but not including the rectum, plus IMA ligation and division. Indications for the procedure are left colon lesions. Morbidities include anastomotic dehiscence.

E. *Low anterior resection*: Removal of the descending colon distal to the splenic flexure, sigmoid colon, upper two-thirds of the rectum, and ligation of IMA and IMV either at the origin or just distal to the origin of the left colic artery. The procedure is indicated for sigmoid and proximal rectal lesions. Morbidities include anastomotic dehiscence and bowel ischemia (secondary to inadequate flow through the marginal artery of Drummond).

F. *Subtotal colectomy*: Removal of right, transverse, descending, and sigmoid colon with ileorectal anastomosis. This procedure is indicated for multiple synchronous colonic tumors and distal transverse colon lesions in patients with a clotted IMA. Morbidities include diarrhea, perineal excoriation, and anastomotic dehiscence.

The surgical treatment of the familial polyposis syndromes is controversial. Traditionally, total abdominal colectomy, proctectomy, and permanent ileostomy was the treatment of choice. Various surgical options have been used in attempts to preserve the rectum. Subtotal colectomy with ileorectal anastomosis has been used, with variable results. This procedure requires careful follow-up as mucosa at risk for polyp formation is left behind in the rectal stump. Total colectomy, mucosal proctectomy, and ileoanal anastomosis has also been advocated as this procedure removes all of the colon and rectal mucosa at risk for developing polyps and thus cancer. The results of this procedure have depended on the experience of the surgical team performing the operation.

Survival

Nodal involvement is the primary determinant of 5-year survival. In node-negative disease, the 5-year survival rate is 90% for patients with T1 and T2 lesions and 80% for those with T3 lesions. Regional nodal involvement decreases survival to about 30% overall; however, in patients with four or fewer positive nodes, survival is 56%.

Adjuvant Therapy

Adjuvant therapy for colon cancer is an evolving and controversial subject. 5-fluorouracil (5-FU) is the most effective single agent for colon carcinoma, with response rates of 15–30% when it is used alone as treatment for patients with advanced disease. Based on early studies that showed some anticancer activity for 5-FU, there have been numerous studies of 5-FU in combination therapies. Adjuvant trials using 5-FU and semustine (MeCCNU) (Gastrointestinal Tumor Study Group [GITSG]) or MeCCNU, vinblastine, and 5-FU (National Surgical Adjuvant Breast and Bowel Project, project C-01) have failed to demonstrate any survival benefit when compared with surgery alone. The failure of these chemotherapeutic combinations led to trials of 5-FU in combination with levamisole, an antihelminthic agent with immunostimulatory properties. The use of levamisole in the adjuvant setting was based on initial studies in patients with advanced stages of colon cancer that showed this agent had some activity when used as single-agent therapy. Prospective randomized studies comparing 5-FU and levamisole to surgery alone were conducted by both the North Central Cancer Treatment Group (NCCTG) and the Intergroup trial (Moertel, et al.) in patients with stage II and III disease. These studies demonstrated a 41% decrease in recurrence and a 33% decrease in mortality for patients with stage III disease compared to surgery alone; the data suggested an improvement in disease-free and overall survival for patients with stage II colon carcinoma as well but did not quite achieve statistical significance in either study. Based on these studies, the National Institutes of Health (NIH) Consensus Conference in 1991 recommended that all patients with stage III colon carcinoma receive adjuvant chemotherapy with 5-FU and levamisole. Adjuvant chemotherapy for patients with stage II colon carcinoma remains controversial.

The addition of leucovorin to 5-FU has been shown to increase antitumor activity in both in vitro and in vivo models. Leucovorin works by stabilizing the 5-FU–thymidylate synthase complex, thus prolonging the inhibition of thymidylate synthase and improving tumor cytotoxicity. Early prospective randomized studies showed an increased survival rate in patients with advanced-stage colon cancer treated with combination 5-FU and leucovorin. This led to numerous prospective randomized trials comparing this combination of agents with various other single-agent and combination regimens in the adjuvant setting. Early results show increased disease-free and overall survival rates for all patients. Subset analysis for patients with stage II and III disease has not yet been done. Other studies are underway to confirm these results and to establish the optimal dosing and scheduling of these agents.

MANAGEMENT OF RECTAL CANCER

There are five goals in the successful management of rectal cancer: (1) cure, (2) local control, (3) restoration of intestinal continuity, (4) preservation of anorectal sphincter function, and (5) preservation of sexual and urinary function. Because of the anatomic constraints of the bony pelvis it may be difficult at times to achieve adequate sphincter, sexual, and urinary function without compromising cure and local control.

Local control is an extremely important aspect of the treatment of the patient with rectal cancer. Up to 25% of patients dying of rectal cancer will have local failure only, while another 50% will have local failure in addition to distant disease. Patients with local failure after treatment for rectal cancer are only rarely salvaged by additional surgery. These patients often suffer greatly with bone and nerve pain, hemorrhage, pelvic sepsis, and bowel and urinary obstruction.

Because of these considerations it is important to provide optimal therapy for patients with rectal cancer initially.

When planning surgical treatment of a rectal cancer, the rectum can be divided into three regions in relation to the anal verge. Tumors in the upper third of the rectum (10–15 cm from the anal verge) behave similarly to cancers in the more proximal bowel. These tumors are adequately treated by anterior or low anterior resection (LAR) with primary anastomosis. Tumors in the middle third of the rectum (5–10 cm from the anal verge) are most often treated with LAR. There has been no survival benefit demonstrated for abdominoperineal resection (APR) over LAR in the management of tumors in this area. However, the ability to successfully perform an LAR for tumors in this area depends on the patient's body habitus, pelvic width, tumor bulk, and associated colonic disease. Most tumors in the distal third of the rectum (0–5 cm from the anal verge) will require APR and permanent colostomy to achieve adequate local control. Occasionally, a very low anterior resection using a stapled anastomosis may be performed. Bowel continuity may also be restored in select patients with a coloanal anastomosis. More recently, local procedures have been performed for early cancers in this region.

In addition to understanding the anatomical site of the tumor, it is important to understand the principles influencing the extent of radical extirpative surgery. Optimal treatment of all malignancies requires an adequate margin of resection. Histologic examination of the bowel wall distal to the gross rectal tumor reveals that only 2.5% of patients will have submucosal spread of disease greater than 2.5 cm. In addition, patients with distal submucosal disease spread greater than 0.8 cm have a poor prognosis and will probably not benefit from more radical surgery. At M. D. Anderson we try to obtain distal negative margins of 2 cm. An adequate lymphadenectomy should be performed for accurate staging and local control. In patients with rectal cancer this procedure involves resection of the mesorectum to the level of the aortic bifurcation. This dissection is facilitated by ligation of the IMA and IMV at the level of the aorta. No benefit in survival or local disease control has been attainable with the use of more radical lymphadectomy. Data suggest that negative lateral (radial) margins are major determinants of survival. Lateral margins can be maximized by sharp dissection outside the mesorectum on the endopelvic fascia. It is important to remember that although a 2-cm distal mucosal margin is adequate, local control of rectal cancer requires maximal extirpation of the mesorectal and lateral pararectal tissues.

Radical Surgical Approaches to Rectal Cancer

Abdominoperineal Resection
The standard treatment for patients with rectal cancer has been the Miles APR. This procedure involves the transab-

dominal resection of the rectum and mesorectum from the level of the inferior mesenteric vessels to the levator muscles, in combination with transperineal excision of the anus and distal rectum. Patients require permanent sigmoid colostomy after APR. It remains the "gold standard" by which other therapies are measured. APR is currently indicated for distal third rectal tumors within 3 cm of the anal verge, tumors involving the anal sphincter musculature, tumors involving the rectovaginal septum, patients with poor continence preoperatively, and patients with diarrheal disorders.

Sphincter-Preserving Surgery
In recent years, the use of adjuvant therapy, the introduction of circular stapling devices, and studies demonstrating the adequacy of 2-cm distal margins have allowed for the safe use of sphincter-preserving surgery for resection of mid- and some distal rectal cancers. LAR is by definition an operation in which the dissection and anastomosis are performed below the peritoneal reflection. It is important to remember that mesorectal and lateral pelvic dissections should be performed as in an APR. As long as a margin of at least 1 cm, but preferably 2 cm, is obtained distal to the gross tumor, anastomosis can be performed if technically feasible. Frozen-section analysis of the distal margin is essential when performing an LAR.

A coloanal anastomosis preserves the sphincter mechanism in patients with low-lying rectal tumors whose negative distal margin of resection is up to but does not include the anal sphincter musculature. The operative dissection is similar to that of LAR and APR, with transection of the distal margin at the level of the levator ani muscles within the abdomen. Through a perineal approach, the remaining anal mucosa is stripped and an anastomosis between the colon and the anus is performed to restore intestinal continuity. At M. D. Anderson we perform a handsewn anastomosis at this level. To provide adequate bowel length and a tension-free anastomosis, the splenic flexure of the colon is completely mobilized. The vascular supply of the left colon is then based on the middle colic artery. We perform a protective diverting ileostomy in all patients undergoing a coloanal anastomosis. Contraindications for an LAR or coloanal anastomosis include tumors involving the anal sphincter musculature, tumors involving the rectovaginal septum, patients with poor continence preoperatively, patients with diarrheal disorders, and unfavorable anatomic constraints (i.e., obesity, narrow pelvis).

Proximal diversion after sphincter preservation is indicated in the following circumstances: (1) anastomosis less than 5 cm above the anal verge; (2) in patients who have received preoperative radiotherapy; (3) in patients on corticosteroids; (4) in any situation where the integrity of the anastomosis is in question; (5) in any case of intraoperative hemodynamic instability.

Local Approaches to Rectal Cancer

Local treatment alone as definitive therapy of rectal cancer was first applied to patients with severe coexisting medical conditions unable to tolerate radical surgery. Currently conservative sphincter-saving local approaches are being more widely considered. Early studies of local excision demonstrate up to a 97% local control rate and 80% disease-free survival for properly selected individuals. Local treatment is best applied to rectal cancers within 10 cm of the anal verge, tumors less than 3 cm in diameter involving less than one-fourth of the circumference of the rectal wall, exophytic tumors, tumors staged less than T2 by EU, and tumors of low histologic grade.

Local therapy of distal rectal cancers can be accomplished by transanal excision, posterior proctectomy, fulguration, or endocavitary irradiation. Transanal excision is the most straightforward approach to removing distal rectal cancers. The deep plane of the dissection is the perirectal fat. Tumors should be excised with an adequate circumferential margin. The defect is then closed primarily. Posterior proctectomy (Kraske procedure) can be used for slightly larger tumors. In this procedure a perineal incision is made just above the anus, the coccyx is removed, and the fascia divided. The rectum can then be mobilized and resection performed. Fulguration uses either standard electrocautery or laser to ablate the tumor. Endocavitary radiation is a high-dose, low-voltage irradiation technique that applies contact radiation to a small rectal cancer through a special proctoscope. Fulguration and endocavitary radiation have the disadvantage of not providing an intact specimen for histologic analysis. While these techniques have been proven safe and effective in retrospective trials, prospective randomized studies are necessary before widespread use of local therapy becomes standard.

While small T1 tumors can be treated with local therapy alone, adjuvant radiotherapy—with or without chemotherapy—appears to be an important component of the treatment of T2 lesions. The risk of occult mesorectal lymph nodes harboring carcinoma is related to the tumor depth of invasion. Adjuvant radiotherapy probably decreases local recurrence rates significantly for a certain percentage of these T2 lesions. However, this question has not been answered by a randomized prospective trial.

Surgery for Locally Advanced Disease

Occasionally patients will present with involvement of adjacent organs (bladder, vagina, ureters, seminal vesicles, etc.). These patients should receive preoperative adjuvant therapy in an attempt to downstage their tumors. If adjacent organ involvement remains after therapy or is encountered unexpectedly at operation, a radical approach to therapy should be undertaken. A tumor should never be shaved off adjacent structures since this approach will result in an unacceptably high rate of local recurrence. Adjacent structures should be resected en bloc as indicated. Whereas a proximal rectal lesion attached to the dome of the bladder may be resected in combination with a partial cystectomy, lesions adherent to the bladder trigone will require pelvic exenteration. Patients in whom this situation may arise should be adequately counseled prior to attempted resection.

Survival after Surgical Therapy

Seventy-five to ninety percent of node-negative rectal cancers are cured by radical surgical resection. Only one-third of patients with regional lymph node metastases will survive 5 years. As mentioned previously 25% of patients who fail will fail in the pelvis alone. However, local failure will occur in up to 75% of patients succumbing to their disease.

The survival rate after local therapy varies from 70 to 86%, with recurrence rates of 10–50%. Many of these patients can be saved with radical surgery after a local recurrence. When analyzing the results of local therapy, it must be remembered that these patients are usually carefully selected for therapy.

Complications of Surgical Therapy for Rectal Cancer

The most common complications encountered intraoperatively during surgery for rectal carcinoma include hemorrhage from the presacral venous plexus, splenic injury, and ureteral injury. The exact incidence of injury to the presacral venous plexus is impossible to obtain; however, it is the most feared and potentially the most lethal intraoperative complication. Iatrogenic splenic injury is usually preventable. These injuries are related to traction on the peritoneum and omentum with avulsion of a portion of the splenic capsule. Ureteral injuries occur in 3–9% of patients undergoing colorectal surgery. The most frequent ureteral injuries occur during division of the lateral ligaments and of the superior rectal vessels.

The most common postoperative complications include perineal wound problems (abscess 11%, hemorrhage 4%), sexual dysfunction (approximately 45%), neurogenic bladder (3.5%), stomal complications (28%), clinically evident anastomotic leak (10–20%), and anastomotic stricture (10%).

Adjuvant Therapy of Locally Advanced Disease

Surgery is the mainstay of therapy for rectal tumors. However, this modality has not provided adequate treatment, as evidenced by the 30–50% recurrence rate after surgery alone. The morbidity of local failure is significant and difficult to manage. Patients may suffer for protracted periods with severe bone and nerve pain, bleeding, and pelvic sepsis. This high local failure rate is likely due to the inability to perform adequate lymphadenectomy and achieve adequate radial margins because of the anatomic constraints of the bony pelvis. Stage is an important prognostic determinant of both local and distant failure. Patients with extension of tumor outside the rectal wall or histologically involved lymph nodes have a 20–40% local recurrence rate. Patients with both positive lymph nodes and extramural tumor extension have local recurrence rates of 40–65%. Patients with these unfavorable tumor characteristics are candidates for adjuvant therapy. Adjuvant radiotherapy has been demonstrated to be effective in decreasing the rate of local recurrence in high-risk patients.

Preoperative Radiotherapy
There are several theoretical advantages to the use of preoperative radiotherapy:

1. A reduction in the size of the tumor increases the potential for sphincter preservation.

2. There is a decreased risk of local failure and distant metastasis from cells shed at operation.

3. There is a decreased risk of late radiation enteritis since the small bowel can be excluded from the radiation field.

4. Some tumors considered unresectable may become resectable with therapy.

5. Tumor cells are well oxygenated when treated preoperatively since there has been no surgical manipulation of the blood supply to the tumor. Well-oxygenated cells are thought to have increased radiosensitivity, and therefore tumor cell killing may be increased.

Despite these advantages, preoperative radiation has not had an impact on overall survival, distant recurrence, or cure rates. However, locoregional control has been improved. Randomized studies have shown a significant decrease in local recurrence with preoperative doses of radiotherapy greater than 34.5 Gy. Additionally, the Jefferson group has reported a 91% sphincter preservation rate for patients with T3 and T4 lesions treated with 45 Gy of preoperative radiotherapy. Local control and overall survival have been acceptable with this approach. Importantly, 10% of patients in this series have achieved a complete pathologic response.

There is some increase in morbidity associated with surgery after preoperative radiotherapy, including delayed wound healing and increased pelvic sepsis. The incidence of these problems can be decreased by waiting 4–6 weeks after completion of radiotherapy before surgery.

Postoperative Radiotherapy
The advantages cited for the use of postoperative radiotherapy include the following:

1. Adequate pathology data are available to evaluate the extent of disease.

2. Patients who will not benefit from therapy are not treated.

3. There is no delay in surgical treatment.

Despite the performance of several large prospective trials, survival, local pelvic control, and extrapelvic recurrence rates have not been improved consistently by radiation doses of 45–50 Gy. In addition, in a large study comparing preoperative to postoperative radiotherapy, there was a significant decrease in local failure seen in the group that received preoperative therapy.

Postoperative Radiotherapy and Chemotherapy

Two large studies of postoperative chemotherapy conducted by GITSG and NCCTG have provided evidence that combination therapy may affect local control and distant failure. In the GITSG trial, there was a decrease in pelvic failure for the group treated by surgery and postoperative chemoradiotherapy (11% versus 24% for surgery alone). In addition, a statistically significant survival advantage was found at 7 years using the combination of resection, radiation, and chemotherapy. The NCCTG trial did not have a surgery alone control. However, there was a significant decrease in pelvic recurrence (14% versus 25%) and a significant decrease in cancer-related deaths for the group treated by resection, radiation, and chemotherapy compared to the group treated with resection and radiotherapy.

The findings from these studies led to the publication of a clinical advisory by the NIH recommending the following adjuvant treatment for patients with Dukes B2 and C rectal carcinoma: "Treatment should be initiated from one to two months after surgery if the patient is fully recovered from the operative procedure, maintaining a reasonable state of nutrition, and has normal hematologic parameters."

Weeks 1 and 5:	5-FU 500 mg/m^2/day × 5 days
Week 9:	Radiation therapy to tumor area and regional nodal distribution. 45 Gy over 4–6 weeks, followed by 5.4-Gy boost in three fractions to the tumor bed. Give 5-FU 500 mg/m^2/day × 3 days during the first and last week of irradiation.
4 and 8 weeks after irradiation:	5-FU 450 mg/m^2/day × 5 days

This regimen is considered to be the current standard of care outside a clinical trial.

M. D. Anderson Experience

Our preferred management of T3–T4 rectal cancer is to use preoperative radiotherapy with a protracted IV infusion of 5-

FU. We deliver 45 Gy of preoperative radiotherapy with standard fractionation. A continuous infusion of 5-FU at a dose of 300 mg/m²/day is given Monday through Saturday. Surgery is performed 6–8 weeks after completion of therapy. A complete pathologic response rate of 30% and an overall response rate of 76% have been seen in patients with T3 lesions. Although the duration of follow-up is short (2 years), only one local recurrence has been seen in 37 patients treated with this approach.

It is important to note that the treatment of rectal cancer is evolving. There are several cooperative trials underway examining the optimal adjuvant therapy for rectal cancer. These trials will attempt to answer several important questions, including the role of preoperative and postoperative therapy, the best agents to use, and the optimal dosing and timing of therapy. We encourage participation in these randomized trials.

RECURRENT AND METASTATIC DISEASE

Two-thirds of patients who undergo curative surgery for colorectal cancer have tumor recurrences. Of the patients who have recurrences, 85% do so during the first 2.5 years after surgery. The remaining 15% recur during the subsequent 2.5 years. The risk of recurrence is higher with stage II or III disease, anaplasia, aneuploidy, or adjacent organ invasion. Recurrences may be local, regional, or distant. Distant disease recurrence, the most common presentation, occurs either alone or concomitantly with locoregional recurrence. Liver involvement occurs in approximately 50% of patients with colon cancer, while lung, bone, and brain involvement occurs in 10%, 5%, and less than 5%, respectively.

CEA is invaluable for postoperative monitoring. It is most useful in patients whose levels are elevated preoperatively and return to normal following surgery. Levels should be determined preoperatively, 6 weeks postoperatively, and then according to the schedule described above in the surveillance section. The absolute level and rate of rise and the patient's clinical status are important in determining prognosis and treatment. Postoperative levels that do not normalize within 6 weeks to 4 months suggest incomplete resection or recurrent disease, although false-positive results do occur. Levels that normalize postoperatively and then start to rise are indicative of recurrence. This may represent occult or clinically obvious disease. A rapidly rising CEA level suggests liver or lung involvement, while a slow, gradual rise is associated with locoregional disease. Despite the reliability of an elevated CEA level in predicting tumor recurrence, 20–30% of patients with locoregionally recurrent tumors have a normal CEA level. Poorly differentiated tumors may not make CEA, which is one explanation for such false-negative results. In contrast, CEA is elevated in 80–90% of patients with hepatic recurrences.

Management of the asymptomatic patient with an elevated CEA level can be challenging. An elevated level should be confirmed by a repeat CEA determination approximately 1 month later. A thorough clinical investigation that includes LFTs; CT scan of the abdomen, pelvis, and chest; colonoscopy; and, if clinically indicated, bone scan or CT of the brain should be performed.

If the metastatic evaluation is negative in the face of an elevated CEA level, a second-look laparotomy should be performed. About 60–90% of patients with asymptomatically elevated CEA levels will have recurrent disease at laparotomy; 55% of these patients will have resectable disease at the time of laparotomy; and 40% will survive 5 years following resection of the recurrence. Early detection of asymptomatic disease results in a higher resectability rate than when resection is performed for symptomatic disease (60% versus 27%). The liver is the most common site of recurrence, followed by adjacent organs, the anastomotic site, and the mesentery. Resectability rates correspond to the level of CEA elevation, with CEA levels less than 11 ng/ml being associated with higher resectability rates.

In recent years, radioimmuno-guided surgery (RIGS) has been used to detect recurrences intraoperatively. This technique is useful in directing the surgeon to disease sites that would otherwise be left behind. In addition, it is especially useful in patients with resectable liver lesions who have extranodal disease that is otherwise not detectable. ^{125}I-labeled monoclonal antibodies directed against CEA are injected 6 weeks before the second-look surgery. The antibodies localize to the tumor sites and can be detected intraoperatively by a handheld gamma probe. Tumor is accurately detected in 81% of patients. Sixteen percent of patients will have tumor that is detected by RIGS alone. Despite this novel modality for detecting and treating disease in the asymptomatic patient, no study has demonstrated a survival advantage with this technique.

Radiolabeled monoclonal antibodies directed against CEA have been approved for imaging the extent and location of extrahepatic metastases. Preliminary studies have shown a sensitivity and specificity that are similar to those of CT in detecting extrahepatic metastases.

Symptomatic recurrences present with a constellation of symptoms ranging from the vague and nonspecific to the clinically overt. The management of recurrent or metastatic disease differs according to the site and type of presentation.

Liver

Close to 70% of patients who die of colon cancer will have hepatic involvement. The liver is the site of metastatic or recurrent disease in 50% of patients and is the primary determinant of patient survival. (See Chapter 11 for the management of colorectal hepatic metastasis.)

Lung

Pulmonary metastases occur in 10% of patients with colorectal cancer. They are most commonly seen in the setting of a large hepatic tumor burden or extensive metastatic disease. Isolated pulmonary metastases occur most commonly with distal rectal lesions, as the venous drainage of the distal rectum bypasses the portal system and allows metastasis to travel directly to the lungs.

The finding of a solitary lesion on a chest radiograph should prompt evaluation with thoracic CT scanning and, for a centrally located lesion, bronchoscopy with biopsy. Peripheral lesions may be amenable to CT-guided needle biopsy. Fifty percent of patients with solitary pulmonary nodules will have primary lung tumors rather than colorectal metastases.

Patients with locally controlled primary tumors, no evidence of metastases elsewhere, and good medical condition are candidates for resection. Unilateral and bilateral pulmonary lesions can be resected. However, if more than one lesion is present in each lung, surgical excision is contraindicated.

The overall 5-year survival rate following resection of pulmonary metastases ranges from 20 to 30%. Two-year survival rates may approach 70%. The interval from resection of the primary lesion to development of pulmonary disease is the most important long-term prognostic factor. Patients with disease-free intervals (the time from resection of the primary tumor to the development of lung metastases) of less than 2 years have a 20-month disease-free survival period following resection of pulmonary metastases. Patients with intervals greater than 2 years have a 40-month disease-free survival period.

Bone and Brain

Metastatic disease to the brain is uncommon and usually occurs after established lung involvement. Symptomatic solitary lesions can be treated by palliative craniotomy and resection. In a very small subpopulation of patients, cranial disease may be the only site of involvement, and excision in this setting may increase survival. Bone metastases are quite uncommon and are best managed with radiation therapy.

Ovary

Three to eight percent of patients have synchronous or metachronous ovarian disease. Bilateral oophorectomy is the treatment of choice in postmenopausal patients with either unilateral or bilateral disease involving the ovaries.

Premenopausal patients with unilateral ovarian disease require oophorectomy. The role of prophylactic oophorectomy in the premenopausal patient is controversial. No study has demonstrated a prolonged survival benefit following prophylactic oophorectomy. Ballantyne et al. reported a median survival of 77% following prophylactic oophorectomy versus 79% in patients who did not undergo oophorectomy. The 5-year disease-free surivival was equivalent for patients with and without oophorectomy (78%).

Pelvis

Local recurrence in the pelvis is a major problem after treatment for rectal cancer. These patients are infrequently saved by additional surgery. Radiation affords good palliation; however, if the patient has previously received adjuvant radiotherapy, external beam radiotherapy may no longer be an option. Radical surgical procedures including pelvic exenteration and sacrectomy may benefit a select group of patients whose disease can be completely extirpated by these procedures. IORT and brachytherapy may be useful adjuvants in the setting of radical surgery for recurrent disease.

SURVEILLANCE

Patients with a history of colon carcinoma require close surveillance. History and physical examination, Hemoccult stool testing, and laboratory tests (complete blood count, CEA determination, LFTs) are performed at M. D. Anderson every 3 months for the first 3 years after surgery, every 6 months during years 4 and 5, and yearly thereafter. Colonoscopy should be performed 3 months after the initial surgery and yearly thereafter. A baseline CT scan of the abdomen and pelvis is obtained 3–4 months after the index procedure. Because of the 47% false-positive rate, the utility of routine CT scanning in surveillance is controversial. However, in the presence of symptoms or abnormal laboratory tests, CT should be performed. A chest radiograph is obtained every 6 months for the first 2 years and yearly thereafter.

UNCOMMON COLORECTAL TUMORS

Lymphoma

Lymphoma is an uncommon tumor that occurs in 0.4% of patients with intestinal lymphoma between the second and eighth decades. Almost all are non-Hodgkin's lymphomas. Twenty-five percent of patients may present with fever, occult blood loss, anemia, a palpable mass, or an acute abdomen. The diagnosis is often made intraoperatively. A history of abdominal pain, fever, and weight loss in a patient who is younger than the expected age for a colorectal tumor should raise the suspicion of intestinal lymphoma.

Abdominal CT and endoscopy with biopsy are the most useful diagnostic tests since lesions are often missed on BE. A thickened bowel, adjacent organ extension, or nodal enlargement may be seen. If the lesion is intraluminal, biopsy will make the diagnosis. Most of these lesions are intermediate- to high-grade B cell lymphomas. If a diagnosis is made preoperatively in an otherwise asymptomatic patient, bone marrow biopsy should be performed.

Surgery is performed in the clinical setting of obstruction, bleeding, or perforation. A thorough exploration is performed and all suspicious nodes or organs are biopsied to assess the stage of disease. The primary intestinal lesion should be resected with negative margins whenever possible. The bowel mesentery should be resected with the tumor so that regional nodes can be pathologically assessed. Intestinal continuity should be restored whenever possible. If a large tumor is found to be unresectable and is not obstructing the bowel, a bypass can be performed. Surgical clips should be placed to facilitate identification of the tumor by the radiation oncologist.

Intestinal lymphoma requires a combined modality approach using surgery and chemotherapy with or without radiation. The overall survival for stage I and II disease is about 80%. This decreases to 35% with advanced disease.

Leiomyosarcoma

Leiomyosarcomas comprise less than 1% of colonic tumors. The peak incidence occurs in the sixth decade. The majority of these tumors present as large intraluminal masses. They may invade the mesenteric and pericolic fat, prostate, vagina, and ischiorectal fossa.

Patients can present with pain, bleeding, obstruction, nausea, vomiting, anemia, tenesmus, or hematuria. A thorough clinical evaluation should be conducted to exclude metastatic disease. Excision with wide surgical margins is the treatment of choice. Colonic tumors are excised with adjacent mesentery. Wide nodal excision is not indicated in the absence of clinically evident disease. Small tumors of the rectum and anal canal can be removed transrectally or endoscopically.

As with other sarcomas, prognosis depends on tumor size, grade, and the presence or absence of adjacent organ involvement. The 5-year survival rate with tumors less than 5 cm is 71% compared to 25% in tumors greater than 5 cm. Survival decreases to 28% at 5 years with adjacent organ involvement. Grade is the most important prognostic factor. Survival with low-grade tumors is 62%, while that with high-grade tumors is only 12%. The liver and peritoneum are the most common sites of recurrence, followed by lymph nodes. Prognosis is poor in recurrent disease. Neither radiation nor chemotherapy are of proven benefit in the management of this disease.

Carcinoid

Carcinoids are neuroendocrine tumors derived from Kulchitsky's cells that are uncommonly found in the colon and rectum. Tumors in this location almost never produce the carcinoid syndrome. Although large tumors may present with bleeding, obstruction, or constipation, tumors less than 2 cm are frequently asymptomatic. Diagnosis is made by endoscopic biopsy. Small lesions (<1 cm) are commonly well differentiated and can be adequately treated with endoscopic excision. Tumors greater than 1 cm have associated lymphatic and distant metastases in 90% and 60% of cases, respectively. Lesions less than 2 cm can be treated with local excision. However, if adequate margins are not present, wider resection is mandatory using standard resection techniques.

Squamous Carcinoma of the Anus

EPIDEMIOLOGY AND ETIOLOGY

Anal cancers constitute 1–2% of all large-bowel malignancies and 2–4% of anorectal cancers. Anal cancer occurs most frequently during the sixth decade of life. Groups reported to be at increased risk of anal cancer include Northern Brazilian females, homosexual males regardless of human immunodeficiency virus (HIV) status, women practicing receptive anal sex, and post-transplantation patients.

Anal cancers are divided into two groups that differ in epidemiology, histology, and prognosis. Anal canal cancers (tumors proximal to the verge) make up 67% of anal cancers. These cancers are three to four times more common in women than men. Anal margin cancers (tumors distal to the anal verge) are more common in males. There are significantly more cases of anal margin cancers in homosexual males.

Anal cancer is associated with poor personal hygiene, chronic anal irritation, infection, and immune suppression. Other risk factors for the development of anal cancer include genital condyloma acuminatum, a history of gonorrhea in men, cigarette smoking, herpes simplex virus type I seropositivity, and a history of *Chlamydia trachomatis* infection. The presence of human papillomavirus (HPV) infection, especially serotypes 16, 18, and 31, has been strongly linked to anal squamous carcinoma. Up to 54% of HIV-positive patients have HPV DNA in their anal canal, which may account for the increased incidence of anal cancers seen in this group.

PATHOLOGY

Over 80% of malignant anal lesions are histologically squamous cell carcinomas. With the exception of melanoma (see below) and small-cell carcinoma, all other histologic subtypes behave similarly and are treated according to their anatomic location. Basaloid carcinoma (basal cell carcinoma with a massive squamous component), mucoepidermoid carcinoma (originating in anal crypt glands), and cloacogenic carcinoma are all variants of squamous carcinoma.

The anal margin is lined by keratinized stratified squamous

epithelium with hair follicles and pigment. The anal canal can be divided into three areas, which overlap considerably. The first is characterized by hairless stratified squamous epithelium and is located between the anal verge and the dentate line. Next is the transitional zone, which is lined with cuboidal and glandular epithelium and is located 1.0–1.5 cm proximal to the dentate line. Finally, there is columnar epithelium, which can be found from the transitional zone proximal to the anorectal ring. Malignant anal tumors may be preceded by or coexist with premalignant dysplasia or anal intraepithelial neoplasia.

The prognosis of anal margin cancers is favorable. Distant metastases from anal margin cancers are rare. When they do occur, metastases most commonly are found in the superficial inguinal lymph nodes (approximately 15% of cases). It is unusual for anal margin cancers to metastasize to mesenteric or internal iliac nodes.

Anal canal cancers are associated with aggressive local growth and if untreated will extend to the rectal mucosa and submucosa, subcutaneous perianal tissue and perianal skin, ischiorectal fat, local skeletal muscle, perineum, genitalia, lower urinary system, and even the pelvic peritoneum and the broad ligament. Historically, mesenteric lymph node metastases have been detected in 30–50% of surgical specimens. Over 50% of patients present with locally advanced disease. The most common sites of distant metastases are the liver, lung, and abdominal cavity. However, most cancer-related deaths are due to uncontrolled pelvic or perineal disease.

DIAGNOSIS

The initial symptoms of anal cancer include bleeding, pain, and local fullness. These symptoms are similar to those caused by the common benign anal diseases, which accompany anal cancer in more than 50% of cases. A detailed history, including that of previous anal pathology and sexual habits, should precede a meticulous physical examination. Physical examination should attempt to identify the lesion, its size and anatomic boundaries, and any associated scarring or condylomata. It is also important to determine the resting and voluntary anal sphincter tone. Occasionally, an examination under general anesthesia may be necessary to complete the local evaluation. Pelvic and abdominal CT scans are important in assessing extent of local disease and distant spread. Proctosigmoidoscopy is essential to assess the proximal extent of disease and to obtain tissue for biopsy. Palpable inguinal lymph nodes should be evaluated by fine-needle aspiration. A chest radiograph should be obtained to rule out the possibility of pulmonary metastases.

STAGING

The current AJCC staging system for anal margin and anal canal cancers is depicted in Tables 10-3 and 10-4.

Table 10-3. AJCC staging of anal canal cancer

Primary tumor (T)

TX	Primary tumor cannot be assessed
T0	No evidence of primary tumor
Tis	Carcinoma in situ
T1	Tumor ≤2 cm in greatest dimension
T2	Tumor >2 cm but not >5 cm in greatest dimension
T3	Tumor >5 cm in greatest dimension
T4	Tumor of any size invades adjacent organ(s)

Lymph nodes (N)

NX	Regional lymph nodes cannot be assessed
N0	No regional lymph node metastasis
N1	Metastasis in perirectal lymph nodes(s)
N2	Metastasis in unilateral internal iliac and/or inguinal lymph node(s)
N3	Metastasis in perirectal and inguinal lymph nodes and/or bilateral internal iliac and/or inguinal lymph nodes

Distant metastasis (M)

MX	Presence of distant metastasis cannot be assessed
M0	No distant metastasis
M1	Distant metastasis

Stage grouping

0	Tis	N0	M0
I	T1	N0	M0
II	T2	N0	M0
	T3	N0	M0
IIIA	T1	N1	M0
	T2	N1	M0
	T3	N1	M0
	T4	N0	M0
IIIB	T4	N1	M0
	Any T	N2	M0
	Any T	N3	M0
IV	Any T	Any N	M1

TREATMENT

Anal Margin Cancer

Small (<5 cm), superficial (T1–T2) anal margin cancers can be treated by a negative-margin wide local excision alone, with a 5-year survival rate greater than 80%. Wide local excision may include parts of the superficial internal and external anal sphincters without compromising anal continence. Even a full-thickness, partial-circumference sphincter resection distal to the puborectalis sling will leave the patient with acceptable anal function.

Elective inguinal lymph node dissection has been abandoned as a primary treatment modality for these tumors. However, prophylactic inguinal irradiation is advocated, especially for

Table 10-4. AJCC staging of anal margin cancer

Primary tumor (T)

TX	Primary tumor cannot be assessed
T0	No evidence of primary tumor
Tis	Carcinoma in situ
T1	Tumor ≤2 cm in greatest dimension
T2	Tumor >2 cm but not >5 cm in greatest dimension
T3	Tumor >5 cm in greatest dimension
T4	Tumor invades deep extradermal structures (i.e., cartilage, skeletal muscle, or bone)

Lymph nodes (N)

NX	Regional lymph nodes cannot be assessed
N0	No regional lymph node metastasis
N1	Regional lymph node metastasis

Distant metastasis (M)

MX	Presence of distant metastasis cannot be assessed
M0	No distant metastasis
M1	Distant metastasis

Stage grouping

0	Tis	N0	M0
I	T1	N0	M0
II	T2	N0	M0
	T3	N0	M0
III	T4	N0	M0
	Any T	N1	M0
IV	Any T	Any N	M1

lesions 5 cm or larger. Lymph node dissection is indicated for residual tumor or for recurrent disease in the inguinal region.

Large and deep anal margin tumors should be treated as anal canal lesions.

Anal Canal Cancer

Until the 1980s, APR with permanent colostomy was the recommended treatment for all anal canal cancers. However, pioneering work by Nigro et al. that has since been confirmed by others has radically changed the approach to this disease. Currently, surgery is reserved for T1 lesions, which may be locally excised; for salvage of patients with an incomplete response to chemoradiotherapy; for locally or regionally (inguinal or iliac lymph nodes) recurrent lesions; for severely symptomatic patients (perineal sepsis, intractable urinary or fecal fistulae, intolerable incontinence); and for temporary fecal diversion in patients with nearly obstructing lesions.

The current regimen for primary treatment of anal canal cancer and large anal margin cancers is chemotherapy (Table 10-5). Complete responses with chemoradiotherapy

Table 10-5. Treatment protocol for anal canal cancer

Days 1–4	5-FU, 750–1,000 mg/m^2 over 24-hour continuous IV infusion
Day 1	Mitomycin C, 10–15 mg/m^2, IV bolus (alternatively, bleomycin, 15 units once a week, or cisplatin, 4 mg/m^2/day with 5-FU dose reduced to 250–300 mg/m^2)
Days 1–35	Radiation therapy 5 days/week for total dose of 45–55 Gy. Boosts of up to 60 Gy may be given to the anus and or inguinal basins
Days 29–32	5-FU, 750–1,000 mg/m^2 over 24-hour continuous IV infusion

can be expected in up to 90% of patients, with 5-year survival rates approaching 85%. Biopsy is performed 6–8 weeks after completion of therapy. Patients with residual disease may be salvaged with radical surgery or second-line chemotherapy. Inguinal lymphadenectomy is reserved for patients who have residual or recurrent disease at this site after chemoradiotherapy.

SURVEILLANCE

Patients should be followed for detection of local and systemic failures as well as for treatment complications. Local inspection, digital examination, anoscopy, and biopsy of any suspicious area are recommended every 3 months for 2 years and twice a year thereafter. Early detection of local recurrence may enable less extensive salvage surgical procedures. Distant failures of epidermoid cancer are responsive to radiotherapy, and up to 30% of patients respond to second-line chemotherapy. Therefore chest radiography, LFTs, and pelvic CT are recommended every 6–12 months for 2–3 years after initial therapy.

Anorectal Mucosal Melanoma

EPIDEMIOLOGY

Primary melanoma of the the anus or rectum is a rare tumor, accounting for 0.4–1.6% of all melanomas and less than 1.0% of all tumors of the anorectum. The overall prognosis for patients with anorectal melanoma is dismal. The reported 5-year survival rate is only 6%, and the median survival time is only 25 months.

PATHOLOGY

Melanomas arising from the true rectum are less common than those developing at the squamocolumnar junction in the anal canal. Nodal metastases in the pelvis are more commonly associated with rectal tumors, whereas inguinal node disease is more likely to result from anal lesions. Most patients present with a clinically localized but advanced polypoid or nodular primary tumor. Prognosis is related to tumor thickness, as with cutaneous melanomas.

DIAGNOSIS

Patients most commonly present with rectal bleeding. Some patients will complain of a painful rectal mass. Occasionally, melanoma will be an incidental pathologic finding after hemorrhoidectomy. Physical examination should include evaluation of the rectal mass as well as palpation of the inguinal nodes. A chest radiograph and LFTs should be performed to determine whether distant metastases are present. Abdominal and pelvic CT scans are helpful in determining the extent of local and regional disease.

TREATMENT

Sphincter-sparing procedures can be attempted if negative margins can be achieved. APR is the treatment of choice for large bulky tumors and recurrent disease. Therapeutic inguinal node dissection is indicated for palpable nodal disease. Because of the high incidence of local recurrence and inguinal nodal disease regardless of treatment used, postoperative adjuvant irradiation of the tumor bed and nodal basins may be warranted.

Selected References

Adam YG, Efron G. Current concepts and controversies concerning the etiology, pathogenesis, diagnosis and treatment of malignant tumors of the anus. *Surgery* 101:253, 1987.

Alexander A. The effect of endorectal ultrasound scanning on the preoperative staging of rectal cancer. *Surg Oncol Clin North Am* 1:39, 1992.

Ballantyne GH, Reigel MM, Wolff BG. Oophorectomy and colon cancer impact on survival. *Ann Surg* 202:209, 1985.

Burnstein MJ. Dietary factors related to colorectal neoplasms. *Surg Clin North Am* 73:13, 1993.

Brister SJ, deVarennes B, Gordon PH. Contemporary operative management of pulmonary metastases of colorectal origin. *Dis Colon Rectum* 31:786, 1988.

Cawthorn SJ, Parums DV, Gibbs NM, et al. Extent of mesorectal spread and involvement of lateral resection margin as prognostic factors after surgery for rectal cancer. *Lancet* 335:1055, 1990.

Cohen AM, Minsky BD, Friedman MA. Rectal Cancer. In VT DeVita, S Hellman, SA Rosenberg (eds), *Cancer: Principles and Practice of Oncology* (4th ed). Philadelphia: Lippincott, 1993.

Cohen AM, Minsky BD, Schilsky RL. Colon Cancer. In VT DeVita, S Hellman, SA Rosenberg (eds), *Cancer: Principles and Practice of Oncology* (4th ed). Philadelphia: Lippincott, 1988.

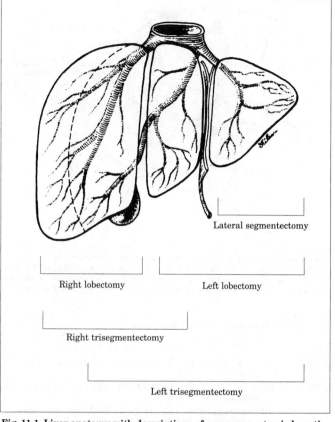

Lateral segmentectomy

Right lobectomy

Left lobectomy

Right trisegmentectomy

Left trisegmentectomy

Fig. 11-1. Liver anatomy with descriptions of common anatomic hepatic resections. (From S Iwatsuki, DG Sheahan, TE Starzl. The changing face of hepatic resection. *Curr Probl Surg* 26:291, 1989.)

chronic hepatitis B virus (HBV) infections. Patients with HCC have a rate of chronic HBV infection that is much higher than that seen in the general population. It has been found that in countries where chronic HBV infection is not endemic, a number of patients with HCC will, in fact, be positive for antibodies to the hepatitis C virus (HCV).

In addition to hepatitis virus infection, a number of other risk factors have been implicated in HCC. Alcohol-related cirrhosis is probably the leading cause of HCC in the United States, Canada, and Western Europe. Dietary intake of aflatoxins is elevated in several countries where the incidence of HCC is high. HCC has also been reported in association with several metabolic disorders, such as hemochromatosis and tyrosinemia. The resultant cirrhosis or chronic hepatocellular injury may be the common etiologic factor.

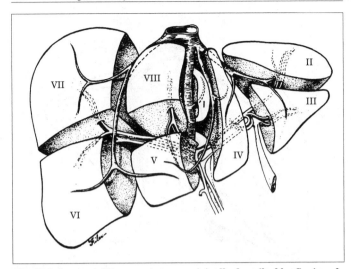

Fig. 11-2. Segmental liver anatomy as originally described by Couinaud. Each of the eight segments is based on its separate and distinct blood supply and biliary drainage. (From S Iwatsuki, DG Sheahan, TE Starzl. The changing face of hepatic resection. *Curr Probl Surg* 26:291, 1989.)

Table 11-1. Hepatic arterial variations

Type I	RHA, MHA, and LHA arise from the CA (55%)
Type II	RHA and MHA arise from the CA, replaced LHA from the LGA (10%)
Type III	MHA and LHA arise from the CA, replaced RHA from the SMA (11%)
Type IV	MHA arises from the CA, replaced RHA from the SMA and replaced LHA from the LGA (1%)
Type V	RHA, MHA, LHA arise from the CA, accessory LHA from the LGA (1%)
Type VI	RHA, MHA, LHA arise from the CA, accessory RHA from the SMA (7%)
Type VII	RHA, MHA, LHA are from the CA, accessory LHA from the LGA, and accessory RHA from the SMA (1%)
Type VIII	Replaced RHA and an accessory LHA; or replaced LHA and an accessory RHA (2%)
Type IX	Absent celiac HA. Entire hepatic trunk arises from the SMA (4.5%)
Type X	Absent celiac HA. Entire hepatic trunk arises from the LGA (0.5%)
Type X (variant)	Double celiac HA (no common HA)

CA = celiac artery; LGA = left gastric artery; LHA = left hepatic artery; HA = hepatic artery; MHA = middle hepatic artery; RHA = right hepatic artery; SMA = superior mesenteric artery.

Men are affected by HCC more frequently than women. In high-incidence areas, the male to female ratio is approximately 4:1, and in low-incidence areas, the ratio is 2:1. Increasing age has also been associated with HCC. More important than the actual age of the patient, however, is the chronicity of the HBV infection or the cirrhosis.

PATHOLOGY

The majority of primary malignancies of the liver are HCC (85–90%), with cholangiocarcinoma, angiosarcoma, and hepatoblastoma being much less common.

The histologic variations of HCC are of little importance in determining the treatment and prognosis of a patient. There are, however, two exceptions. The first, fibrolamellar carcinoma (FLC), is found in younger patients and is thought to carry a better prognosis. The second exception is adenomatous hyperplasia. This premalignant lesion develops within a regenerating nodule in a cirrhotic liver. Therefore complete resection of adenomatous hyperplasia is curative.

HCC will frequently spread by local extension to the diaphragm and adjacent organs and into the portal and hepatic veins. Metastatic spread occurs most often to regional lymph nodes (periportal), lungs, bone, adrenals, and brain.

CLINICAL PRESENTATION

Most patients with HCC have a history of HBV infection, alcoholic liver disease, or cirrhosis. Common presenting symptoms include upper abdominal pain or discomfort, a palpable right upper quadrant mass, weight loss, ascites, or other sequelae of portal hypertension. Jaundice is relatively uncommon. On physical examination, one may find firm, nodular hepatomegaly, a hepatic rub, or an arterial bruit in the right upper quadrant. Numerous paraneoplastic complications have been described, including hypoglycemia, hypercalcemia, erythrocytosis, and hypertrophic pulmonary osteoarthropathy.

DIAGNOSIS

Certain laboratory and radiologic findings should raise one's suspicion for HCC. Alpha-fetoprotein (AFP) is elevated in 50–90% of all patients with HCC, with the highest levels usually found in those with large tumors or rapidly growing tumors. Consequently, a patient with a small HCC may have minimal or even no elevation of AFP. Transient increases in AFP may also be seen in benign chronic liver diseases such as cirrhosis. Serum AFP measurements are used to monitor patients for tumor recurrence, as levels should fall to normal after curative resection.

Radiologic confirmation of a mass in the liver can be made by either ultrasound (US) or computed tomography (CT). US, which is as sensitive and specific as CT for detecting small lesions (<3 cm in diameter), has the advantage of being relatively inexpensive. As a result, US has been used extensively as a screening tool in regions where the incidence of HCC is high.

Conventional CT is able to detect larger lesions in the liver and to assess the presence of extrahepatic disease. Sensitivity can be improved by using CT angiography, in which a contrast agent is injected into the hepatic artery during the study. The blood supply to HCC is derived almost entirely from the hepatic artery; thus, the tumor will appear as a hyperdense area on the scan. The accuracy of the study depends on the uniform distribution of contrast agent to both lobes of the liver. Unfortunately, this is not always possible in a diseased, cirrhotic liver or with variant hepatic arterial anatomy.

More recently, CT with arterial portography (CTAP) has proved to be the best method to study mass lesions in the liver. In CTAP, a contrast agent is injected into the superior mesenteric artery or the splenic artery prior to the scan, and delayed images are then taken when contrast has entered into the portal venous system. Since it is not well perfused by the portal system, HCC is seen as a low-density area against the surrounding liver parenchyma. The sensitivity of CTAP in identifying liver lesions is reported to be as high as 97%.

Although not available in the United States, lipiodol has been used in Asia and Europe to aid in evaluating small HCCs. Lipiodol, an oily derivative of the poppy seed combined with iodine contrast medium, is retained by HCC cells. It is injected into the hepatic artery, and a CT scan is performed 1–2 weeks later. Lesions as small as a few millimeters can be detected using this technique.

The histologic diagnosis of HCC can be obtained by percutaneous needle biopsy or fine-needle aspiration of the mass, usually under US guidance. The risk of hemorrhage following this procedure is not insignificant, as most HCCs are hypervascular, and patients may have ascites or some degree of coagulopathy. Tumor seeding of the biopsy track, a rare event, has been reported. Therefore a preoperative liver biopsy is unnecessary unless the work-up has demonstrated the lesion to be unresectable and tissue is needed to plan appropriate alternative therapy.

The evaluation of the patient is completed with a chest radiograph to exclude pulmonary metastases. Further studies, such as a CT scan of the brain or bone scan, are not indicated unless there is clinical suspicion of metastases to these areas.

STAGING

The current American Joint Committee on Cancer (AJCC) staging system for HCC is shown in Table 11-2.

Eisenberg B, DeCosse JJ, Harford F, et al. Carcinoma of the colon and rectum: The natural history reviewed in 1704 patients. *Cancer* 49:1131, 1982.

Fisher B, Wolmark N, Rockette H, et al. Postoperative adjuvant chemotherapy or radiation therapy for rectal cancer: Results from the NSABP Protocol R-01. *J Natl Cancer Inst* 90:21, 1988.

Gerard A, Buyse M, Nordlinger B. Preoperative radiotherapy as adjuvant treatment in rectal cancer: Final results of a randomized study of the European Organization for Reseach and Treatment of Cancer (EORTC). *Ann Surg* 208:606, 1988.

Gastrointestinal Tumor Study Group. Prolongation of the disease free interval in surgically treated rectal carcinoma. *N Engl J Med* 312:1465, 1985.

Grinnell RS, Lane N. Benign and malignant adenomatous polyps and papillary adenomas of the colon and rectum: An analysis of 1856 tumors in 1335 patients. *Surg Gynecol Obstet* 106:519, 1958.

Gunderson LL. Adjuvant irradiation of rectal cancer. *Int J Rad Oncol Biol Phys* 13:5, 1987.

Haggitt RC, Glotzbach RE, Soffer EE, et al. Prognostic factors in colorectal carcinomas arising in adenomas: Implications for lesions removed by endoscopic polypectomy. *Gastroenterology* 89:328, 1985.

Hautefeuille P, Valleur P, Perniceni T. Functional and oncologic results after coloanal anastomosis for low rectal carcinoma. *Ann Surg* 207:61, 1988.

Hermanek P. Evolution and pathology of rectal cancer. *World J Surg* 6:502, 1982.

Jessup JM, Bothe A, Stone MD, et al. Preservation of sphincter function in rectal carcinoma by a multimodality treatment approach. *Surg Oncol Clin North Am* 1:137, 1992.

Jones DJ, James RD. Anal cancer. *Br Med J* 305:169, 1992.

Kemeny N, Cohen A, Bulino JR, et al. Continuous intrahepatic infusion of floxuridine and leucovorin through an implantable pump for the treatment of hepatic metastases for colorectal carcinoma. *Cancer* 65:2446, 1990.

Localio SA, Eng K, Coppa GF. Abdominosacral resection for midrectal cancer: A fifteen year experience. *Ann Surg* 198:320, 1983.

Lynch HT, Watson P. Extracolonic cancer in hereditary non-polyposis colorectal cancer. *Cancer* 71:677, 1993.

Mandel JS, Bond JH, Bradely M, et al. Sensitivity, specificity and positive predictivity of the Hemoccult test in screening for colorectal cancers: The University of Minnesota's Colon Cancer Control Study. *Gastroenterology* 97:597, 1989.

Martin EW, Cooperman M, et al. Sixty second look procedures indicated primarily by rise in serial carcinoembryonic antigen. *J Surg Res* 28:389, 1980.

Mendenhall WM, Million RR, Bland KI. Initially unresectable rectal adenocarcinoma treated with preoperative irradiation and surgery. *Ann Surg* 205:41, 1987.

Milson JW. Pathogenesis of colorectal cancer. *Surg Clin North Am* 73:6, 1993.

Moertel CG, Fleming TR, MacDonald JS, et al. Levamisole and fluorouracil for adjuvant therapy of resected colon carcinoma. *N Engl J Med* 322:352, 1990.

Mohiuddin M, Marks G. Preoperative radiation therapy as the key to extending sphincter preservation in rectal cancer. *Int J Radiat Oncol Biol Phys* 10(Suppl 2):90, 1984.

Nigro ND, Sydel HG, Considine B, et al. Combined preoperative radiation and chemotherapy for squamous cell carcinoma of the anal canal. *Cancer* 51:1286, 1983.

NIH Consensus Conference. Adjuvant therapy for patients with colon and rectal cancer. *JAMA* 264:1444, 1990.

Nivatvongs S, Rojanasakul A, Reiman HM, et al. The risk of lymph node metastases in colorectal polyps with invasive adenocarcinoma. *Dis Colon Rectum* 34:323, 1991.

Ota DM, Skibber R, Rich TA. MD Anderson Cancer Center experience with local excision and multimodality therapy for rectal cancer. *Surg Oncol Clin North Am* 1:147, 1992.

Papillon J, Gerard JP. Role of radiotherapy in anal preservation for cancer of the lower third of the rectum. *Int J Radiat Oncol Biol Phys* 19:1219, 1990.

Parks AG, Percy JP. Resection and sutured coloanal anastomosis for rectal carcinoma. *Br J Surg* 69:301, 1982.

Philipshen SJ, Heilweil M, Quan SHQ, et al. Patterns of pelvic recurrence following definitive resections of rectal cancer. *Cancer* 53:1354, 1983.

Quirke P, Durdey P, Dixon MF, et al. Local recurrence of rectal adenocarcinoma due to inadequate surgical resection. *Lancet* 11:996, 1986.

Quirke P, Scott N. The pathologist's role in the assessment of local recurrence in rectal carcinoma. *Surg Oncol Clin North Am* 1:1, 1992.

Ross MI, Stern SJ, Wanebo HJ. Mucosal Melanoma. In CM Balch, AN Houghton, GM Milton, et al (eds), *Cutaneous Melanoma* (2nd ed). Philadelphia: Lippincott, 1992. Pp 331–333.

Salvati EP, Rubin RJ, Eisenstat TE, et al. Electrocoagulation of selected carcinoma of the rectum. *Surg Gynecol Obstet* 166:393, 1988.

Sardi A, Workman M, Mojzisik C, et al. Intraabdominal recurrence of colorectal cancer detected by radioimmunoguided surgery (RIGS system). *Arch Surg* 124:55, 1989.

Shank B, Cohen AM, Kelsen D. Cancer of the Anal Region. In VT DeVita, S Hellman, SA Rosenberg (eds), *Cancer: Principles and Practice of Oncology* (4th ed). Philadelphia: Lippincott, 1993. Pp 1006–1022.

Sindelar WF, Hoekstra HJ, Kinsella TJ. Surgical approaches and techniques in intraoperative radiotherapy for intraabdominal, retroperitoneal and pelvic neoplasms. *Surgery* 103:247, 1988.

Sischy B. The use of endocavitary irradiation for selected carcinomas of the rectum: Ten years' experience. *Radiother Oncol* 4:97, 1985.

Stein BL, Coller JA. Management of malignant colorectal polyps. *Surg Clin North Am* 73:47, 1993.

Stryker SJ, Wolff BG, Culp CE. Natural history of untreated colonic polyps. *Gastroenterology* 93:1009, 1987.

Surtees P, Ritchie JK, Phillips RKS. High versus low ligation of the inferior mesenteric artery in rectal cancer. *J Surg* 77:618, 1990.

Tierney RP, Ballantyne GH, Modlin IM. The adenoma to carcinoma sequence. *Surg Gynecol Obstet* 171:81, 1990.

Vanek VW, Whitt CL, Abdu RA. Diagnosis and preoperative management of colorectal carcinoma. *Contemp Surg* 32:39, 1988.

Walsh PC, Schlegel PN. Radical pelvic surgery with preservation of sexual function. *Ann Surg* 208:391, 1988.

Williams NS, Dixon MF, Johnston D. Reappraisal of the 5 centimeter rule of distal excision for carcinoma of the rectum: A study of distal intramural spread and of patients' survival. *Br J Surg* 70:150, 1983.

Winawer SJ, Andrews M, Flehinger B, et al. Progress report on controlled trial of fecal occult blood testing for the detection of colorectal neoplasia. *Cancer* 45:2959, 1980.

Wolmark N, Rockette H, Fisher B, et al. The benefit of leucovorin modulated fluorouracil as postoperative adjuvant therapy for primary colon cancer: Results from National Surgical Adjuvant Breast and Bowel Project Protocol C-03. *J Clin Oncol* 11:1879, 1993.

Wolmark N, Fisher B. An analysis of survival and treatment failure following abdominoperineal and sphincter saving resection in Duke's B and C rectal carcinoma. *Ann Surg* 204:480, 1976.

Hepatobiliary Cancers

Alan M. Yahanda

Surgical Anatomy of the Liver

A basic knowledge of the anatomy of the liver is essential to the management of hepatic or biliary tract neoplasms. On the most elementary level, the liver can be divided into right and left lobes (Fig. 11-1) by an imaginary line drawn between the gallbladder bed and the vena cava (Cantlie's line). The left lobe is further divided by the falciform ligament into the medial segment (that portion between the falciform ligament and Cantlie's line) and the lateral segment (that portion to the left of the falciform ligament). The right lobe is divided into anterior and posterior segments.

Most surgeons further conceptualize the segmental anatomy of the liver in the manner described by Couinaud. Each of the eight segments of the liver is defined by its distinct and separate arterial and portal vascular supplies and its hepatic venous and biliary drainage (Fig. 11-2). A thorough understanding of these vascular structures and their locations within the liver is mandatory to perform a safe hepatic resection.

Anatomic variations of the hepatic artery are frequent. At the University of Texas M. D. Anderson Cancer Center, hepatic arterial variants are divided into ten types (Table 11-1). By far the most common types are I, II, and III, constituting approximately 76% of all cases.

Liver resections can be classified as a *trisegmentectomy* (removal of the right lobe and the medial segment of the left lobe, or removal of the left lobe and either the anterior or posterior segment of the right lobe), a *lobectomy* (removal of the entire left or right lobe), a *segmentectomy* (removal of an anatomic segment of the liver, based on Couinaud's segmental anatomy), and a *subsegmental* or *nonanatomic resection* (see Fig. 11-1). An additional type of resection is a *total hepatectomy*, which obviously can be done only in the setting of liver transplantation.

Primary Hepatocellular Carcinoma

EPIDEMIOLOGY

Primary hepatocellular carcinoma (HCC) is relatively rare in the United States, with an annual incidence of less than 5 cases per 100,000. It is ranked as the twenty-second most common type of cancer in the country. Globally, however, HCC stands as one of the most common and deadly of all tumors. This striking geographic variation in the incidence of HCC is thought to be related to the varying prevalence of

Table 11-2. AJCC staging system for primary liver cancer

Primary tumor (T)

Tx	Primary tumor cannot be assessed
T0	No evidence of tumor
T1	Solitary tumor ≤2 cm without vascular invasion
T2	Solitary tumor ≤2 cm with vascular invasion; or multiple tumors ≤2 cm, limited to one lobe without vascular invasion; or solitary tumor >2 cm without vascular invasion
T3	Solitary tumor >2 cm with vascular invasion; or multiple tumors ≤2 cm, limited to one lobe with vascular invasion; or multiple tumors, any >2 cm, limited to one lobe, with or without vascular invasion
T4	Multiple tumors in more than one lobe; or tumor involving a major branch of the portal or hepatic vein(s)

Regional lymph nodes (N)

Nx	Regional lymph nodes cannot be assessed
N0	No regional lymph node metastasis
N1	Regional lymph node metastasis

Distant metastasis (M)

Mx	Presence of distant metastasis cannot be assessed
M0	No distant metastasis
M1	Distant metastasis

Stage grouping

Stage I	T1	N0	M0
Stage II	T2	N0	M0
Stage III	T3	N0	M0
	T1–3	N1	M0
Stage IVa	T4	Any N	M0
Stage IVb	Any T	Any N	M1

Source: OH Beahrs et al. *Manual for Staging Cancer* (3rd ed). Philadelphia: Lippincott, 1988.

EVALUATION OF OPERATIVE RISK

Before contemplating major surgery, let alone hepatic resection, in a patient with a diseased liver, one must first determine whether the patient has adequate liver function to tolerate surgery and anesthesia. In addition, one must try to predict whether the remaining liver will have adequate hepatic function following resection of the tumor. This assessment has been plagued by the lack of specific tests to determine hepatic function and hepatic reserve. Traditionally, the Child-Pugh classification or its modifications have been applied to liver resection in the same manner they were originally used in portosystemic shunt surgery. The parameters measured in this classification scheme give a rough estimation of the gross synthetic and detoxification capacity of the liver. Numerous studies have validated this system as a predictor of survival in cirrhotic patients. To better evaluate liver function, several other tests have been devised, including the urea-nitrogen synthesis rate, galactose elimination capacity, indocyanine green

(ICG) clearance, and bromsulphalein and aminopyrine breath tests. A ratio of liver function to liver volume can be determined by radionuclide imaging using technetium-labeled N-pyridoxyl-5-methyltryptophan; the uptake of tracer by the anticipated liver remnant is compared with that of the whole liver. A more invasive, but more accurate, method is to determine the ICG clearance rate of the liver remnant by injecting the dye directly into the hepatic artery supplying that particular portion of the liver.

Despite modern surgical techniques and perioperative care, hepatic resection carries an operative mortality as high as 20%. The majority of perioperative deaths are due to liver failure, hemorrhage, and sepsis.

The preoperative evaluation of liver function at M. D. Anderson is based primarily on the Child-Pugh classification scheme. The age of the patient is taken into consideration, as elderly patients (>70 years) do not tolerate major hepatic resection well. Coexisting medical problems such as ischemic heart disease and chronic obstructive pulmonary disease are investigated, as these are known to be poor prognostic factors. The CTAP and accompanying arteriogram are used to determine the presence and extent of cirrhosis and portal hypertension. We do not use any other tests, such as the aminopyrine breath test or ICG clearance, in the preoperative work-up of liver function.

SURGICAL THERAPY

The definitive treatment for resectable HCC remains surgery. Unfortunately, of the patients presenting with HCC, only 10–30% will be eligible for surgery, and of those patients who undergo exploration, only 50–70% will have a resection with curative intent. The criteria that render a tumor to be unresectable include (1) the presence of extrahepatic disease, (2) evidence of severe hepatic dysfunction, (3) an extensive tumor that would leave too little liver remaining following extirpation, and (4) tumor involvment of the portal vein or vena cava. The latter criterion has become more a relative contraindication, as many surgeons are now resecting portions of involved portal vein and hepatic artery.

The operative approach to the patient with a potentially resectable HCC should begin with a thorough surgical exploration of the abdomen, searching for any evidence of extrahepatic disease. In particular, care is taken to evaluate the periportal lymph nodes, as well as the nodes in the hepatoduodenal ligament. The liver is then completely mobilized to allow full examination of the organ. Intraoperative US should be used to define both the size of the tumor and its relationship to the major vascular and biliary structures.

Once the tumor has been determined to be resectable, the decision must then be made as to how much liver to remove. This will depend, in part, on the size of the mass, the number of nodules, the tumor's proximity to vascular structures, and the severity of the liver disease. Most surgeons believe a 1-cm margin of uninvolved tissue around a tumor is adequate. Larger HCCs, especially those in cirrhotic livers, should have the widest margin possible that will leave a sufficient amount of remnant tissue. In such cases, it may be necessary to compromise on the 1-cm tumor-free margin. A segmentectomy is usually practical only for small tumors. Several series have demonstrated that for HCCs smaller than 3 cm, the best operation is a segmentectomy. More radical surgeries for these lesions are accompanied by higher operative morbidity and mortality without any reduction in the recurrence rate or improvement in survival. On the other hand, lesser operations, such as wedge resections, should be discouraged as they are associated with high rates of recurrence. The extent of the resection is often limited by the concomitant presence of cirrhosis and impaired liver function. In these cases, nonanatomic or subsegmental resections are useful to preserve as much liver as possible.

Recurrence rates following hepatic resection range between 30% and 70% in the literature. The site of the recurrence is usually intrahepatic. Tumor size and number are by far the most significant factors predicting tumor recurrence. Other risk factors include capsular or vascular invasion by tumor cells, high histologic grade, presence of cirrhosis, and tumor located deep in the liver.

Survival data vary depending on the patient population. In those series in which all stages are evaluated, the 5-year survival rate following hepatic resection is 15–30%. Better survival rates have also been reported in patients with small HCCs. Zhou et al. achieved a 100% 5-year survival rate in patients with stage I disease treated by radical resection.

The role of orthotopic liver transplantation (OLT) in the treatment of HCC is still not completely defined. In theory, total hepatectomy seems advantageous, as it would remove the entire diseased organ, thereby reducing recurrences and improving survival. In the larger series reported in the literature, the survival rates for patients undergoing OLT for HCC range from 15 to 35% at 5 years and are no better, or are even worse, than those reported for subtotal resection. Likewise, the tumor recurrence rates with OLT are similar to those for subtotal hepatic resection. There are, however, several subpopulations for which OLT may confer improved survival. The Pittsburgh group found that when HCC was associated with cirrhosis, OLT provided a significant survival advantage over subtotal resection at each tumor stage. This survival advantage was absent in the noncirrhotic patients. The Pittsburgh group more recently reported a small series in which patients with advanced HCC first underwent at least three cycles of intra-arterial chemotherapy before OLT. Although the follow-up was short, the 1-year survival rate was 91% in the treated patients. This result was in contrast to patients undergoing OLT without chemotherapy, who had a 1-year survival rate of 43%.

Cryosurgery has been advocated as an alternative to resection for HCC. With this technique, liquid nitrogen is circulated through a metal probe placed in the tumor. Each freezing takes 15–20 minutes, and multiple areas may be treated, particularly for larger tumors. This technique has generally been reserved for patients with unresectable tumors, although it can be used in combination with a resection. Cryosurgery has the advantage of treating only the tumor and not the surrounding liver parenchyma. Its disadvantage is that it necessitates both an anesthetic and a laparotomy. Survival rates are about 10% at 5 years.

The management of previously resected HCC that recurs in the liver is difficult. Most often, further liver resection is not possible without subjecting the patient to certain postoperative liver failure. Most patients should be treated with surgical therapies that do not require resection, such as cryosurgery, or nonoperative therapies such as percutaneous ethanol injection or chemoembolization. As mentioned previously, OLT can be considered in highly selected cases.

CHEMOTHERAPY

Systemic chemotherapy has little activity against HCC. The results of single-agent clinical trials demonstrate response rates under 20%. The most active agent appears to be doxorubicin, with an overall response rate, pooled from several trials, of 19%. Multiagent chemotherapeutic regimens have been equally disappointing.

A variety of regional treatments have been studied in an effort to improve the poor results with systemic chemotherapy. Intra-arterial infusion of chemotherapeutic agents is advantageous for several reasons. As mentioned previously, the blood supply to HCC is derived from the hepatic arteries. Intra-arterial infusion allows the delivery of high concentrations of cytotoxic drugs directly to the tumor. In addition, since these agents are metabolized in the liver, their systemic levels can be minimized.

Numerous studies have been performed using intra-arterial infusion of single and multiple chemotherapeutic agents. While there appears to be some survival benefit from intra-arterial therapy, there have been few prospective trials comparing it with standard IV systemic chemotherapy. Intra-arterial doxorubicin, alone or in combination with other agents, has produced the best response rates.

Hepatic artery ligation or occlusion has been used as a palliative treatment for unresectable HCC. It can offer significant symptomatic relief in some patients. This palliation, however, is usually transient, as collateral vessels quickly revascularize the liver.

Transcatheter arterial embolization (TAE) is basically a combination of both intra-arterial infusion chemotherapy and hepatic artery occlusion. Chemotherapeutic agents are either infused into the liver prior to embolization or impregnated in the gelatin sponges used for the embolizaton. Lipiodol has also been used in conjunction with TAE. When it is combined with cytotoxic drugs or radionuclides and injected into the hepatic artery, lipiodol will remain selectively in HCC tissue for an extended period, delivering locally concentrated therapy. The treatment protocols that have produced the highest survival rates are TAE with gelatin sponges containing the chemotherapeutic agent or TAE with gelatin sponges and lipiodol mixed with the chemotherapeutic agent. There was a slight survival difference in favor of those treated by the former regimen, with 2-year survival rates of 55% and 43%, respectively.

Percutaneous ethanol injection (PEI) has been used with some success in cirrhotic patients who are ineligible for surgery. With this technique, US is used to direct the placement of a needle in the tumor. Through this needle, 8–10 ml of 95% ethanol is injected. These treatments are repeated once or twice a week on an outpatient basis. Several studies have documented survival rates following this treatment that are similar, or even better than, those with hepatic resection. The largest series reported is by Livarghi et al., who treated 207 cirrhotic HCC patients using PEI. These patients were deemed to have unresectable tumors or to be at too high a surgical risk, or they refused surgery. The majority of the patients were Child's class A (66%) and had lesions less than 5 cm in diameter. The 3-year survival rates for patients with single and multiple lesions were 63% and 31%, respectively. Some Japanese surgeons are using PEI as the primary treatment for small HCC (<3 cm in diameter) with excellent survival rates.

RADIOTHERAPY

External beam radiotherapy has limited use in the treatment of HCC. The dose that can be safely delivered to the liver is about 30 Gy; higher doses cause radiation hepatitis. Radiotherapy can, however, provide palliative, symptomatic relief in cases of unresectable HCC. Alternatively, locally concentrated doses of radiation can be delivered with intra-arterial infusion of lipiodol or antiferritin antibodies that are coupled with radioactive iodine.

MULTIMODALITY THERAPY

Combinations of surgical and nonsurgical therapies are currently the state of the art in the treatment of HCC. Some tumors that were previously considered unresectable can now be rendered resectable with intra-arterial chemotherapy and radiotherapy. A variety of chemotherapeutic agents have been studied in the neoadjuvant setting, including doxorubicin, 5-fluorouracil (5-FU), mitomycin C, and cisplatin. Furthermore, tumor recurrence may be prevented by the administration of adjuvant intra-arterial chemotherapy following surgical resection, ethanol injection, or cryosurgery.

Metastasis to the Liver

Virtually every malignant tumor has been known to metastasize to and proliferate in the liver. The bulk of these metastases are from gastrointestinal primary tumors, especially from the colon and rectum. In collected series of resected noncolorectal metastases to the liver, there are few 5-year survivors. The exceptions to this appear to be metastases from endocrine tumors, Wilms' tumor, and, to a lesser extent, renal cell carcinoma. In the case of endocrine tumors, even a subtotal resection of gross disease can lead to significant palliation by decreasing the volume of hormone-secreting tumor. Given that the vast majority of metastases to the liver considered for resection are from colorectal primary tumors, the remainder of this discussion is concerned with their management.

EPIDEMIOLOGY AND ETIOLOGY

Of the 150,000 patients newly diagnosed with colon cancer each year, approximately 50% will have recurrences within 5 years following surgical resection of the primary tumor. Of those who have recurrences, only 20% will have the liver as the sole or predominant site, and fewer still will have lesions amenable to surgical resection. It has been estimated that fewer than 5,000 patients a year are potential candidates for resection of their liver metastases.

The discovery of metastatic disease in the liver is made at the time of the initial presentation for the primary lesion (synchronous lesions) in 25–50% of patients. The remainder will have their metastatic disease found some time following resection of the primary (metachronous) lesions. Metachronous lesions are associated with a Dukes C primary tumor in 60–75% of cases, and the disease-free interval is usually less than 2 years.

CLINICAL PRESENTATION

Symptoms or clinical signs suggesting metastatic disease in the liver are usually late occurrences. Consequently, findings such as ascites, jaundice, right upper quadrant pain, and elevation of liver function values are associated with a poor prognosis.

DIAGNOSIS

In the vast majority of patients, metastases to the liver are found through routine postoperative carcinoembryonic antigen (CEA) screening or radiologic imaging following resection of their colorectal primary tumor. Any patient with a rising CEA level should undergo a thorough diagnostic evaluation, including a chest radiograph and a contrast-enhanced CT scan of the abdomen and pelvis. In addition, the colon should be examined by either a barium enema or, preferably, colonoscopy to exclude the presence of a metachronous colon or rectal primary tumor as the source of the rising CEA.

DETERMINING RESECTABILITY

In cases in which the initial evaluation suggests the metastatic disease is isolated to the liver, one must then determine whether the patient is a candidate for surgical resection. Patients should be further studied using CTAP to better visualize small lesions that might have been missed by standard CT. The rationale for CTAP in this setting is the same as for primary tumors of the liver; metastatic lesions derive the majority of their blood supply from the hepatic artery, not the portal vein. At the time of CTAP, visceral angiography is performed to exclude tumor encasement of major blood vessels and the presence of any hepatic arterial anomalies.

For patients who have had their primary cancer removed without treatment of their synchronous liver metastases, median survivals of 4.1–12.0 months are reported, with a rare long-term survivor. Given that some patients will live prolonged periods even without surgery, are the patients surviving following resection those who would have done well even without treatment?

Many investigators have attempted to identify that group of patients who will benefit from hepatic resection. From these studies, several factors that impact on resectability can be gleaned. Absolute contraindications to hepatic resection include the presence of common bile duct or celiac lymph node involvement and the presence of four or more metastatic lesions (even if all are located within the same lobe); each of these are associated with a poor prognosis. The presence of extrahepatic metastases has traditionally been considered another contraindication to hepatic resection. Hughes et al. found that patients with extrahepatic metastases resected simultaneously with the hepatic resection did not have reduced overall survival. The disease-free survival, however, was significantly shorter. Therefore at M. D. Anderson, we think that in the presence of extrahepatic metastases, hepatic resection should be considered only if all metastases (hepatic and extrahepatic) can be removed safely and completely with negative surgical margins. Other relative contraindications to hepatic resection include patient age greater than 70 years, presence of coexisting serious medical problems, preoperative CEA level over 200 ng/ml, metastatic lesions greater than 8 cm in diameter, and the presence of bilobar disease.

In patients whose liver metastases are deemed to be resectable by preoperative evaluation, there is no need to seek histologic identification of the mass prior to exploration. Percutaneous biopsy of lesions under US or CT guidance may be necessary prior to initiation of alternative therapies in patients for whom surgical resection is not indicated.

EVALUATION OF OPERATIVE RISK

Patients undergoing surgery for metastases to the liver differ from those with HCC in that cirrhosis is not as frequently present. This does not relieve the surgeon of the responsibility of determining the preoperative condition of the liver parenchyma and the expected adequacy of hepatic reserve following resection of the tumor. The preoperative evaluation of liver function is the same as outlined for patients with HCC.

SURGICAL THERAPY

Once the metastases have been determined to be potentially resectable, the patient should undergo a thorough exploratory laparotomy. Particular attention should be paid to the presence of any extrahepatic disease and enlarged portal and celiac lymph nodes. The colon should be examined for any local recurrences of the primary tumor. The liver is examined, first by visual inspection and palpation, then by intraoperative US. This study will help define the relationship of the tumor(s) to the portal veins, hepatic veins, and vena cava. In addition, it can identify small lesions that were not palpable or demonstrable on preoperative imaging studies. Suspicious areas can be sampled by fine-needle aspiration under US guidance. Complete exploration combined with intraoperative US will determine that nearly half of all patients have unresectable disease. In a prospective trial conducted by the Gastrointestinal Tumor Study Group (GITSG), 42% of patients who underwent surgical exploration were found to have unresectable tumors, and only 46% underwent curative resection. Over two-thirds of the patients had tumors deemed unresectable due to anatomic constraints, such as the proximity of the tumor to major blood vessels or the presence of bilobar disease.

The type of resection performed will depend on the size, number, and location of the lesions. In all cases, the resection must achieve at least a 1-cm tumor-free margin. Thinner margins are invariably associated with local recurrences and shorter survival. Solitary lesions smaller than 4 cm can usually be extirpated with either a nonanatomic resection or a segmentectomy. Larger lesions should be approached with an anatomic lobectomy, if at all possible. Lesser procedures for these lesions result in a poor prognosis, probably because of the inability to achieve an adequate tumor-free margin around the large tumor. Lesions that are situated in proximity to major intrahepatic vascular structures are best removed with a lobectomy even though they may be small.

The presence of bilobar metastases is not necessarily a contraindication to resection. Patients with multiple unilobular metastases have no survival advantage or prolongation of disease-free survival compared with patients with a comparable number of bilobar metastases. What dictates resectability will be the amount of normal, functioning liver parenchyma that will remain following removal of the lesions. Small lesions are best treated with multiple segmentectomies; these can be safely performed in up to three isolated segments. Larger bilobar lesions or those involving more than three segments should be removed with a triseg-mentectomy if their locations and the patient's hepatic reserve will allow such a major procedure.

The operative mortality reported in most major series ranges from 5 to 10%. Postoperative complications occur in 12 to 43% of all patients. The most common sources of morbidity are hepatic failure, bile leak (biloma or biliary fistula), intra-abdominal hemorrhage, and subphrenic or intra-abdominal abscess. In most reported series of hepatic resection for col-orectal metastases, the 5-year survival rate ranges from 25 to 40%.

Despite surgical removal of all gross tumor, the majority of patients will have a tumor recurrence following hepatic resection. In the two large series compiled by Hughes and Scheele, the recurrence rates were 70% and 61%, respective-ly. Results from the GITSG study were better, with a report-ed recurrence rate of 49%. The patterns of recurrence have been described in detail by Hughes, et al. Of 607 patients treated with hepatic resection, 316 had initial recurrences at one site. The liver (47%) and lung (23%) were the most com-mon sites of initial recurrence. Analysis of late recurrences showed a similar distribution, with involvement of the liver in 43% of patients and the lungs in 31%. In only 16% of patients was the late recurrent disease in the liver alone. As a result, those patients who have recurrences following hepatic resection for liver metastases are seldom candidates for further resective surgery. Synchronous liver metastases found at the time of surgery for a primary tumor should, in general, not be resected in the same operation. The exception would be a solitary, small, peripherally located lesion in a healthy, hemodynamically stable patient that could be ade-quately excised with a wedge resection. Lesions that are larger or that will require a major hepatic resection are best approached during a second operation after further evalua-tion and staging. A delay of weeks to months between surg-eries has not been shown to have a negative impact on sur-vival. Obviously, at the time of the initial operation, a thor-ough exploration should be conducted to rule out the pres-ence of extrahepatic metastases. The liver should also be examined by intraoperative US, if available.

CHEMOTHERAPY

Systemic chemotherapy has been studied extensively in the treatment of liver metastases from colorectal carcinoma. Clinical trials using single or multiple chemotherapeutic agents have been disappointing, with response rates ranging from 0 to 45%. In addition, the duration of the responses has been short. Almost all regimens are based on 5-FU, an agent that has been one of the most active against colorectal can-cer.

Patients with unresectable metastatic disease confined to the liver may be considered for regional chemotherapy, administered via a hepatic arterial infusion (HAI) pump. This option is attractive because it allows infusion of high concentrations of drug to the tumor while limiting systemic toxicity.

Prior to implantation of the HAI pump, it is imperative that the possibility of extrahepatic or nodal metastases be excluded. In addition, a good quality arteriogram is necessary for the proper positioning of the catheter. Once the decision has been made to proceed with pump placement, a cholecystectomy should first be performed to prevent the development of chemical cholecystitis, a well-described complication of HAI. In the presence of normal hepatic arterial anatomy, the infusion catheter is placed into the gastroduodenal artery (GDA), in a retrograde direction, with its tip just at the take-off of this artery from the common hepatic artery. The right gastric artery and any accessory arteries distal to the GDA should be ligated to prevent inadvertent perfusion of extrahepatic tissues. The pump is usually positioned in a subcutaneous pocket in the right lower quadrant of the abdomen with the catheter inserted through the anterior abdominal wall. Following placement of the catheter, a fluorescein dye study should be performed through the catheter. A Wood's lamp is used to confirm that no extrahepatic perfusion is present. Prior to the initiation of chemotherapy, a radionuclide pump study is performed during the postoperative period to reconfirm the proper functioning of the catheter.

Variant hepatic arterial anatomy must be recognized and defined clearly on the preoperative arteriogram. When present, accessory lobar vessels are ligated to prevent inhomogeneous perfusion of drug to that lobe. Replaced hepatic arteries are managed in several ways. Two catheters can be placed—one to infuse the main hepatic artery and the other to supply the replaced vessel. One or two infusion pumps may need to be used. The method used at M. D. Anderson is to ligate the replaced vessel and use a single catheter to infuse the main hepatic artery. The lobe with the ligated accessory artery will rapidly develop collateral flow from the other lobe, allowing it to be perfused with the drug.

Although 5-FU is the favored drug in systemic chemotherapy, its first-pass clearance by the liver is low. Consequently, the relative increase in hepatic exposure to the drug by HAI is estimated to be only 5- to 10-fold. A related pyrimidine antagonist, floxuridine (fluorodeoxyuridine [FUDR]), has a much higher extraction on the first pass through the liver. The estimated increase in exposure of the liver to this drug when delivered by HAI is 100- to 400-fold, making it an ideal drug for this use.

Interest in HAI increased after the development of the totally implantable Infusaid pump. This device allows both continuous and bolus injection of drug into the hepatic artery. Initial studies using this delivery system for the infusion of FUDR demonstrated remarkable response rates—as high as 83%. There have since been five major randomized trials comparing the efficacy of HAI to standard IV chemotherapy (Table 11-3). All studies showed significantly better response rates for patients receiving HAI chemotherapy. Because of differences in study design and length of follow-up, survival data are not as easily compared. All studies showed a tendency for longer survival in patients treated with HAI; however, only the French multicenter trial demonstrated a statistically significant improvement in survival rate. In this study, the 1-year survival rates for HAI and IV regimens were 64% and 44%, respectively.

The efficacy of HAI therapy can be further evaluated by the patterns of responses and failures. In a Memorial Sloan-Kettering Cancer Center study, 82% of patients in the IV group had disease progression in the liver compared with 37% in the HAI group. On the other hand, 56% of patients who received HAI developed extrahepatic disease compared with 37% of patients who received IV chemotherapy. These data demonstrate, once again, that regional control of the disease alone may not be adequate, as the majority of people treated with HAI ultimately die of extrahepatic disease.

This problem has been the impetus for several studies aimed at reducing the rate of extrahepatic failure in patients receiving HAI. One approach has been to infuse IV chemotherapy concomitantly with HAI infusion. Safi et al. compared patients treated with intrahepatic FUDR with those treated with both intrahepatic and IV FUDR. Both groups had comparable response rates and survival durations; however, the rates of extrahepatic failure differed between the two treatment groups. Extrahepatic metastases developed in 61% of patients in the HAI group and in 33% of patients in the HAI/IV group. Another approach that has been taken at M. D. Anderson is to alternate administration of FUDR and 5-FU via the HAI pump. The use of 5-FU not only reduces the toxicity to the liver but also, because of the lower first-pass clearance of that drug by the liver, allows significant systemic levels to be attained. This treatment has resulted in a 50% response rate and a prolongation of survival compared with intrahepatic FUDR alone.

There has been only one prospective, randomized study evaluating the use of HAI as an adjunct to surgical resection of hepatic metastases. Wagman et al. randomized patients with solitary, resectable lesions to receive surgery or surgery plus postoperative HAI with FUDR. A second group with multiple resectable lesions was randomized to surgery plus HAI or HAI alone. Patients from groups treated with surgery plus HAI had a longer disease-free interval; however, they did not have longer survivals.

Although HAI significantly decreases the systemic toxicity of chemotherapy, it is by no means a benign procedure. The locally concentrated dose of drug is associated with a number of complications including chemical hepatitis, biliary sclerosis, gastritis, and gastric or duodenal ulcer disease. Permanent hepatic damage can be averted by careful moni-

Table 11-3. Major randomized trials comparing hepatic arterial infusion (HAI) and IV chemotherapy for liver metastases from colorectal cancer

Study	No. of patients	HAI		IV	
		Response		Response	
		Agent	(%)	Agent	(%)
MSKCC	162	FUDR	50	FUDR	20
NCI	64	FUDR	62	FUDR	17
NCOG	115	FUDR	42	FUDR	10
Mayo	69	FUDR	48	5-FU	21
France	163	FUDR	43	5-FU	9

MSKCC = Memorial Sloan-Kettering Cancer Center (N Kemeny, et al. *Ann Intern Med* 107:459, 1987); NCI = National Cancer Institute (AE Chang et al. *Ann Surg* 206:685, 1987); NCOG = Northern California Oncology Group (DC Hohn et al. *J Clin Oncol* 7:1646, 1989); Mayo = Mayo Clinic (JK Martin et al. *Arch Surg* 125:1022, 1990); France = multicenter French cooperative study (P Rougier et al. *J Clin Oncol* 10:1112, 1992.)
5-FU = 5-fluorouracil; FUDR = floxuridine.

toring of liver function during chemotherapy and prompt reduction of the dose should evidence of chemical hepatitis be noted.

Cancer of the Extrahepatic Bile Duct

EPIDEMIOLOGY AND ETIOLOGY

Cancer of the extrahepatic bile duct (cholangiocarcinoma) is extremely rare. In most reported series, the male to female incidence ratio is equal and patients are in their seventh decade. There is no significant geographic variation in the prevalence of the tumor.

The etiology of cholangiocarcinoma is unknown. Several diseases are associated with an increased incidence of such tumors: sclerosisng cholangitis, ulcerative colitis, choledochal cysts, and infection with *Clonorchis sinensis*. The common cancer-causing factor in all of these conditions is unclear, although chronic inflammation of the bile duct probably plays a role.

PATHOLOGY

Histologically, cholangiocarcinoma can be classified as papillary, nodular, or sclerosing adenocarcinomas. The papillary variety has a better prognosis than the other two types. Papillary tumors are usually well differentiated and can present with multiple lesions within the duct. The worst prognosis is associated with the sclerosing type, which is usually poorly differentiated.

The majority of cholangiocarcinomas are located in the proximal portion of the duct. A tumor arising at the confluence of the right and left hepatic ducts is termed a Klatskin's tumor, following the description of 13 such lesions by Klatskin in 1965.

Cholangiocarcinomas are slow growing and most often spread by local extension or metastasize to regional lymph nodes. Lesions of the proximal and middle thirds of the extrahepatic bile duct can compress, constrict, or invade the underlying portal vein or hepatic artery. In addition, proximal tumors can invade the liver parenchyma. It has been appreciated that hilar cholangiocarcinomas will involve the parenchyma of the caudate lobe in as many as 36% of patients. Distant metastases from cholangiocarcinomas are rare.

There are a number of pathologic findings important in predicting the outcome of patients with cholangiocarcinoma. These factors include infiltration to the serosa of the bile duct, lymph node metastases, vascular invasion, and perineural invasion.

CLINICAL PRESENTATION

The most common presenting symptom in patients with cholangiocarcinoma is obstructive jaundice. Rarely, a very proximal tumor may block a segmental or lobar bile duct without the occurrence of clinical jaundice. Other symptoms that may occur are pruritus, weight loss, fatigue, vague abdominal pain, and nausea. A patient may present with cholangitis and sepsis resulting from contamination of the obstructed bile. Except for the jaundice, the physical findings in a patient with bile duct cancer are nonspecific. In cases of middle or distal duct obstruction, a distended gallbladder may be palpable.

DIAGNOSIS

When extrahepatic bile duct obstruction is suspected, the first radiologic test that should be performed is US, as it can provide information about the level and nature of an obstructing lesion. CT is as sensitive as US in demonstrating bile duct dilation. Because of its higher cost, however, CT should not be used routinely as the initial diagnostic test. Should the US demonstrate extrahepatic bile duct dilation that is not a result of common bile duct stones, a CT should be obtained. CT has the advantage of being able to identify the actual tumor mass more often than US. In addition, CT is better able to define the relationship of the tumor to surrounding structures and to evaluate the remainder of the abdomen for metastatic spread.

The actual location of the tumor and, more important, its proximal extent must be defined before planning any surgical intervention. This goal can be accomplished one of two ways: percutaneous transhepatic cholangiography (PTC) or endoscopic retrograde cholangiopancreatography (ERCP). If the point of obstruction is thought to be proximal, PTC is the preferred method for visualizing the biliary tract. For suspected distal bile duct lesions, ERCP is superior, as it will enable one to image both the bile duct and the pancreatic duct.

The work-up for a suspected cholangiocarcinoma is completed with visceral angiography and portography. As mentioned previously, these tumors have a tendency to involve the portal vein and the hepatic artery by local invasion. Evidence of encasement of these vascular structures would suggest that the lesion is unresectable.

Obtaining tissue to confirm the diagnosis of bile duct cancer is difficult because of the location of such tumors and their small size. Fine-needle aspiration can be done under US or CT guidance. Cytologic evaluation of bile and of bile duct brushings is also possible, although the sensitivity of these tests is only about 30% and 40%, respectively. In most cases, the decision to operate is based on the preoperative radiologic examinations, not histologic confirmation.

The differential diagnosis for focal stenosis or obstruction of the bile duct is given in Table 11-4. Although the list is extensive, choledocholithiasis and cholangiocarcinoma are the most common causes.

STAGING

The current AJCC staging system for cholangiocarcinoma is shown in Table 11-5.

SURGICAL THERAPY

The definitive therapy for all extrahepatic bile duct carcinomas is surgical resection; however, only a fraction of these lesions will ultimately be resectable. Overall resectability rates range from 10 to 85%, depending on the series. Lesions of the lower third of the bile duct have the best rates of resectability, followed by those of the middle third. Proximal cholangiocarcinomas are technically difficult to approach, resulting in the lowest rate of resectability among bile duct tumors. Standard criteria that render a tumor unresectable are (1) encasement of the hepatic artery or portal vein, (2) lymph node involvement outside the hepatic pedicle, (3) distant metastases, (4) bilateral tumor extension into secondary hepatic ducts, or (5) bilateral extension of tumor into hepatic parenchyma.

The need for preoperative biliary drainage had been debated at length in the literature. Earlier reports noted that preoperative hyperbilirubinemia was a poor prognostic indicator and that normalization of the bilirubin level prior to surgery was associated with reduced morbidity and mortality. More recent studies, however, have found no benefit from, or have found deleterious effects of, preoperative biliary drainage. Nevertheless, Cameron advocates routine, preoperative placement of biliary drainage catheters to facilitate identifi-

Table 11-4. Differential diagnosis for focal bile duct obstruction

Malignant lesions
    Primary cholangiocarcinoma
    Mucoepidermoid carcinoma
    Direct invasion
        Hepatoma
        Gallbladder carcinoma
        Pancreatic carcinoma
        Retroperitoneal sarcoma
    Metastases to hilar or periportal lymph nodes
    Lymphoid tumors (Hodgkin's and non-Hodgkin's lymphoma)
Benign lesions
    Choledocholithiasis
    Sclerosing cholangitis
    Iatrogenic bile duct stricture
    Mirizzi's syndrome
    Idiopathic focal stenosis
    Tuberculosis
    Clonorchis or *Ascaris* infestation

cation and dissection of the bile duct during surgery and to aid the intraoperative placement of larger, softer Silastic transhepatic stents.

Resectable lesions of the lower third of the bile duct are best treated with a pancreaticoduodenectomy. The proximal bile duct should be resected to the point that the surgical margin is negative for tumor. Occasionally, this may require removal of the majority of the extrahepatic biliary tract with a high hepaticojejunostomy. The operative approach for a pancreaticoduodenectomy at M. D. Anderson is outlined in Chapter 12.

Lesions of the middle third of the bile duct are in proximity to the hepatic artery and the portal vein and have a tendency to invade these structures. If such a tumor has been deemed resectable, it is best treated by local excision and regional lymph node dissection. All efforts should be made to achieve a microscopically negative margin. Care must be taken not to disrupt the soft tissues containing the blood supply to the remaining proximal bile duct to which the hepaticoenteric anastomosis will be performed, or one will risk a postoperative bile duct stricture. Biliary drainage is reestablished using a Roux-en-Y hepaticojejunostomy.

The surgical management of proximal cholangiocarcinomas is controversial. Numerous reports have suggested that radical excision of the duct and any involved liver improves survival and quality of life. However, some surgeons think the morbidity and mortality associated with major hepatic resection for this tumor are too high to justify its use. Part of the controversy involves the necessity of resecting the caudate lobe (segment I) en bloc with the bile duct. Proponents of this approach state that pathologic examination of resected specimens demonstrates direct invasion of tumor into the liver parenchyma or the bile ducts of the caudate lobe in as many

Table 11-5. AJCC staging system for cancer of the extrahepatic bile duct and gallbladder

Primary tumor (T)

Tx   Primary tumor cannot be assessed
T0   No evidence of primary tumor
Tis   Carcinoma in situ
T1   Tumor invades the mucosa or muscle layer
T1a   Tumor invades the mucosa
T1b   Tumor invades the muscle layer
T2   Tumor invades the perimuscular connective tissue
T3   Tumor invades adjacent structures

Regional lymph nodes (N)

Nx   Regional lymph nodes cannot be assessed
N0   No regional lymph node metastasis
N1   Metastasis in the cystic duct, pericholedochal, and/or hilar lymph nodes (hepatoduodenal ligament)
N2   Metastasis in the peripancreatic, periduodenal, periportal, celiac, superior mesenteric, and/or posterior pancreaticoduodenal lymph nodes

Distant metastasis (D)

Mx   Presence of distant metastasis cannot be assessed
M0   No distant metastasis
M1   Distant metastasis

Stage grouping

Stage	T	N	M
Stage 0	Tis	N0	M0
Stage I	T1	N0	M0
Stage II	T2	N0	M0
Stage III	T1–2	N1–2	M0
Stage IVa	T3	Any N	M0
Stage IVb	T3	Any N	M1

Source: OH Beahrs et al. *Manual for Staging Cancer* (3rd ed). Philadelphia: Lippincott, 1988.

as 35% of patients. In addition, the site of tumor recurrence following bile duct resection is often the caudate lobe. Therefore several surgeons have recommended routine caudate lobectomy with bile duct excision. Other surgeons think the caudate lobe should be removed only if it is invaded by the tumor, citing equivalent survival data for those who had caudate lobectomy and those with similar lesions who did not. A final area of controversy is the use of total hepatectomy and OLT for tumors with bilateral extension into secondary intrahepatic biliary ducts. Thus far, there is no convincing evidence that liver transplantation is of benefit to these patients.

The surgical approach to proximal bile duct tumors at M. D. Anderson depends on their location relative to the confluence of the right and left bile ducts and on their proximal extension. Lesions in this region are classified according to the scheme described by Bismuth and Corlette (Fig. 11-3). Type I and II lesions are treated by local excision and local lymph

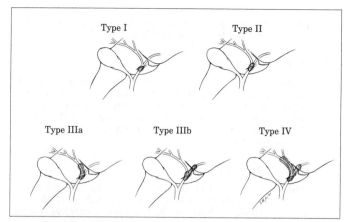

Fig. 11-3. Classification of extrahepatic bile duct tumors according to the location of the obstructing lesion (Bismuth classification).

node dissection. We do not perform routine caudate lobe resections for type II tumors unless invasion into the lobe can be demonstrated. Type IIIa and IIIb lesions undergo local excision and either right or left hepatic lobectomy, respectively. Type IV lesions are not considered resectable. We do not advocate the use of OLT in patients with such advanced disease.

Despite aggressive surgical management, the majority of patients with bile duct carcinoma will succumb to their tumors. Survival rates are the best for lesions of the distal bile duct. Langer et al. reported mean survival times of 37, 32, and 28 months for patients with tumors in the distal, middle, and upper thirds of the bile duct, respectively. Reported 5-year survival rates range from 7 to 50% depending on the tumor location, with distal lesions being associated with higher rates. Patients with negative lymph nodes and clear surgical margins have the best prognoses.

The optimal palliation for patients with unresectable tumors is unclear. If the tumor has been deemed unresectable prior to exploration, the bile duct can be intubated either percutaneously or endoscopically. The use of metallic in-dwelling stents, which are more durable than traditional stents, has made this option more appealing. If the tumor has been found to be unresectable at the time of exploration, the duct can be intubated using either transhepatic Silastic stents or a T tube following dilation of the lesion. When technically feasible, operative biliary bypass with or without concomitant tumor resection provides the best survival and quality of life for patients with unresectable tumors. Unresectable lesions at the bile duct confluence, especially Bismuth type III and IV lesions, can be particularly difficult to palliate. A left intrahepatic cholangioenteric anastomosis has been used with success in these situations. In this technique, the left hepatic duct branch is located between segments III and IV and is drained into a Roux-en-Y limb of jejunum.

CHEMOTHERAPY

There are no clearly effective chemotherapeutic agents for the treatment of cholangiocarcinoma. Single-agent trials using 5-FU have demonstrated response rates under 15%. Other agents, such as doxorubicin, mitomycin C, and cisplatin, used alone or in combination with 5-FU, have been no more successful.

RADIOTHERAPY

Radiotherapy has been demonstrated to be effective in the palliation of patients with unresectable bile duct cancers. Doses of 40–60 Gy have resulted in median survival rates of 12 months, as well as symptomatic improvement. At M. D. Anderson, postoperative chemoradiation is given to patients with resected bile duct cancers. Patients receive continuous-infusion 5-FU concomitantly with 54 Gy of radiation to the tumor bed. Although patient numbers are small and follow-up time is short, initial results suggest a prolongation of survival in treated patients when compared with untreated, historical controls. Intraoperative radiotherapy (IORT) has also been used at our institution in combination with external beam radiation. Again, due to the small numbers of patients treated at this and other institutions, no firm conclusion can be drawn regarding the benefit of IORT. There does appear to be a prolongation of survival in the limited number of patients who have received this therapy.

Periampullary Carcinoma

James Cusack

PATHOLOGY

Adenocarcinoma accounts for 95 percent of malignancies of the periampullary area and may develop from four different tissues of origin at this site: head of pancreas, ampulla of Vater, distal bile duct, and periampullary duodenum. Although the modes of presentation and treatment are similar, the prognosis for each of these malignancies is different. The 5-year survival rate for adenocarcinoma of the head of the pancreas is reported as 18%; of the ampulla, 36%; of the distal bile duct, 34%; and of the periampullary duodenum, 33%. Determination of the tissue of origin is therefore critical, because it affects management decisions regarding potential for cure and extent of resection necessary to obtain tumor-free resection margins.

Determination of the tissue of origin may be made from fine-needle aspiration biopsy or endoscopic biopsy and is based on mucin production and the degree of cellular differentiation.

Anatomic information based on thin-section CT and endoscopic retrograde cholangiopancreatography may also contribute to the determination of the tissue of origin. Detection of a mutation in the Kirsten(Ki)-*ras* proto-oncogene, which occurs in 75–90% of pancreatic adenocarcinomas, may be helpful in differentiating these neoplasms from other periampullary tumors.

Locoregional spread of periampullary adenocarcinoma results from lymphatic invasion and direct tumor extension to adjacent soft tissues. In a prospective study of regional lymph node metastases in patients undergoing pancreaticoduodenectomy for periampullary adenocarcinoma, Cubilla et al. found significant variability in both the frequency of lymph node metastases and the pattern of lymph node involvement, depending on the tissue of origin. Ampullary lesions metastasized to regional lymph nodes in only 33% of cases, typically involving only a single lymph node in the posterior pancreaticoduodenal group. Duodenal adenocarcinomas had an intermediate risk of nodal metastasis, with metastases to several lymph nodes in different subgroups of the paraduodenal area. Pancreatic adenocarcinoma, with its propensity to invade the rich lymphatic network of the pancreas and its ability to directly invade adjacent tissues, had the highest frequency of lymph node involvement (88%); metastases typically involved multiple lymph nodes, multiple subgroups, and distant sites.

TREATMENT

The standard Whipple pancreaticoduodenectomy is thought to provide adequate tumor clearance in the case of nonpancreatic periampullary carcinoma because disease spread is usually localized. Although biopsy-proved paraduodenal lymphadenopathy is thought by most surgeons to preclude curative resection in patients with pancreatic adenocarcinoma, one may appropriately consider en bloc resection in patients with duodenal, ampullary, or distal bile duct tumors in the presence of regional lymph node metastasis if the disease is confined to the field of resection. A detailed description of operative technique is provided in Chapter 12.

The effectiveness of locoregional control of periampullary adenocarcinoma by surgery alone and the potential benefits of adjuvant chemoradiation continue to be examined. In a retrospective review of 41 patients with periampullary carcinoma, Willett et al. identified patients with "low-risk" pathologic features (tumor limited to ampulla or duodenum, well- or moderately well-differentiated histology, negative resection margins, and uninvolved lymph nodes) who had significantly better 5-year actuarial local control and survival rates—100% and 80%, respectively. In contrast, patients with "high-risk" pathologic features (tumor invasion of pancreas, poorly differentiated histology, positive resection margins, and involved lymph nodes) had 5-year actuarial local control and survival rates of 50% and 38%, respectively.

Based on these findings, the authors have proposed a course of preoperative chemoradiation to improve local disease control and survival rates in patients with locally advanced, poorly differentiated tumors.

Gallbladder Cancer

EPIDEMIOLOGY AND ETIOLOGY

Although carcinoma of the gallbladder is a rare tumor, it is actually the most common malignancy of the biliary system and the fifth most common cancer of the gastrointestinal tract. The tumor has been reported in almost all age groups but is most often found in patients in their seventh and eighth decades. There is a striking difference in the incidence of the tumor between the sexes; females are affected three to four times as often as males.

The exact etiology of carcinoma of the gallbladder is not known; however, there are several entities with which it is frequently associated. Cholelithiasis is found in the vast majority of gallbladders resected for carcinoma. Furthermore, gallbladder carcinoma can be found in 1–2% of all cholecystectomy specimens, a rate that is several times higher than that reported in autopsy studies. Chronic cholecystitis, especially cases in which the gallbladder is calcified ("porcelain gallbladder"), has also been associated with an increased risk of cancer, with an incidence as high as 61%.

PATHOLOGY

Adenocarcinoma of the gallbladder is a slow-growing tumor that usually arises in the fundus. Grossly, the gallbladder is firm and the walls are thickened. The tumor has a tendency to invade surrounding structures including the liver, bile duct, and duodenum. The papillary subtype of gallbladder carcinoma characteristically grows intraluminally and spreads intraductally. It is a less aggressive tumor that, consequently, carries a better prognosis.

Lymph node metastases are found in 50–75% of gallbladder carcinoma cases. The cystic duct node, at the confluence of the cystic and hepatic ducts, is the initial focus of regional lymphatic spread. Invasion of the liver, either by direct extension or via draining veins that empty into segments IV and V, is seen in more than 50% of patients. Distant hematogenous spread is rare and is usually seen only in the later stages of the disease.

CLINICAL PRESENTATION

In most series, the most common presenting complaint is abdominal pain. Nausea, vomiting, weight loss, and jaundice are other common symptoms. The majority of patients have had symptoms for 3 months or less prior to presentation. On physical examination, patients may have right upper quadrant pain with hepatomegaly or a palpable, distended gallbladder. In advanced cases, patients may have jaundice, cachexia, and ascites.

DIAGNOSIS

Unfortunately, no laboratory or radiologic tests are routinely accurate in making the diagnosis of gallbladder carcinoma. That inconsistency, along with the paucity of clinical signs and symptoms, has made the tumor's preoperative diagnosis difficult. In fact, a correct preoperative diagnosis of gallbladder cancer is made in fewer than 10% of cases in most series. In the Roswell Park experience, none of the 71 patients reported were correctly diagnosed preoperatively. The most common preoperative diagnoses are acute and chronic cholecystitis and malignancies of the bile duct or pancreas.

In the rare event a diagnosis of gallbladder carcinoma is suspected preoperatively, US or CT may demonstrate a mass with local hepatic extension or suspicious portal adenopathy. Angiography may demonstrate encasement of the cystic or hepatic arteries or the portal vein. There may also be increased vascularity around the gallbladder. Cholangiography is of value in jaundiced patients because it allows the determination of the location and extent of biliary obstruction.

The most common staging system used for carcinoma of the gallbladder, as described by Nevin, is based on the depth of invasion and the spread of tumor (Table 11-6). The standard AJCC staging scheme, shown for comparison in Table 11-5, is more cumbersome. The bulk of the literature on gallbladder cancer uses the Nevin staging system.

SURGICAL THERAPY

The surgical treatment for gallbladder carcinoma is dictated by the stage of the tumor. In fact, in developing his staging system, Nevin found that survival was inversely correlated with the depth of invasion and the extent of spread. Patients with tumor confined to the mucosa and muscularis (stages I and II) all survived 5 or more years, whereas those who had transmural involvement or spread to lymph nodes (stages III and IV) had a 5-year survival rate of only 10%. None of the stage V patients survived beyond 1 year.

The majority of patients with gallbladder carcinoma present with advanced disease (stage V). Standard criteria that make a tumor unresectable include (1) distant hematogenous or lymphatic metastases, (2) peritoneal implants, or (3) invasion of tumor into major vascular structures such as the celiac or superior mesenteric arteries, vena cava, or aorta. Tumors involving the hepatic artery or portal vein have been extirpated with an en bloc vascular resection and recon-

Table 11-6. Nevin's staging system for gallbladder carcinoma

Stage I	Intramucosal involvement only
Stage II	Involvement of the mucosa and muscularis
Stage III	Transmural involvement of gallbladder wall
Stage IV	Metastases to the cystic duct lymph nodes
Stage V	Involvement of the liver by direct extension or metastasis, or metastases to any other organ

struction, but such an extensive procedure would not be considered standard therapy. The dismal prognosis for patients with stage V cancers has made many surgeons advocate palliative procedures rather than resection.

The optimal treatment for patients with stage III and IV tumors is an extended cholecystectomy. The components of this procedure are a cholecystectomy, regional lymph node dissection in the hepatoduodenal ligament, and a wedge resection of the gallbladder bed (including at least a 3-cm margin of normal parenchyma). Using this operative approach, Morrow reported mean survival times for patients with stage III and IV tumors of 48 and 5 months, respectively. Similarly, the Roswell Park group noted a median survival time of 13 months for patients with stage III cancers and 5.3 months for those with stage IV lesions. There are advocates of more extensive hepatic resection for stage IV disease, but the poor prognosis of these patients does not justify the more morbid operation.

Stage I carcinoma of the gallbladder can be adequately treated with cholecystectomy alone, with 5-year survival rates as high as 100% in several series. Hepatic resection and lymphadenectomy are not justified for patients with stage I disease.

The management of stage II tumors is not so clearly defined. Several studies suggest that cholecystectomy alone is sufficient treatment. On the other hand, a number of groups report higher rates of recurrence and lower survival rates for stage II patients treated with cholecystectomy alone. The treatment philosophy at M. D. Anderson involves extended cholecystectomy for most patients diagnosed with stage II disease. Patients with stage II disease not offered extended cholecystectomy include patients with tumors based on the anterior, or serosal, surface of the gallbladder (away from the liver) and patients in whom the medical risk of the procedure outweighs the potential benefit.

NONOPERATIVE THERAPY

The use of single and multiple chemotherapeutic agents either as primary therapy or as adjuvant therapy has been disappointing. Radiotherapy has shown some promise when used in the postoperative adjuvant setting, although most series are small. IORT has also been used with some success.

At M. D. Anderson, patients with gallbladder cancer are treated postoperatively with a combination of continuous-infusion chemotherapy and external beam radiation in a manner similar to treatment for patients with cholangiocarcinoma. It is too early to draw any conclusions regarding the impact of this regimen on survival.

Selected References

Bismuth H, Nakache R, Diamond T. Management strategies in resection for hilar cholangiocarcinoma. *Ann Surg* 215:31, 1992.

Blumgart LH, Kelley CJ. Hepaticojejunostomy in benign and malignant high bile duct stricture: Approaches to the left hepatic ducts. *Br J Surg* 71:257, 1984.

Cady B, Stone MD, McDermott WV, et al. Technical and biological factors in disease-free survival after hepatic resection for colorectal cancer metastases. *Arch Surg* 127:561, 1992.

Cameron JL, Broe P, Zuidema GD. Proximal bile duct tumors: Surgical management with Silastic transhepatic biliary stents. *Ann Surg* 196:412, 1982.

Cameron JL, Pitt HA, Zinner MJ, et al. Management of proximal cholangiocarcinomas by surgical resection and radiotherapy. *Am J Surg* 159:91, 1990.

Cubilla, AL, Fortner J, Fitzgerald PJ. Lymph node involvement in carcinoma of the head of the pancreas area. *Cancer* 41:880, 1978.

Di Bisceglie AM, Rustgi VK, Hoofnagle JH, et al. Hepatocellular carcinoma. *Ann Intern Med* 108:390, 1988.

Gagner M, Rossi RL. Radical operations for carcinoma of the gallbladder: Recent status in North America. *World J Surg* 15:344, 1991.

Hohn DC, Stagg RJ, Friedman MA, et al. A randomized trial of continuous intravenous versus hepatic intraarterial floxuridine in patients with colorectal cancer metastatic to the liver: The Northern California Oncology Group Trial. *J Clin Oncol* 7:1646, 1989.

Hughes KS, et al. Resection of the liver for colorectal carcinoma metastases: A multi-institutional study of indications for resection. *Surgery* 103:278, 1988.

Hughes KS, Simon R, Songhorabodi S, et al. Resection of the liver for colorectal carcinoma metastases: A multi-institutional study of patterns of recurrence. *Surgery* 100:278, 1986.

Iwatsuki S, Sheahan DG, Starzl TE. The changing face of hepatic resection. *Curr Probl Surg* 26:283, 1989.

Iwatsuki S, Starzl TE, Sheahan DG, et al. Hepatic resection versus transplantation for hepatocellular carcinoma. *Ann Surg* 214:221, 1991.

Kanematsu T, Matsumata T, Shirabe K, et al. A comparative study of hepatic resection and transcatheter arterial embolization for the treatment of primary hepatocellular carcinoma. *Cancer* 71:2181, 1993.

Karl RC, Morse SS, Halpert RD, et al. Preoperative evaluation of patients for liver resection: Appropriate CT imaging. *Ann*

Surg 217:226, 1993.

Kemeny N, Daly J, Reichman B, et al. Intrahepatic or systemic infusion of fluorodeoxyuridine in patients with liver metastases from colorectal carcinoma: A randomized trial. *Ann Intern Med* 107:459, 1987.

Klatskin G. Adenocarcinoma of the hepatic duct at its bifurcation within the portahepatis: An unusual tumor with distinctive clinical and pathological features. *Am J Med* 38:241, 1965.

Langer JC, Langer B, Taylor BR, et al. Carcinoma of the extrahepatic bile ducts: Results of an aggressive surgical approach. *Surgery* 98:752, 1985.

Livarghi T, Bolondi L, Lazzaroni S, et al. Percutaneous ethanol injection in the treatment of hepatocellular carcinoma in cirrhosis: A study on 207 patients. *Cancer* 69:925, 1992.

MacIntosh EL, Minuk GY. Hepatic resection in patients with cirrhosis and hepatocellular carcinoma. *Surg Gynecol Obstet* 174:245, 1992.

McPherson DAD, Benjamin IS, Hodgson HJF, et al. Preoperative percutaneous transhepatic biliary drainage: The results of a controlled trial. *Br J Surg* 71:371, 1984.

Morrow, CE, et al. Primary gallbladder carcinoma: Significance of serosal lesions and results of aggressive surgical treatment and adjuvant chemotherapy. *Surgery* 94:709, 1983.

Nagorney DM, van Heerden JA, Ilstrup DM, et al. Primary hepatic malignancy: Surgical management and determinants of survival. *Surgery* 106:740, 1989.

Nevin JE, Moran TJ, Kay S, et al. Carcinoma of the gallbladder: Staging, treatment and prognosis. *Cancer* 37:141, 1976.

Ogura Y, Mizumoto R, Tabaya M, et al. Surgical treatment of carcinoma of the hepatic duct confluence: Analysis of 55 resected carcinomas. *World J Surg* 17:85, 1993.

Order SE, Stillwagon GB, Klein JL, et al. Iodine-131 antiferritin, a new treatment modality in hepatoma: A Radiation Therapy Oncology Group Study. *J Clin Oncol* 3:1573, 1985.

Pitt HA, Somes AS, Lois JF, et al. Does preoperative percutaneous biliary drainage reduce operative risk or increase hospital cost? *Ann Surg* 201:545, 1985.

Rich TA. Adjuvant Therapy for Primary Biliary and Pancreatic Cancer. In JE Niederhuber (ed), *Current Therapy in Oncology.* St. Louis: Mosby-Year Book, 1993.

Rougier P, Laplanche A, Huguier R, et al. Hepatic arterial infusion of floxuridine in patients with liver metastases from colorectal carcinoma: Long-term results of a prospective randomized trial. *J Clin Oncol* 10:1112, 1992.

Safi F, Bittner R, Rosher R, et al. Regional chemotherapy for hepatic metastases of colorectal carcinoma (continuous intraarterial versus continuous intraarterial/intravenous therapy): Results of a controlled clinical trial. *Cancer* 64:379, 1989.

Scheele J, Stangl R, Altendorf-Hofmann A. Hepatic metastases from colorectal carcinoma: Impact of surgical resection on the natural history. *Br J Surg* 77:1241, 1990.

Shirai Y, Yoshida K, Tsukada K, et al. Inapparent carcinoma of the gallbladder: An appraisal of a radical second operation after simple cholecystectomy. *Ann Surg* 215:326, 1992.

Silk YN, Douglass HO, Nava HR, et al. Carcinoma of the gallbladder: The Roswell Park experience. *Ann Surg* 210:751, 1989.

Sitzmann JV, Abrams R. Improved survival for hepatocellular cancer with combination surgery and multimodality treatment. *Ann Surg* 217:149, 1993.

Sitzmann JV, Coleman JA, Pitt HA, et al. Preoperative assessment of malignant hepatic tumors. *Am J Surg* 159:137, 1990.

Stagg RJ, Venook AP, Chase JL, et al. Alternating hepatic intraarterial floxuridine and fluorouracil: A less toxic regimen for treatment of liver metastases from colorectal cancer. *J Natl Cancer Inst* 83:423, 1991.

Stain SC, Baer HU, Denison AR, et al. Current management of hilar cholangiocarcinoma. *Surg Gynecol Obstet* 175:579, 1992.

Steele G Jr, Bleday R, Mayer RJ, et al. A prospective evaluation of hepatic resection for colorectal carcinoma metastases to the liver: Gastrointestinal Tumor Study Group protocol 6584. *J Clin Oncol* 9:1105, 1991.

Steele G Jr, Ravikumar TS. Resection of hepatic metastases from colorectal cancer: Biologic perspectives. *Ann Surg* 210:127, 1989.

Suenaga M, Nakao A, Harada A, et al. Hepatic resection for hepatocellular carcinoma. *World J Surg* 16:97, 1992.

Wagman LD, Kemeny MM, Leong L, et al. A prospective, randomized evaluation of the treatment of colorectal cancer metastatic to the liver. *J Clin Oncol* 8:1885, 1990.

Wanebo HJ, Castle WN, Fechner RE. Is carcinoma of the gallbladder a curable lesion? *Ann Surg* 195:624, 1982.

Willett CG, Warshaw AL, Convery K, Compton CC. Patterns of failure after pancreaticoduodectomy for ampullary carcinoma. *Surg Gynecol Obstet* 176:33, 1993.

Yu YQ, Xu DB, Zhou XD, et al. Experience with liver resection after hepatic arterial chemoembolization for hepatocellular carcinoma. *Cancer* 71:62, 1993.

Zhou X, Tang Z, Yu Y, et al. Clinical evaluation of cryosurgery in the treatment of primary liver cancer: Report of 60 cases. *Cancer* 61:1889, 1988.

Zhou XD, Tang ZY, Yu YQ, et al. Solitary minute hepatocellular carcinoma: A study of 14 patients. *Cancer* 67:2855, 1991.

Pancreatic Adenocarcinoma

George M. Fuhrman, David H. Berger, and
Barry W. Feig

Epidemiology

Pancreatic cancer is the eighth most common malignancy
and the fourth leading cause of adult cancer death in the
United States. In 1993, 27,700 new cases of adenocarcinoma
of the pancreas were diagnosed in the United States and
25,000 patients died of this aggressive malignancy. Recently,
the incidence of pancreatic cancer has been increasing by
300–500 new cases per year. Only 3% of all patients diagnosed with pancreatic cancer can expect to survive 5 years.

The etiology of pancreatic adenocarcinoma and the reason
for the alarming increase in incidence are uncertain.
Epidemiologic studies report cigarette smoking increases the
risk of developing pancreatic cancer threefold. Coffee, alcohol, organic solvents, and petroleum products have been
linked epidemiologically to pancreatic cancer. However, none
of these agents are conclusively causal. Diabetes mellitus
and chronic pancreatitis are complications of the neoplasm
rather than etiologic factors. Since a high-risk group of
patients has not been identified, there is presently no role for
screening programs.

Staging

The current American Joint Committee on Cancer Staging
(AJCC) staging for pancreatic cancer is listed in Table 12-1.

Clinical Presentation

The presenting signs and symptoms of patients with pancreatic cancer are shown in Table 12-2. The most common presenting symptoms are weight loss, pain, and jaundice.

Pain is initially of low intensity, visceral in origin, and poorly localized to the upper abdomen. This pain may mimic peptic ulcer disease. Severe pain localized to the lower thoracic
or upper lumbar area is more characteristic of advanced disease due to invasion of the celiac and superior mesenteric
plexus.

Anorexia and weight loss are common in pancreatic cancer
patients. Weight loss results from malabsorption and
decreased caloric intake. The sudden onset of diabetes mellitus in nonobese adults older than 40 years warrants evaluation for pancreatic cancer.

Painless jaundice as the sole presenting symptom is more
frequently seen with ampullary or distal bile duct tumors but

Table 12-1. AJCC staging of pancreatic cancer

T1	No direct tumor extension beyond pancreas			
T2	Limited extension to duodenum, bile duct, or stomach			
T3	Advanced extension (surgically unresectable)			
N0	Regional lymph nodes negative			
N1	Regional lymph nodes positive			
M0	No distant metastases			
M1	Distant metastases			
Stage I	T1–2	N0	M0	Resectable tumor
Stage II	T3	N0	M0	Locally advanced tumor
Stage III	T1–3	N1	M0	Nodal metastases
Stage IV	T1–3	N0–1	M1	Distant metastases

Table 12-2. Presenting signs and symptoms of patients with carcinoma of the head of the pancreas

Sign or symptom	Percentage of patients
Weight loss	90
Pain	75
Malnutrition	75
Jaundice	70
Anorexia	60
Pruritis	40
Courvoisier's sign	33
Diabetes mellitus	15
Ascites	5
Gastric outlet obstruction	5

can be present with adenocarcinoma of the head or uncinate process of the pancreas. Courvoisier's sign, a palpable gallbladder at presentation, is seen in less than one-third of patients.

Management

An algorithm for the management of pancreatic adenocarcinoma is shown in Fig. 12-1.

PREOPERATIVE EVALUATION

Once the suspicion of pancreatic cancer is raised, radiologic confirmation should be attempted. Several large reviews of pancreatic cancer note delays in diagnosis of greater than 2 months from the onset of symptoms in the majority of patients. Ultrasound should be the initial diagnostic test in the jaundiced patient to confirm extrahepatic biliary ductal dilatation and to assess the pancreatic head and liver.

Computed tomography (CT) remains the test of choice to evaluate the extent of disease and to assess tumor resectabil-

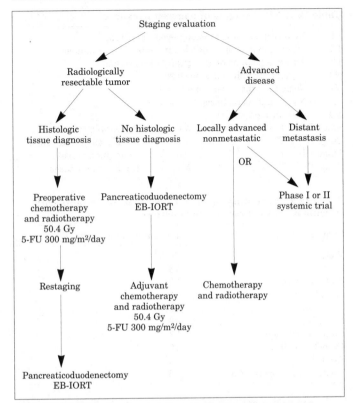

Fig. 12-1. Algorithm for the management of pancreatic carcinoma. (EB-IORT = electron beam intraoperative radiotherapy; 5-FU = 5-fluorouracil.)

ity. Thin-section CT scanning through the pancreas with an IV bolus injection of contrast can delineate the pancreatic mass, the relationship of the tumor to the superior mesenteric artery and vein and to the celiac axis, the patency of the portal vein, and the presence of distant metastatic disease. At the University of Texas M. D. Anderson Cancer Center, thin-section CT scanning correctly makes the diagnosis of pancreatic cancer in 95% of patients. Furthermore, 86% of patients deemed resectable by thin-section contrast-enhanced CT scanning have proved to be resectable at laparotomy.

Endoscopic retrograde cholangiopancreatography (ERCP) is used to differentiate choledocholithiasis from malignant obstruction of the distal common bile duct when a mass is not seen on CT. We do not routinely use ERCP in the diagnostic evaluation of the patient with a potentially resectable pancreatic neoplasm.

Angiography has been used to demonstrate encasement of

the celiac or mesenteric vessels; however, this information is readily obtained by thin-section contrast-enhanced CT scan. Currently, the only indication for routine angiography in the work-up of these patients is to exclude the possibility of aberrant arterial anatomy. This information prevents iatrogenic arterial injury of a replaced right hepatic artery. At M. D. Anderson, angiography is used in the evaluation of pancreatic carcinoma patients operated on prior to referral in whom dissection is often more difficult.

Percutaneous CT-guided needle biopsy of pancreatic neoplasms is an effective method of obtaining cytologic confirmation of the diagnosis. The possibility of shedding cancer cells into the peritoneal cavity during this procedure is theoretic. A study at M. D. Anderson examining peritoneal cytology after percutaneous fine-needle aspiration biopsy has documented the presence of tumor-positive peritoneal cytology in two of 30 patients. The significance of this finding is uncertain: One of the two patients continues to be disease-free 12 months after operation. Percutaneous needle biopsy should be considered in cases where pretreatment cytologic confirmation of the diagnosis is important, such as in patients being considered for preoperative multimodality therapy as part of a clinical trial.

Historically, preoperative biliary tract drainage was done in an attempt to lower the serum bilirubin level. It was believed that this approach would provide benefit by improving immunologic, hepatic, and renal function. However, randomized prospective trials in this country have failed to demonstrate a reduction in operative morbidity or mortality following routine preoperative biliary drainage. Currently, decompression can be recommended only as part of a clinical trial for patients with a total bilirubin level above 20 mg/dl or for patients with symptomatic jaundice who are to be treated with preoperative radiation or chemotherapy.

PATHOLOGY

Approximately 90% of pancreatic exocrine tumors arise from the pancreatic ductules, and 80% of these tumors are adenocarcinoma. Pancreatic adenocarcinomas arise in the head of the gland in 60–70% of cases. The remainder of the tumors are located in the body or tail, or diffusely throughout the pancreas.

Pancreatic adenocarcinoma grossly, on cut section, is firm and white with poorly defined margins. An associated surrounding area of pancreatitis is often present and can make pathologic diagnosis difficult. An intense desmoplastic reaction is identifiable on both gross and microscopic examination. Histologically, identification of mucin production is helpful in diagnosing an adenocarcinoma. Perineural invasion can be identified in the majority of specimens. The degree of differentiation reported on microscopic examination is based on the degree of formation of tubular glandular structures.

SURGICAL TREATMENT

Surgical resection of carcinoma of the pancreatic head remains the only potentially curative treatment modality. Five surgical techniques are used to resect pancreatic cancer: (1) the standard pancreaticoduodenectomy, modified from Whipple's initial description in 1935; (2) pylorus-preserving pancreaticoduodenectomy; (3) total pancreatectomy; (4) regional pancreatectomy; and (5) the M. D. Anderson extended resection.

The current standard of therapy for carcinoma of the head of the pancreas is either the Whipple procedure or the pylorus-preserving pancreaticoduodenectomy. A systematic approach to these operations is necessary to accurately assess resectability and to minimize morbidity and mortality.

Thorough abdominal exploration should precede resection. There is no role for resection of adenocarcinoma in the presence of metastatic disease. Exploration includes intraoperative inspection and palpation of the liver, peritoneal surfaces, para-aortic lymphatics, and root of the mesentery for spread of tumor. The right colon and terminal ileum are fully mobilized and the lesser sac is opened to expose the anterior surface of the pancreas and superior mesenteric vein (SMV) at the inferior border of the pancreas. The gastroepiploic vein or middle colic vein can be followed proximally to permit identification of the SMV. The duodenum is mobilized (Kocher's maneuver) until the vena cava and renal veins are visualized. The relationship of the tumor to the superior mesenteric artery (SMA) is then assessed by palpation. Cholecystectomy is performed to facilitate the evaluation and dissection of the structures within the gastroduodenal ligament. At this point the dilated common bile duct is divided proximal to the cystic duct. This maneuver allows identification of the portal vein and its relationship to the pancreas. Careful inspection and palpation of periportal lymph nodes is performed and suspicious nodes are evaluated by frozen-section examination. The hepatic artery is followed proximally to the gastroduodenal artery, which is ligated at its origin. The stomach, or first portion of the duodenum for pylorus preservation, is then divided. Although the common bile duct and proximal gastrointestinal tract have been divided, resection can still be aborted at this point and a double bypass performed.

The proximal jejunum is dissected from its mesentery and divided. The pancreas overlying the SMV-portal vein confluence is divided. Venous branches to the uncinate process and pancreatic head are ligated. Tumors arising from this portion of the pancreas can be adherent to the SMV. The specimen is now attached only to the retroperitoneum and the SMA. To complete the dissection, the SMA is skeletonized to its origin. The tissue dissected from the SMA origin represents the retroperitoneal margin. The surgeon should be aware of two proximal branches from the superior mesenteric artery: the inferior pancreaticoduodenal artery, which is ligated, and the possibility of an aberrant right hepatic artery, which should be preserved.

The concept of pylorus-preserving pancreaticoduodenectomy was introduced by Traverso and Longmire in 1978 in an attempt to eliminate the postgastrectomy syndromes seen after antrectomy. There are sufficient follow-up data available demonstrating that pylorus preservation does not adversely affect local control or survival. This operation technically differs from a standard Whipple procedure only in the preservation of the blood supply to the proximal duodenum. This can be accomplished by carefully preserving the right gastroepiploic arcade after ligation of the right gastroepiploic artery and vein close to their origin. The right gastric artery can be spared in some cases to provide additional blood supply to the duodenum. The most significant morbidity of pylorus preservation is transient gastric stasis. Operative time and blood loss are slightly reduced compared to classic pancreaticoduodenectomy.

Routine total pancreatectomy as definitive therapy for adenocarcinoma of the head of the pancreas has been advocated by some authors. They cite the possible multicentric nature of pancreatic cancer and the avoidance of a pancreatic anastomosis as justification for this approach. However, the incidence of pathologic documentation of multicentricity of pancreatic adenocarcinoma is less than 10% and does not justify the additional operative morbidity and life-long insulin dependence due to total pancreatectomy. The significant operative morbidity and mortality from pancreaticoduodenectomy is historically attributed to pancreaticojejunal anastomotic leak. However, anastomotic complications are rare in centers experienced with this operation. Also, more effective management of pancreatic anastomotic leakage with hyperalimentation, percutaneous drainage, and somatostatin analogue has reduced the magnitude of this problem. Total pancreatectomy is only indicated, in our opinion, if there is tumor at the pancreatic margin on serial frozen sections or if the pancreas is not suitable for an anastomosis.

Regional pancreatectomy includes an extensive retroperitoneal and hepatoduodenal lymph node dissection and sleeve resection of the SMV-portal venous confluence. Superior mesenteric and hepatic arterial resections have also been included by proponents of this more radical approach. The potential oncologic gain of regional pancreatectomy has been limited by increased morbidity and mortality.

Extended resection, the preferred method of resection at M. D. Anderson, includes a standard pancreaticoduodenectomy with antrectomy, a regional lymphadenectomy, and selective inclusion of a venous resection. We believe venous resection should be considered when the lesion has been deemed resectable, the pancreatic neck is divided, and while dissecting the uncinate process from the SMV the tumor is found to be adherent to the posterior-lateral portion of the vein. We believe vein resection is preferable to shaving the tumor from the portal-superior mesenteric venous confluence. In addition, we perform venous resection for any tumor involving the SMV-portal venous confluence as long as the vein has been demonstrated to be patent by preoperative CT. Venous resection is facilitated by ligation of the splenic vein at its junction with the SMV.

Intraoperative decision making in the surgical treatment of pancreatic cancer can challenge the most experienced surgeon. The morbidity and mortality associated with pancreaticoduodenectomy are greater than those seen after other operations. Patients and their families must be informed preoperatively of the required complex postoperative care and potential complications of pancreaticoduodenectomy. This is most critical when there is no preoperative histologic confirmation of the diagnosis. Neoplasms of the pancreatic head can obstruct the pancreatic duct, resulting in pancreatitis, which makes definitive diagnosis difficult. An intraoperative transduodenal biopsy that reveals inflammation does not exclude the possibility of malignancy. Occasionally a surgeon will suspect that a malignancy exists but will be unable to establish radiologic or histologic confirmation. Every large series of pancreatic resections includes a few patients resected for benign disease. The potential morbidity of an unnecessary pancreatic resection is preferred to leaving a potentially curable lesion in situ. Repeated biopsy to obtain histologic confirmation of malignancy is inadvisable due to the risk of pancreatic fistula, pancreatitis, and hemorrhage. Patients should be aware of the potential need to perform a resection without histologic confirmation of malignancy.

An unsuspected pancreatic mass encountered at laparotomy requires thoughtful management. The initial step in the treatment of such a patient involves a thorough search for distant disease and appropriate biopsy. If no metastases are detected, a transduodenal biopsy of the mass should be attempted. A negative biopsy result should not lead to repetitive biopsies; the abdomen should be closed after the pathology that prompted laparotomy is addressed. If the operation was performed for jaundice, a loop cholecystojejunostomy will provide palliation of biliary obstruction and will not interfere with a future pancreatic resection. Pancreaticoduodenectomy without preoperative counseling of the patient and family is not indicated.

SURGICAL RESULTS

Aggressive surgical resection of pancreatic head tumors has come under intense scrutiny, although presently, pancreaticoduodenectomy remains the only procedure capable of curing adenocarcinoma of the pancreatic head. Many physicians have adopted a nonoperative or palliative approach to pancreatic cancer due to the previously reported high operative morbidi-

Table 12-4. Five-year survival, morbidity, and mortality after curative pancreaticoduodenectomy for adenocarcinoma of the pancreatic head

Author	Morbidity (%)	Mortality (%)	Survival (%)
Trede (Mannheim, Germany)	18	0	24
Cameron (Johns Hopkins)	36	2	19
Grace (UCLA)	26	2	13
Geer (Memorial Sloan-Kettering)	27	3	24

Table 12-3. Postoperative complications associated with pancreaticoduodenectomy

Sepsis	13%
Pancreatic fistula	10%
Biliary fistula	5%
Renal failure	13%
Gastrointestinal hemorrhage	10%
Pancreatitis	2%
Cardiac	5%
Myocardial infarction	
Congestive heart failure	
Arrhythmia	
Pulmonary	7%
Infection	
Embolus	

ty and mortality rates associated with the surgical procedure. However, postoperative morbidity rates that were greater than 50% in reports from the late 1960s are now less than 25% in the most recently reported series. The most common complications are listed in Table 12-3. Postoperative mortality rates have also decreased, from a high of greater than 20% in the early series to as low as 3% in the most recent reviews.

Despite the improvement in morbidity and mortality, there has been little change in long-term patient survival. The 5-year survival rate following curative pancreaticoduodenectomy for carcinoma of the pancreatic head remains less than 25%, with a median survival of 20 months (Table 12-4).

Body and tail tumors are often considered to have a poorer prognosis than lesions of the pancreatic head, as these tumors frequently go undetected until they are locally advanced or metastatic. A Mayo Clinic report suggests that the rare patient with body or tail lesions amenable to resection for cure have similiar long-term survival rates to patients who have undergone complete resection of the more common carcinoma of the pancreatic head. At M. D. Anderson, we have resected one adenocarcinoma of the pancreatic body over the past 36 months, during which time we performed 50 pancreaticoduodenectomies for adenocarcinoma of the pancreatic head.

At M. D. Anderson we advocate an aggressive surgical

approach in combination with multimodality therapy for patients with localized pancreatic head lesions. Assuming a nonoperative approach to lesions of the pancreatic head would eliminate the opportunity to cure patients with tumors of the ampulla of Vater and distal common bile duct, which have a better prognosis. These lesions are usually indistinguishable preoperatively from adenocarcinoma of the pancreatic head.

ADJUVANT THERAPY

Since the 5-year survival rate of patients with resected pancreatic cancer is poor, it is imperative to examine the potential benefit of adjuvant therapy in this disease. Autopsy series indicate that 85% of patients will experience recurrences in the field of resection. Furthermore, approximately 70% of patients will have metastasis to the liver. Therefore, adjuvant therapy must address the possibility of distant disease (chemotherapy) as well as the possibility of local-regional recurrence (radiotherapy). The initial studies examining adjuvant therapy of pancreatic cancer were based on results from studies on patients with advanced disease.

Most widely used chemotherapeutic agents have limited activity against pancreatic cancer. 5-fluorouracil (5-FU) is the only active agent, and its effect is marginal. Most studies report an overall response of 15–28% in patients with advanced disease. No combination chemotherapeutic regimen has been found to be more effective than 5-FU alone. Studies of 5-FU have demonstrated the ability of this agent to act as a radiosensitizer—that is, to improve tumor responses to radiotherapy.

External beam radiotherapy is beneficial in the treatment of patients with unresectable pancreatic cancer. Combined 5-FU and radiation therapy have been reported to significantly increase survival in patients with locally advanced disease. In a study at the Mayo Clinic patients with unresectable pancreatic cancer were randomized to receive high-dose, postoperative radiotherapy (60 Gy) alone; high-dose, postoperative radiotherapy (60 Gy) plus concomitant 5-FU; or standard-dose, postoperative radiotherapy (40 Gy) and 5-FU. Patients receiving 5-FU and radiotherapy experienced a significant survival advantage compared with patients who received radiotherapy alone. Patients who received the higher dose of radiotherapy did not derive an additional survival advantage.

The combination of postoperative external beam radiotherapy and concomitant 5-FU as adjuvant therapy after resection was investigated by the Gastrointestinal Tumor Study Group (GITSG). Patients were randomized to receive surgery alone or surgery followed by radiotherapy (40 Gy delivered in two 20-Gy courses) and 5-FU (500 mg/m^2 by IV bolus delivered daily for the initial 3 days of each radiotherapy course and continued weekly for 2 years). Median survival was 20 months in the group that received adjuvant therapy; this was significantly longer than the 11-month median survival seen in patients treated with surgery alone.

Preoperative chemoradiation has been advocated to avoid treatment delay and to ensure that all resected patients receive multimodality therapy. In the GITSG study of post-operative adjuvant therapy, 24% of the patients had a delay in the initiation of adjuvant therapy because of prolonged recovery following pancreatic resection. Other potential benefits of preoperative chemoradiation include the opportunity to increase the efficacy of radiotherapy by delivering treatment to well-oxygenated cells not made hypoxic by surgical dissection and the potential for downstaging of tumors initially considered unresectable. Patients with unresectable tumors who experience significant responses to treatment would thus become candidates for potentially curative resection. Currently this approach is being studied prospectively at M. D. Anderson. Our preliminary experience with preoperative radiotherapy and 5-FU has demonstrated a significant histologic treatment effect in all resected specimens. Preoperative chemoradiation has not increased operative morbidity or mortality.

Electron beam intraoperative radiotherapy (EB-IORT) can be used to boost the radiation dose to the pancreatic bed and surrounding high-risk lymph node basins. EB-IORT for locally advanced unresectable tumors has been reported to reduce symptoms from advanced disease and prolong survival. A National Cancer Institute controlled prospective trial of adjuvant radiotherapy for pancreatic cancer examined the benefit of IORT (20 Gy) in addition to external beam radiotherapy (50 Gy) following resection. Although IORT did not have an impact on overall survival in this small study, patients who received IORT experienced prolonged disease-free survival and improved local control. At M. D. Anderson complications are not increased in patients undergoing resection and EB-IORT.

The current M. D. Anderson approach to patients with resectable pancreatic cancer is preoperative chemoradiation (5-FU and 50.4 Gy external beam radiotherapy), followed by en bloc resection of the tumor and draining lymph nodes and EB-IORT (10 Gy) to the pancreatic bed. Patients with a microscopic positive margin at the SMA origin on frozen section receive 15 Gy of EB-IORT following resection (Fig. 12-2).

SURVEILLANCE

Patients should be seen at 3-month intervals following curative resection of pancreatic adenocarcinoma. Follow-up visits should include a thorough history and physical examination, a complete blood count, serum electrolyte determination, and liver function tests. A chest x-ray and abdominal CT should be obtained at 6- to 12-month intervals, or earlier if symptoms develop.

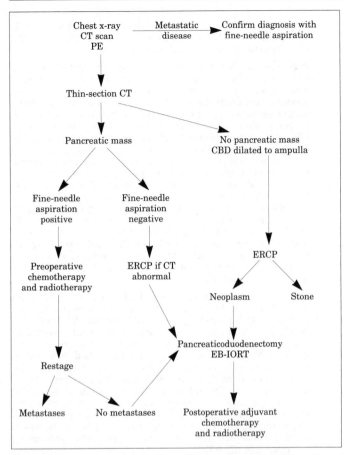

Fig. 12-2. Management of the patient with jaundice and extrahepatic ductal dilatation at M. D. Anderson. (PE = physical examination; CBD = common bile duct; ERCP = endoscopic retrograde cholangiopancreatography; EB-IORT = electron beam intraoperative radiotherapy.)

There have been numerous attempts to identify a tumor marker for pancreatic cancer. The most frequently measured antigens, CEA, CA 19-9, and pancreatic-oncofetal antigen (POA), have not been shown to predict recurrence following resection of pancreatic adenocarcinoma.

Postoperatively, all patients receive some form of enteral nutritional supplementation via a jejunostomy tube for at least 6 weeks. Nutritional status should be carefully assessed at each clinic visit, including a serum albumin level, dietary history, and evaluation of general body habitus.

Patients must also be evaluated for signs of malabsorption resulting from pancreatic enzyme insufficiency. This is readily treatable with pancreatic enzyme replacement.

PALLIATION

Patients with unresectable or recurrent pancreatic cancer frequently require palliative treatment for biliary obstruction, gastric outlet obstruction, and pain. Historically, palliation for these patients was undertaken at laparotomy after determining that a tumor was unresectable. Operative biliary bypass, gastric bypass, and splanchnicectomy are proven, effective methods of achieving palliation. However, with the advent of improved diagnostic techniques, unresectability can often be determined prior to laparotomy. Biliary diversion can then be achieved either endoscopically or percutaneously. Gastric outlet obstruction occurs in only 10–15% of patients and is often a preterminal event that does not mandate operative correction. CT-guided alcohol splanchnicectomy is an effective option in the palliation of pain for the occasional patient unresponsive to narcotics. Therefore the surgeon can avoid laparotomy in most patients with limited life expectancy.

Biliary Obstruction

Jaundice is a common presenting symptom in patients who have carcinoma of the head of the pancreas. Prolonged biliary obstruction leads to coagulopathy, hepatic dysfunction, malabsorption, and altered bile salt metabolism. Patients often complain of severe, disabling pruritis. Relief of biliary obstruction results in significant palliation of these problems and improvement in overall patient well being. It is helpful to group pancreatic cancer patients into four separate categories when considering operative versus nonoperative biliary decompression:

1. Patients in poor health who would not tolerate laparotomy and are clearly best served by nonoperative palliative measures.

2. Patients with concomitant gastric outlet obstruction who require laparotomy for palliation of that symptom; the benefit of avoiding the complications of a stent or transhepatic drain warrants the limited additional morbidity of adding an operative biliary bypass.

3. Patients undergoing operation for resection but who are found to have unsuspected unresectable disease; these patients are also best served by an operative biliary bypass.

4. Patients who have unresectable pancreatic cancer on diagnostic evaluation and are an acceptable medical risk for laparotomy; these patients are candidates for operative or nonoperative management, depending on the judgment of the surgeon and the expertise of the available endoscopist or invasive radiologist. At M. D. Anderson these patients are

successfully managed with nonoperative palliative measures.

Surgical biliary diversion can be accomplished by either choledochoenteric or cholecystoenteric bypass. A Roux limb requires an additional anastomosis and longer operative time compared to using a simple loop of small bowel for biliary bypass. Roux reconstruction is required when an unresectable tumor prevents a loop from reaching the right upper quadrant without tension. Although the possibility of recurrent obstruction due to tumor progression exists after choledochoduodenostomy, this procedure is a simple and viable option. Most authorities advocate either loop choledochojejunostomy or cholecystojejunostomy for surgical palliation of malignant biliary obstruction. Cholecystojejunostomy has the advantage of being simple to perform; however, the possibility of recurrent biliary obstruction after this procedure also exists. The advantage of choledochojejunostomy is that it provides a more proximal biliary anastomosis and therefore obstruction by progressive extension of tumor is less likely. The high operative mortality and short median survival associated with each procedure are due to the aggressive nature of the malignancy rather than the technique used. The choice of surgical option ultimately depends on local tumor considerations and the surgeon's experience.

Nonoperative palliative biliary decompression can be accomplished endoscopically or percutaneously. Experienced endoscopists report a success rate greater than 90%. In randomized studies comparing endoscopic biliary decompression with conventional surgical bypass, the procedures have resulted in identical survival and relief of jaundice. Total hospital stay is also similar for the two procedures because of the need for occasional readmissions to change stents after endoscopic decompression. Percutaneous transhepatic biliary drainage has provided successful palliation in 80–90% of patients. External catheters are being replaced by newer indwelling endoprostheses, which are associated with a lower rate of infectious complications. Hemobilia has been seen in up to 12% of percutaneously treated patients. Although endoscopic biliary decompression is the preferred method of nonoperative palliation, the choice of technique depends on the expertise available.

Gastric Outlet Obstruction

Patients with pancreatic cancer rarely present with duodenal obstruction. Furthermore, less than 15% of patients will require operative correction of gastric outlet obstruction prior to death. Clearly, patients with unresectable disease and gastric outlet obstruction require a gastrojejunostomy for palliation. Controversy exists as to whether all patients undergoing palliative laparotomy should undergo prophylactic gastroenterostomy. Complications resulting from the additional operative time and additional anastomosis are minimal. However, the incidence of subsequent duodenal obstruction in asymptomatic patients who undergo only biliary bypass is low. In addition, the development of gastric outlet obstruction is often a preterminal event not requiring treatment. At M. D. Anderson patients with symptoms of duodenal obstruction or operative or radiographic evidence of impending gastric outlet obstruction undergo palliative gastrojejunostomy at the time of biliary bypass.

Pancreatic Pain

Pain is the most disabling symptom of advanced pancreatic carcinoma. It occurs in the majority of patients during the course of their disease. Sophisticated surgical neurotomies have been described but require prolonged operative time and are rarely used today. Pancreaticojejunostomy has been advocated by some for relief of pain caused by proximal pancreatic duct obstruction; however, acceptance of this extensive and potentially morbid procedure has been limited.

Chemical splanchnicectomy is a much simpler approach and has been reported to provide pain relief in up to 80% of patients. This procedure can be performed surgically or percutaneously with CT guidance by injection of phenol and alcohol around the celiac axis. Limited morbidity is associated with this procedure. A randomized prospective trial of intraoperative celiac plexus alcohol injection versus placebo injection in patients with unresectable tumors is underway at The Johns Hopkins Hospital. This study should better define the role of chemical splanchnicectomy in the management of patients with pain from advanced pancreatic cancer.

Cystic Neoplasms

Cystic neoplasms of the pancreas account for approximately 1% of all pancreatic cancers and 10% of all pancreatic cystic lesions. Classically, these tumors are large, located in the distal pancreas, and affect women three times more frequently than men. The diagnosis of a cystic neoplasm must be considered in patients with radiographic evidence of a pancreatic cyst and no prior symptoms or history of pancreatitis.

Cystic neoplams with a serous epithelial lining (serous cystadenoma) have no malignant potential. When a mucinous epithelial lining is present in the cyst wall, the lesion is frankly malignant (mucinous cystadenocarcinoma) or premalignant (mucinous cystic neoplasm).

It is often impossible to distinguish malignant from benign cystic neoplasms preoperatively or intraoperatively, as the epithelial lining is often incomplete. Therefore all cystic neoplasms should be resected for potential cure. Patients with malignant cystic neoplasms who undergo complete resection have a 40–60% 5-year survival rate.

Selected References

Crist DW, Sitzman JV, Cameron JL. Improved hospital morbidity, mortality, and survival after the Whipple procedure. *Ann Surg* 206: 358, 1987.

Dalton RR, Sarr MG, van Heerden JA. Carcinoma of the body and tail of the pancreas: Is curative resection justified? *Surgery* 111:489, 1992.

Fortner JG. Regional pancreatectomy for cancer of the pancreas, ampulla, and other related sites. *Ann Surg* 199:418, 1984

Geer RJ, Brennan MF. Prognostic indicators for survival after resection of pancreatic adenocarcinoma. *Am J Surg* 165:68, 1993.

Grace PA, Pitt HA, Tompkins RK, et al. Decreased morbidity and mortality after pancreatoduodenectomy. *Am J Surg* 151:141, 1986.

Hatfield ARW, Tobias R, Terblanche J, et al. Preoperative external biliary drainage in obstructive jaundice: A prospective controlled trial. *Lancet* 2:896, 1982.

Howard JM, Jordan GL, Reber HA (eds). *Surgical Diseases of the Pancreas.* Philadelphia: Lea & Febiger, 1987.

Itani KM, Coleman RE, Akwari OE, et al. Pylorus-preserving pancreaticoduodenectomy: A clinical and physiologic appraisal. *Ann Surg* 204:655, 1986.

Kalser MH, Ellenberg SS. Pancreatic cancer, adjuvant combined radiation and chemotherapy following curative resection. *Arch Surg* 120:899, 1985.

Lillemoe KD, Sauter PK, Pitt HA, et al. Current status of surgical palliation of periampullary carcinoma. *Surg Gynecol Obstet* 176:1, 1993.

Moertel CG, Frytak S, Hahn RG, et al. Therapy of locally unresectable pancreatic carcinoma: A randomized comparison of high dose (6000 rads) radiation alone, moderate dose radiation and 5-fluorouracil. *Cancer* 48:1705, 1981.

Moosa AR, Scott MH, Lavelle-Jones M. The place of total and extended total pancreatectomy in pancreatic cancer. *World J Surg* 8:895, 1984.

Shepherd HA, Royle G, Ross APR. Endoscopic biliary endoprosthesis in the palliation of malignant obstruction of the distal common bile duct: A randomized trial. *Br J Surg* 75:1166, 1988.

Sindelar WF, Kinsella TJ. Randomized trial of intraoperative radiotherapy in resected carcinoma of the pancreas. *Radiat Oncol Biol Physiol* 12:148, 1986.

Trede M, Schwall G, Saeger H. Survival after pancreaticoduodenectomy. 118 consecutive resections without an operative mortality. *Ann Surg* 211:447, 1990.

Warshaw AL, Compton CC, Lewandrowski K, et al. Cystic tumors of the pancreas. *Ann Surg* 212:432, 1990.

Warshaw AL, Swanson RS. Pancreatic cancer in 1988. *Ann Surg* 208:541, 1988.

Pancreatic Endocrine Tumors and Multiple Endocrine Neoplasia

Douglas S. Tyler

Overview

Pancreatic endocrine tumors have a prevalence of approximately one case per 200,000 population in clinical studies but are found in almost one in 100 unselected autopsy cases. The tumors tend to arise in the islet cells of the pancreas but can also be located in the small bowel, especially the duodenum, and the adrenal glands. Although the islet cells are thought to be of neural crest origin, more recent studies suggest they may be of endodermal origin.

Islet cell tumors are usually divided into tumors that are functioning and those that are nonfunctioning. Over 75% of the islet cell tumors diagnosed clinically are functioning and frequently secrete more than one hormone. The tumors are considered entopic if they produce hormones or peptides usually found within the pancreas (e.g., insulinomas, glucagonomas, somatostatinomas, and PPomas) or ectopic if the hormones or peptides are not native to the normal pancreas (e.g., gastrinomas, VIPomas, GRFomas, and neurotensinomas). An overview of the characteristics of pancreatic endocrine tumors is shown in Table 13-1.

The diagnosis of pancreatic endocrine tumors is usually made by the recognition of the clinical syndrome caused by excess hormone production. However, PPomas and nonfunctioning islet cell tumors do not secrete hormones that produce clinical syndromes. As a result, these two tumors present like ductal adenocarcinoma of the pancreas.

Histologic diagnosis of the islet cell tumor can be obtained with computed tomography (CT)-guided fine-needle aspiration. Resectability is defined by absence of metastatic disease and no invasion of the superior mesenteric or hepatic arteries. In general, islet cell tumors are more indolent than ductal adenocarcinoma and carry a better prognosis.

Gastrinoma: Zollinger-Ellison Syndrome

In 1955 Zollinger and Ellison described a syndrome characterized by a severe atypical form of peptic ulceration, gastric hypersecretion, gastric hyperacidity, and a non–insulin-producing islet cell tumor of the pancreas. They theorized that a humoral factor arising from the tumor was responsible for the syndrome. Several years later, the hormone gastrin was discovered and found to be the underlying cause of the syndrome.

Table 13-1. Characteristics of pancreatic endocrine neoplasms

Tumor name	Main hormone	Cell type	Syndrome	Percentage malignant	Main pancreatic location	Extrapancreatic locations	Percentage associated with MEN-I
Gastrinoma	Gastrin	D	Peptic ulcers Diarrhea	60–90	Head	Duodenum (30–40%) Other (10–20%)	25
Insulinoma	Insulin	B	Hypoglycemia	10–15	Body, tail	Rare	10
VIPoma	Vasoactive intestinal peptide	H	Watery diarrhea Hypokalemia	60–80	Body, tail	Adrenal (10%)	Rare
Glucagonoma	Glucagon	A	Hyperglycemia Dermatitis	60–70	Body, tail	Rare	Rare
Somatostatinoma	Somatostatin	D	Hyperglycemia Steatorrhea Gallstones	90	Head	Proximal intestine (44%)	Never
GRFoma	Growth hormone releasing peptide		Acromegaly	30		Lung (53%) Intestine (10%) Other (7%)	Rare
PPoma	Pancreatic polypeptide	PP	None	>60	Head	Rare	Occasional
Nonfunctioning	None		None	>60	Head	Rare	

MEN-I = multiple endocrine neoplasia type I syndrome.

Table 13-2. Clinical situations in which Zollinger-Ellison syndrome should be suspected and screened for

Recurrent peptic ulcers
Failure of peptic ulcer to heal on medical therapy
Postoperative peptic ulcer
Postbulbar peptic ulcer
Multiple upper gastrointestinal ulcers
Family history of peptic ulcer disease
Peptic ulcer occurring with diarrhea
Diarrhea that persists with no clear etiology
Family history of known MEN-I, pancreatic islet tumor, pituitary
   adenoma, or parathyroid adenoma
Presence of another pancreatic endocrine tumor
Prominent gastric or duodenal rugal folds associated with ulcer
   disease

MEN-I = multiple endocrine neoplasia type I syndrome.

EPIDEMIOLOGY

Less than 0.1% of patients with duodenal ulcer disease and about 2% of patients with recurrent ulcers after appropriate medical therapy will have a gastrinoma. Approximately 75% of gastrinomas occur sporadically; the remaining 25% are associated with the multiple endocrine neoplasia type I syndrome (MEN-I). The mean age at onset of symptoms is 60 years, and about 60% of those diagnosed with Zollinger-Ellison syndrome are male. Gastrinomas that occur as part of MEN-I are more often benign, multicentric, and extrapancreatic and occur at an earlier age than sporadic gastrinomas.

CLINICAL PRESENTATION

High levels of gastrin stimulate the gastric parietal cells to secrete a large volume of gastric acid, which not only leads to the severe ulcer disease but also injures the small-bowel mucosa well past the ligament of Treitz, resulting in various degrees of malabsorption. Profuse watery diarrhea occurs in up to 50% of patients due to the combination of acid hypersecretion and small-bowel mucosal injury. In addition to secreting gastrin, the majority of gastrinomas also secrete at least one other peptide hormone, such as insulin, pancreatic polypeptide (PP), or glucagon.

The clinical manifestations of gastrinomas are related predominantly to the elevated levels of gastrin. Ninety percent of patients have endoscopically documented ulcerations of the upper gastrointestinal (GI) tract. Most of these ulcers are accompanied by abdominal pain, with bleeding occurring in 30–50% and perforation occurring in 5–10%. As many as 50% will have secretory diarrhea, with 10% having it as their only manifestation of the syndrome. Patients with Zollinger-Ellison syndrome are often initially misdiagnosed, as shown by the fact that the mean duration of symptoms before diagnosis is more than 6 years. Clinical situations in which Zollinger-Ellison syndrome should be suspected are listed in Table 13-2.

Table 13-3. Prognosis in patients with Zollinger-Ellison syndrome

Clinical situation	No. of patients	5-year survival (%)	10-year survival (%)
All patients	271	63.5	51.8
No tumor found at exploration	45	94.2	87.2
Tumor resected	114	83.6	72.9
Tumor incompletely resected	32	71.0	20.0
Unresectable	67	36.3	—
MEN-I present	108	76.2	68.7
MEN-I absent	274	61.2	56.2

MEN-I = multiple endocrine neoplasia type I syndrome.

BIOCHEMICAL DIAGNOSIS

The diagnosis of gastrinoma requires confirmation with laboratory studies. A fasting serum gastrin measurement is the first test obtained. A level over 1,000 pg/ml is usually diagnostic of a gastrinoma and is seen in about 30% of patients. The majority of patients with gastrinomas have fasting gastrin levels in the 200–1,000 pg/ml range (normal 100–200 pg/ml). Typically, patients with gastrinomas have a basal acid output of greater than 15 mEq/hour or greater than 5 mEq/hour if they have had a previous ulcer operation aimed at reducing gastric acid secretion. A basal acid output–maximal acid output ratio greater than 0.6 also helps support the diagnosis of gastrinoma.

Provocative testing using the secretin stimulation test helps confirm the diagnosis in patients with borderline gastrin elevation and gastric acid secretion. After an overnight fast, the patient is given 2 units of secretin per kilogram of body weight IV. An increase in the serum level of gastrin by more than 200 pg/ml over baseline levels is diagnostic of gastrinoma. Patients with either antral G-cell hyperplasia or hypertrophy do not respond to secretin.

TUMOR LOCALIZATION

Tumor localization has become increasingly important in recent years with the demonstration that resection of gastrinomas is associated with an excellent prognosis and is frequently curative (Table 13-3). In addition, identification of metastatic disease prior to surgery can save a patient an unnecessary exploration. A number of tests have been used for the localization of gastrinomas preoperatively, including CT scans, magnetic resonance imaging (MRI), abdominal ultrasound, selective visceral angiography, selective venous sampling of portal venous tributaries, intra-arterial secretin with hepatic venous sampling for gastrin, endoscopy, and endoscopic ultrasound. CT scanning with thin sections and IV bolus contrast is usually the initial imaging study of choice as it has the highest overall sensitivity (50%) and specificity (95%) in localizing primary gastrinomas and is approximately equal to MRI scanning in identifying metastatic gastrinoma. If the location of the tumor is still in question after CT, visceral angiography should be performed. Studies suggest that the sensitivity and specificity of visceral angiography is close to if not better than with CT scanning. Both of these studies are good at excluding metastatic disease. Endoscopy rarely identifies gastrinomas, although endoscopic ultrasound holds some promise.

The use of venous sampling to localize gastrinomas is controversial. In the hands of an experienced radiologist, this test is able to localize gastrinomas about 90% of the time. However, while venous sampling is as sensitive as CT and angiography in tumor localization, it is not as specific. Since most gastrinomas are found in the gastrinoma triangle (an anatomic area bound by the neck of the pancreas medially, the junction of the second and third portion of the duodenum inferiorly, and the junction of the cystic duct and common bile duct superiorly), many surgeons think venous sampling provides only information that is already known. Another localizing study is the intra-arterial secretin test with hepatic venous sampling for gastrin. This test can be easily performed during the patient's localizing arteriogram.

TREATMENT

Once the diagnosis of gastrinoma is made, the first step is to control the gastric acid hypersecretion. Prior to the advent of H_2-blockers, total gastrectomy was the treatment of choice because tumor localization could be achieved only about 5% of the time. Although it carried significant morbidity and mortality rates, total gastrectomy was extremely effective in preventing the acid-related complications of gastrinomas. Within the last 15–20 years, the development of powerful antisecretory agents along with improved methods of tumor localization have significantly altered the approach to patients with gastrinomas.

H_2-blockers initially control acid secretion in most patients with gastrinomas, but over time most of these individuals require increasing dosages. In addition, anywhere from 0 to 65% of patients will fail to respond to this form of medical therapy (depending on the series). On the other hand, omeprazole, a gastric proton pump inhibitor, is associated with a lower failure rate (0–7.5%) and a more convenient dosing schedule. The long-term side effects of omeprazole are not clear. As more experience is gained with omeprazole, it is becoming increasingly the drug of first choice. Octreotide acetate, the somatostatin analogue, may also be useful in decreasing the release of gastrin and other peptide hormones from gastrinomas.

Total gastrectomy is now reserved for patients with unresectable tumors who are noncompliant with medical therapy or do not have access to routine follow-up. Other ulcer operations designed to reduce acid secretion, such as a highly selective vagotomy, are reserved for patients who become refractory to medical management and have either an unresectable tumor or one that cannot be located.

In a patient with a sporadic gastrinoma, surgical exploration with attempted curative resection should follow localization studies regardless of whether the tumor is identified preoperatively. Since as many as 10–40% of tumors may not be localized prior to surgery, a standardized approach to exploration needs to be undertaken. With this approach, a gastrinoma can be identified in approximately 30–50% of patients with negative preoperative localizing studies. The exploration should be done through a bilateral subcostal incision. Approximately 40% of the tumors will be in the duodenum, another 40% will be found superficially on or around the pancreas, and about 10–15% will be within the substance of the pancreas. Therefore complete mobilization of the pancreas to allow inspection and palpation of the gland is required. Any lymph node or suspicious mass should be evaluated by frozen-section examination. Intraoperative ultrasound may be helpful in identifying intrapancreatic lesions. If no tumor is identified, a longitudinal duodenotomy should be made in the second portion of the duodenum. Intraoperative endoscopy with transillumination of the duodenal wall may be done to identify duodenal gastrinomas prior to making the duodenotomy. Once the duodenum is opened, careful bimanual examination of the bowel wall, along with its eversion, helps identify duodenal gastrinomas, which are frequently located submucosally. When the tumor is small (<2 cm), duodenal gastrinomas can be resected with a small margin of normal tissue, while pancreatic gastrinomas are usually enucleated. Larger tumors usually require some form of pancreatic resection such as a pancreaticoduodenectomy or distal pancreatectomy.

Despite extensive preoperative localizing studies and careful surgical exploration, up to one-third of patients have no tumor identified at laparotomy. "Blind" pancreatic resection is not recommended. If the patient's acid hypersecretion is well controlled medically, then no further intraoperative treatment needs to be done. Patients with Zollinger-Ellison syndrome in whom no tumor is found have an excellent prognosis, with 5- and 10-year survival rates of more than 94% and 87%, respectively (see Table 13-3). If gastric hypersecretion is a problem despite medical management or the patient is receiving high dosages of H_2-blockers, consideration should be given to performing a highly selective vagotomy. Total gastrectomy should be considered in patients who have had previous life-threatening complications from their ulcer disease despite appropriate medical management.

The role of surgery in patients with Zollinger-Ellison syndrome and MEN-I is more controversial. Resection of gastrinomas in patients with MEN-I rarely results in normal serum gastrin levels, suggesting that the probability of curing these patients with surgery is extremely low. As a result, many authorities have recommended that patients with MEN-I and gastrinomas do not undergo exploration. Other groups feel that resection of localized tumors may help reduce the risk of metastatic disease; therefore they recommend that patients with MEN-I undergo localizing studies and that exploration be carried out only if the gastrinoma is visualized. The prognosis for patients with Zollinger-Ellison syndrome based on surgical outcome is shown in Table 13-3.

METASTATIC DISEASE

Now that medical treatment of gastric acid hypersecretion in Zollinger-Ellison syndrome is so effective, patients rarely die from complications related to peptic ulcer disease. As a result, patients live longer, only to die from metastatic disease. The larger series of gastrinoma patients report a 50–90% incidence of metastatic disease. A number of therapeutic options exist for patients with advanced disease depending on their symptoms. Chemotherapy results have been inconsistent. The most promising regimen appears to be a combination of streptozocin and 5-fluorouracil, with or without doxorubicin; this combination gives response rates of 50–70%. Complete responders to chemotherapy are rare no matter what agents are used. The somatostatin analogues appear effective in controlling symptoms of gastrinomas but show a disappointing objective tumor response rate of 10–20%. Interferon has also been used and shown some early promising results in patients refractory to chemotherapy.

Patients with isolated liver metastases have been treated with hepatic artery embolization, which may help decrease the size of these usually well-vascularized tumors. The role of local treatments for metastatic disease has been questioned in view of the finding that 12% of patients with liver metastases also have bone metastases. Tumor debulking surgery has been advocated by some as a method of prolonging life expectancy; however, those in whom gross tumor is left behind do not benefit from debulking.

Insulinomas

EPIDEMIOLOGY

In most series, insulinomas are the most common islet cell tumors of the pancreas, with a reported incidence of 0.8–0.9 cases per 1 million population per year. These tumors occur slightly more often in women than in men. The average age at presentation is between 40 and 50 years.

CLINICAL PRESENTATION

The clinical symptoms of insulinomas are due to the hypoglycemia induced by excess insulin secretion. A list of the

Table 13-4. Symptoms associated with insulinomas and their frequency

Symptoms	Frequency (%)
Neuroglycopenic symptoms	
Visual disturbances	59
Confusion	51
Altered consciousness	38
Weakness	32
Seizures	23
Symptoms related to hypoglycemic catecholamine release	
Sweating	43
Tremulousness	23
Tachycardia	23

common symptoms and their frequency is shown in Table 13-4. GI symptoms including hunger, nausea, weight gain, and vomiting are also reported occasionally.

BIOCHEMICAL DIAGNOSIS

The original diagnostic criteria for an insulinoma is known as Whipple's triad and was proposed by Whipple, who initially described the syndrome. This triad consists of (1) symptoms of hypoglycemia at fasting, (2) documentation of blood glucose levels less than 50 mg/dl, and (3) relief of symptoms following administration of glucose. However, Whipple's triad has proven not to be very specific.

The most reliable method of diagnosing an insulinoma is the provocative test of fasting. Blood glucose and insulin levels are measured every 4–6 hours during the fast. Eighty percent of patients with insulinoma become symptomatic within 24 hours of starting the fast, and almost all will be symptomatic if the fast is continued for 72 hours. The presence of an elevated insulin level higher than 6 μU/ml along with concurrent hypoglycemia and an insulin-glucose ratio greater than 0.3 confirm the diagnosis. Measurement of the beta-cell products C-peptide and proinsulin is important because they both are usually elevated in patients with insulinoma. Patients who are surreptitiously administering insulin to themselves will usually have low levels of C-peptide and proinsulin. Patients taking oral hypoglycemics will have normal or elevated levels of C-peptide and proinsulin, so differentiation from an insulinoma is made by measurement of plasma levels of sulfonylureas.

TUMOR LOCALIZATION

Once the diagnosis is confirmed, localization studies are carried out. The majority of insulinomas are 10–15 mm in diameter and are evenly distributed throughout the pancreas. About 10% of insulinomas are multicentric. There are no histologic criteria of malignancy for insulinomas; therefore the diagnosis of a malignant tumor is based on the demonstration of metatstatic disease, which is noted in 10% of cases. Dynamic CT scanning is usually the first localizing study done because it can detect about two-thirds of the primary tumors and the majority of metastatic lesions. When no tumor is seen with the CT scan, visceral angiography with digital subtraction techniques is successful in visualizing lesions about 60–90% of the time. Selective portal venous sampling is reserved mainly for patients whose tumors cannot be visualized with CT or angiography. Portal venous sampling is able to define the general area of the tumor in 90% of patients overall and about 75% of patients in whom other localizing tests are negative.

TREATMENT

When localization is accomplished, surgical exploration is carried out. Even in the few patients whose tumor is not localized with the above studies, surgical exploration is currently recommended. Many such patients have a small benign tumor that can be identified with intraoperative ultrasound by surgeons experienced in pancreatic surgery.

At exploration, the pancreas must be completely mobilized as described previously for intrapancreatic gastrinomas. Small insulinomas located away from the main pancreatic duct can be enucleated. Small lesions in close proximity to the main pancreatic duct can be enucleated, but this requires the use of intraoperative ultrasound to avoid injury to the duct. Distal pancreatectomy is recommended for small lesions near the pancreatic duct to minimize the risk of a pancreatic fistula. Large lesions in the head of the pancreas may require pancreaticoduodenectomy, while those in the body and tail can be treated with a distal pancreatectomy. Insulinomas are identified about 95% of the time at initial exploration. As with gastrinomas, blind resection of the pancreas is not recommended when no tumor is identified. In experienced hands, a second exploration using intraoperative ultrasound has a greater than 90% chance of identifying and resecting the lesion. If no tumor is identified at the second exploration, then pancreatic biopsy is recommended to rule out beta-cell hyperplasia, a condition that can be treated by subtotal pancreatectomy.

METASTATIC DISEASE

Patients with malignant metastatic disease should be considered for resection of the primary tumor and accessible metastatic lesions. Approximately 65% of patients with malignant tumors will have recurrences at a mean of about 2.8 years. Median disease-free survival is approximately 5 years in patients with malignant insulinoma who undergo curative resection. Although the chances for cure after resection are low in patients with malignant insulinoma, hypoglycemic symptoms may improve in patients whose disease is not well controlled by medical therapy.

Palliation can be achieved with medical therapy as well as surgery. Diazoxide can control the endocrine symptoms of insulinomas in 50–70% of patients by inhibiting the beta-cell's release of insulin. Octreotide controls symptoms in 40–60% of patients. Of the chemotherapeutic agents used for patients with metastatic disease, streptozocin, dacarbazine, and doxorubicin have the best response rates.

VIPoma

EPIDEMIOLOGY

Although not a normal product of pancreatic islet cells, vasoactive intestinal peptide (VIP) can be secreted by islet cell tumors. The syndrome of excessive VIP secretion is associated with watery diarrhea, hypokalemia, and either hypochlorhydria or achlorhydria. First described in association with islet cell tumors in 1958, the syndrome has many names including Verner-Morrison syndrome, pancreatic cholera, and WDHA (watery diarrhea, hypokalemia, and achlorhydria). Subsequently, it has been realized that only 80% of so-called VIPomas are located in the pancreas. Ten percent of the tumors are located elsewhere (retroperitoneum, lung, or esophagus) and 10% of the cases are due to islet cell hyperplasia. To date, only about 200 well-documented cases of VIPoma have been described, and in most cases the tumor is malignant.

CLINICAL PRESENTATION

Patients usually present with excessive secretory diarrhea that is aggravated by oral food intake and averages 3–5 liters per day. The patients become hypokalemic secondary to fecal potassium loss. The presence of a VIPoma is confirmed by demonstrating an elevated serum VIP level in the setting of secretory diarrhea. Interestingly, VIP may not be responsible for all the symptoms associated with the syndrome: Peptide histadine-isoleucine and prostaglandins have been implicated as contributing factors in some studies.

TUMOR LOCALIZATION

Preoperative localization should include chest and abdominal CT scans followed by mesenteric arteriography if the tumor location is still in question.

TREATMENT

Preoperative preparation should include adequate rehydration and correction of electrolyte imbalances. Octreotide is the preferred drug to use preoperatively to help decrease circulating VIP and help control the diarrhea. Steroids and indomethacin also may be helpful. At exploration, the majority of tumors are located in the distal pancreas and are amenable to a complete resection by a distal pancreatectomy. A careful evaluation of both adrenals is mandatory if no tumor is found in the pancreas. About 50% of the time, metastatic disease is found outside the pancreas at exploration. If curative resection is not possible, then surgical debulking is often indicated to help ease the clinical symptoms.

Streptozocin and interferon are currently the most active chemotherapeutic agents for advanced disease.

Glucagonoma

Glucagonomas arise from the A cells in the pancreatic islets of Langerhans. The syndrome caused by this tumor is due to excess secretion of glucagon.

CLINICAL PRESENTATION

Patients with glucagonoma usually present with mild diabetes that rarely requires insulin administration and a severe dermatitis called *necrolytic migratory erythema*. The skin rash is most often located on the lower abdomen, perineum, perioral area, and/or feet. Other symptoms often seen with this syndrome include malnutrition, anemia, weight loss, glossitis, and venous thrombosis.

BIOCHEMICAL DIAGNOSIS

The diagnosis is confirmed by documenting the presence of an elevated fasting serum glucagon level, almost always greater than 500 pg/ml (normal 0–150 pg/ml).

TUMOR LOCALIZATION

CT scanning is the first localization study. Most tumors are large at the time of diagnosis, ranging from 5 to 10 cm, and occur most often in the body and tail of the pancreas.

TREATMENT

Surgical exploration should be undertaken in any patient whose tumor is thought to be resectable. Sixty-eighty percent of patients will have metastatic disease diagnosed by preoperative studies or at the time of exploration. Patients who are symptomatic due to metastatic disease frequently benefit from surgical resection. Patients with widely metastatic disease in whom surgical debulking is not possible can often benefit from medical therapy. Octreotide has been successful in controlling the diabetes and dermatitis in 60–90% of patients. Dacarbazine and streptozocin have had some success in treating unresectable or recurrent glucagonomas.

Somatostatinomas

Somatostatinomas arise from the D cells of the islets of Langerhans and are among the rarest endocrine neoplasms, with an estimated yearly incidence of one in 40 million. The syndrome associated with these tumors is marked by hyperglycemia, cholelithiasis, steatorrhea, and diarrhea. Early diagnosis is difficult because symptoms are frequently nonspecific. Most of these lesions are located in the head of the pancreas. Over 90% of the lesions are malignant, and metastatic disease is found in the majority of cases. Patients taken to surgery for attempted curative resection should also have a cholecystectomy performed due to the high incidence of cholelithiasis.

Miscellaneous Functioning Tumors

Many islet cell tumors previously thought to be nonfunctioning have been found to secrete PP. Since this substance can now be measured, these tumors are referred to as *PPomas*. (Interestingly, 25–75% of all functioning pancreatic endocrine tumors secrete PP.) When an elevated level of PP is detected in conjunction with a pancreatic mass, the diagnosis of PPoma is made by excluding the possibility of other functioning islet cell tumors. The excess secretion of PP is not associated with any clearly defined clinical syndrome, and thus these tumors are usually large at the time of diagnosis, presenting with symptoms related to local growth. Surgical excision is the treatment of choice for resectable tumors. PPomas are usually located in the head of the pancreas and are almost always malignant. Sixty percent are metastatic at the time of diagnosis. The 5-year overall survival rate is 44%.

Growth hormone-releasing factor (GRF) is another hormone that has recently been identified as a tumor product. Referred to as *GRFomas*, tumors that secrete GFR are located in the pancreas 30% of the time, lung 55% of the time, and intestine 15% of the time. About 30% of the lesions are malignant. Patients usually present with acromegaly, but these tumors also may secrete other products. Forty percent of patients have Zollinger-Ellison syndrome, and 40% have Cushing's syndrome. Although octreotide can significantly suppress the levels of circulating growth hormone in this syndrome, surgical excision, if possible, is the treatment of choice.

Other uncommon islet cell tumors include those that secrete neurotensin, adrenocorticotropic hormone (ACTH), or a parathyroid hormone (PTH)-like peptide.

Table 13-5. Features of multiple endocrine neoplasia (MEN) syndromes

MEN-I	MEN-IIa	MEN-IIb
Hyperparathyroidism	Medullary thyroid carcinoma	Medullary thyroid carcinoma
Pancreatic endocrine tumors	Pheochromocytoma	Pheochromocytoma
Pituitary adenomas	Hyperparathyroidism	Multiple neuromas and ganglioneuroma
Adrenal adenomas		Skeletal deformities
Thyroid nodules		

Nonfunctioning Tumors

Twenty to fifty percent of pancreatic islet tumors are found to be nonfunctioning in that they do not secrete any detectable levels of hormones. Instead of a well-defined clinical syndrome, the presentation of these tumors is similar to that of pancreatic ductal adenocarcinoma. Common symptoms include abdominal pain, weight loss, and jaundice. Most of these tumors are found in the head of the pancreas, and the majority are malignant. Diagnosis can be made by CT-guided fine-needle aspiration as well as by the characteristic hypervascular appearance on arteriography. Following localization studies, operative exploration for attempted curative resection is indicated. The prognosis for patients with nonfunctioning islet cell tumors is significantly better than for those with pancreatic ductal adenocarcinoma, with the overall 5-year survival rate in the former group approaching 50%. Chemotherapy with streptozocin and 5-fluorouracil has shown some favorable responses.

Multiple Endocrine Neoplasia

OVERVIEW

There are currently three well-defined MEN syndromes (MEN-I, MEN-IIa, and MEN-IIb), characterized by a familial predisposition to develop tumors in various endocrine glands either metachronously or synchronously. An overview of the three syndromes is given in Table 13-5.

MEN-I

MEN-I, also known as Wermer's syndrome, is characterized by the development of parathyroid hyperplasia, pituitary tumors, and pancreatic islet cell tumors. Adenomas of the adrenal gland and thyroid can also occur. MEN-I is inherited in an autosomal dominant pattern, with the predisposing gene being located on chromosome 11. The gene is transmitted with nearly 100% penetrance, but there is significant variability in the degree of gene expression. The clinical manifestations of the syndrome usually develop in the third or fourth decade and can vary significantly depending on the endocrine tissue involved and the hormones produced.

Forty percent of patients with MEN-I develop adrenal tumors. Therefore prior to surgical resection of endocrine tumors, all MEN-I patients need to be screened by measuring urinary excretion of glucocorticoids, mineralocorticoids, catecholamines, vanillylmandelic acid, metanephrines, and sex hormones.

Hyperparathyroidism

Hyperparathyroidism is the most common endocrine abnormality seen in MEN-I and is usually the first to develop. Almost all patients develop hyperparathyroidism secondary to four-gland hyperplasia.

The clinical presentation is similiar to that seen in sporadic hyperparathyroidism, with most patients being asymptomatic. The diagnosis is made by measuring the serum calcium, phosphate, and PTH levels.

There is some controversy over the appropriate surgical procedure in these patients. Many surgeons perform a three and one-half gland parathyroidectomy. With this technique, there is a 40–50% incidence of persistent or recurrent hyperparathyroidism, as well as a 25% incidence of hypoparathyroidism. Our preferred technique is to perform a four-gland excision and autotransplant pieces of the least hyperplastic gland into the brachioradialis muscle in the forearm. With this technique, the incidence of hypoparathyroidism is only about 5%. Although roughly 50% of patients develop graft-dependent hyperparathyroidism, it can be effectively managed by removing several pieces of parathyroid tissue from the forearm under local anesthesia. This technique saves the patients a neck re-exploration.

Because there is a 15% incidence of thyroid neoplasms in patients with MEN-I, the thyroid needs to be examined carefully at the time of neck exploration as well as followed closely postoperatively.

Pancreatic Tumors

The second most common neoplasms associated with MEN-I are the pancreatic islet cell tumors, which occur in approximately 60% of MEN-I patients. The clinical syndrome associated with these tumors results from the hormone secreted by them. The most common islet cell tumors are gastrinomas, followed by insulinomas. Rarely, glucagonomas, PPomas, VIPomas, and somatostatinomas are found. In general MEN-I–associated pancreatic endocrine tumors are multifocal; they may be located outside the pancreas, as is often the case with gastrinomas. The treatment of these tumors has been discussed in previous sections. Symptoms related to excess hormone production can be treated medically. Surgical correction of primary hyperparathyroidism should be performed first, because this may help decrease calcium-induced hormone release from pancreatic endocrine tumors. In general, surgery is not recommended for treatment of pancreatic tumors in MEN-I patients unless a localized tumor can be identified on preoperative studies or symptoms cannot be controlled medically as occurs frequently with insulinomas in MEN-I.

Pituitary Neoplasms

Pituitary neoplasms occur in 30–50% of MEN-I patients, with benign prolactin-producing adenomas being the most common. Symptoms may be related directly to the tumor, such as headache and diplopia, or be related to the specific hormone overproduced. Excess prolactin causes galactorrhea and amenorrhea in women and impotence in men. Tumors may also produce growth hormone (30%) or ACTH (<10%), leading to acromegaly or Cushing's disease, respectively. Bromocriptine, a dopamine agonist, can be used to treat prolactinomas medically. Transsphenoidal hypophysectomy is reserved for patients who fail to respond to bromocriptine and who have non–prolactin-secreting tumors. All patients with MEN-I should be followed periodically with measurement of serum prolactin and growth hormone levels.

MEN-II

MEN-II consists of two syndromes, each inherited in an autosomal dominant pattern with 100% penetrance but variable expression. Both syndromes are marked by the presence of medullary thyroid carcinoma (MTC) and pheochromocytoma. In MEN-IIa, patients frequently also develop hyperparathyroidism secondary to four-gland hyperplasia. Patients with MEN-IIb tend to have a characteristic facies and marfanoid habitus. MEN-IIb is also marked by the development of multiple neuromas on the lips, tongue, and oral mucosa. In addition, IIb patients have a high incidence of skeletal abnormalities as well as diffuse ganglioneuromatosis of the GI tract, which can lead to a number of GI motility problems. There are several unique features of the neoplasms seen in the MEN syndromes.

Medullary Thyroid Carcinoma

MTC makes up about 5–10% of all thyroid malignancies. The vast majority—approximately 80 percent—of these tumors occur sporadically, without any previous family history. The remaining 20% are familial, usually associated with either MEN-IIa or MEN-IIb. MTC can occur in the familial setting without any other associated syndromes. Some features of sporadic and familial MTC are shown in Table 13-6. In the setting of MEN-II, MTC is usually the first endocrine abnormality to occur. MTC arises from the parafollicular or C cells

Table 13-6. Features of sporadic versus familial medullary thyroid carcinoma

Features	Sporadic	Familial
Proportion of cases	80%	20%
Age of onset	40–60 yrs	10–30 yrs
Location	Unilateral	Bilateral

of the thyroid and as a result has the capability to secrete not only calcitonin but also a variety of other hormonally active substances such as serotonin, ACTH, prostaglandins, and melanin.

Clinical Presentation
MTC is often detected when it is clinically occult in patients screened for MEN-II. About 30% of the patients with MTC present with watery diarrhea, usually secondary to the stimulatory effect of high plasma calcitonin levels on intestinal fluid and electrolyte secretion. Symptoms such as hoarseness, dysphagia, and repiratory difficulty may be related to locally advanced disease. Presenting symptoms may also be secondary to metastatic disease, which is most commonly seen in the lungs, liver, and bones.

Diagnosis
The diagnosis of MTC can be made either pathologically using fine-needle aspiration or with a series of laboratory tests. When there is a palpable lesion, fine-needle aspiration can be performed. Histologically MTC frequently shows sheets of uniformly round or polygonal cells separated by fibrovascular stroma. Immunohistochemical staining for calcitonin in the tumor cells is the most reliable way to confirm the diagnosis. Laboratory measurements for serum calcitonin are also important and usually demonstrate marked elevation, especially in patients with palpable tumors. Patients with clinically occult tumors, however, may have normal or minimally elevated serum calcitonin levels.

Provocative tests can be used to identify those patients who have MTC. The original provocative test for diagnosing MTC was the calcium infusion test. With this test patients with MTC show a marked rise in calcitonin as compared with healthy persons, who have no rise at all. A more rapid method for making the diagnosis is the pentagastrin stimulation test. Pentagastrin is given by IV bolus, and serum calcitonin levels are measured within the next 5 minutes. Patients with MTC show a marked rise in serum calcitonin levels, often higher than in the calcium infusion test. More recently, it has been shown that the highest stimulated serum calcitonin levels can be obtained with the sequential administration of calcium followed by an IV bolus of pentagastrin. Stimulated values of calcitonin above 300 pg/ml suggest MTC. Plasma values above 1,000 pg/ml are diagnostic. Most authorities recommend that members of families at risk for MTC undergo provocative screening beginning at age 5 years and continuing through age 45.

Treatment

Once the diagnosis of MTC is made, patients should be screened for pheochromocytoma and hyperparathyroidism. If a pheochromocytoma is found, it should be treated first (see Chapter 14). Surgery for the MTC is then done 2 weeks later. If hyperparathyroidism is diagnosed, it can be treated at the time of neck exploration for the MTC.

The appropriate treatment for MTC is total thyroidectomy and central neck dissection. In the MEN-II syndromes, MTC is frequently multicentric and bilateral and metastasizes early to the cervical lymph nodes. The central neck dissection, which removes the lymphatic tissue between the jugular veins, the hyoid bone, and the sternal notch, helps eradicate microscopic metastatic disease. Patients with palpable lymphadenopathy should also undergo a functional neck dissection on the side of the enlarged pathologic nodes. Patients can be followed postoperatively with provocative testing to identify residual or recurrent MTC. Overall, the prognosis of MTC is good, with 80–90% 10-year survival rates being reported. In general, the course of the MTC determines the prognosis for patients with MEN-II. The average life expectancy for this group of patients is more than 50 years.

Metastatic Disease

Controversy exists over the appropriate management of patients with stimulated elevations of plasma calcitonin levels in the postoperative period. Such a finding implies the presence of residual disease in the neck or mediastinum or of undetected metastatic disease. Some clinicians think that these patients should be followed with observation only because MTC is slow-growing and the chance for cure with repeat neck exploration is low. Others recommend repeat neck exploration after selective catherization of the neck veins and determination of stimulated plasma calcitonin levels. In experienced hands, a 30–40% normalization of plasma calcitonin levels by provocative testing can be achieved after repeat exploration. There are currently few options for patients with advanced disease: radioactive iodine ablation, thyroid suppression, radiotherapy, and chemotherapy have not been shown to be very effective for MTC. Because of the indolent nature of the tumor, many physicians do not treat metastatic disease aggressively.

Pheochromocytoma

Pheochromocytoma associated with MEN-II usually appears between the ages of 10 and 30 years and is usually diagnosed concurrently or shortly after MTC. The pheochromocytomas associated with MEN-II are usually bilateral (60–80% of the time), limited to the adrenal medulla, and almost always benign. It appears that the adrenal gland becomes hyperplastic before the pheochromocytoma develops.

The work-up and management of pheochromocytoma is discussed in more detail in Chapter 14. It should be remembered that patients with MEN-II should have a I-131 M-iodo-benzylguanidine (MIBG) scan preoperatively in addition to other localizing studies. In this population of patients, the MBIG not only is the most sensitive (94%) and specific test (almost 100%), it also can help determine whether bilateral pheochromocytomas are present.

Because many years can separate the development of pheochromocytomas in opposite adrenal glands in MEN-II, some controversy exists over the optimal surgical procedure for patients who are initially found to have a unilateral pheochromocytoma. Although some surgeons recommend bilateral adrenalectomy in patients with MEN-II because up to 80% of these patients will develop bilateral tumors, a more conservative approach is followed by most to avoid as long as possible the need for lifetime glucocorticoid and mineralocorticoid replacement. This approach involves unilateral adrenalectomy and examination of the contralateral adrenal at the time of exploration. If no abnormality is found, the unaffected adrenal is left intact and the patient is followed closely for evidence of a contralateral tumor.

Hyperparathyroidism

Hyperparathyroidism is the third and most variable component of the MEN-IIa syndrome. Most often the patients are asymptomatic and the diagnosis is made on routine follow-up laboratory tests. Occcasionally, patients present with kidney stones. In patients with MEN-II, a work-up for hyperparathyroidism should be undertaken before neck exploration for MTC. If, at the time of exploration, the calcium levels are normal and the parathyroid glands appear normal, no parathyroidectomy is performed. If calcium and serum PTH levels are elevated or if the glands appear grossly abnormal and are hyperplastic on biopsy specimens at the time of neck exploration for MTC, a total parathyroidectomy should be performed. Transplantation of approximately one-half of the most normal-appearing parathyroid gland into the forearm should be carried out. If normal parathyroid tissue should become devascularized in the course of performing a total thyroidectomy for MTC in a patient with MEN-II, parathyroid autotransplantation should also be performed. Patients with MEN-IIa should have the autotransplant performed into the brachioradialis muscle of the forearm because the gland could become hyperplastic in the future and this placement facilitates later removal. In patients with MEN-IIb, since hyperparathyroidism rarely develops, the devascularized parathyroid glands can be transplanted into the sternocleidomastoid muscle in the neck.

Selected References

GASTRINOMAS

Harmon JW, Norton JA, Collen MJ. Removal of gastrinomas for the control of Zollinger-Ellison syndrome. *Ann Surg* 200:396, 1984.

Norton JA, Doppman JL, Collen MJ, et al. Prospective study of gastrinoma localization and resection in patients with Zollinger-Ellison syndrome. *Ann Surg* 204:468, 1986.

Norton JA, Doppman JL, Gardner JD, et al. Aggressive resection of metastatic disease in selected patients with malignant gastrinoma. *Ann Surg* 203:352, 1986.

Norton JA, Doppman JL, Jensen RT. Curative resection in Zollinger-Ellison syndrome: Results of a 10 year prospective study. *Ann Surg* 215:8, 1992.

Pipeleers-Mirichal M, Somers G, Willems G, et al. Gastrinomas in the duodenums of patients with multiple endocrine neoplasia type I and the Zollinger-Ellison syndrome. *N Engl J Med* 322:723, 1990.

Thompson JC, Lewis BG, Wiener I, Townsend CM Jr. The role of surgery in Zollinger-Ellison syndrome. *Ann Surg* 197:594, 1983.

Wolfe MM, Jensen RT. Zollinger-Ellison syndrome: Current concepts in the diagnosis and management. *N Engl J Med* 317:1200, 1987.

Zollinger RM, Ellison EC, O'Dorisio T, Sparks J. Thirty years' experience with gastrinoma. *World J Surg* 8:427, 1984.

ISLET CELL TUMORS

Gower WR, Fabri PJ. Endocrine neoplasms (non-gastrin) of the pancreas. *Semin Surg Oncol* 6:98, 1990.

Howard TJ, Stabile BE, Zinner MJ, et al. Anatomic distribution of pancreatic endocrine tumors. *Am J Surg* 159:258, 1990.

Legaspi A, Brennan MF. Management of islet cell carcinoma. *Surgery* 104:1018, 1988.

Maton PN. The use of long-acting somatostatin analogue, octreotide acetate, in patients with islet cell tumors. *Gastroenterol Clin North Am* 18:897, 1989.

Sloan DA, Schwartz RW, Kenady DE. Surgical therapy for endocrine tumors of abdominal origin. *Curr Opinion Oncol* 5:100, 1993.

Thompson GB, van Heerden JA, Grant CS, et al. Islet cell carcinomas of the pancreas: A twenty-year experience. *Surgery* 104:1011, 1988.

Venkatesh S, Ordonez NG, Ajani J, et al. Islet cell carcinoma of the pancreas. *Cancer*.65:354, 1990.

MULTIPLE ENDOCRINE NEOPLASIA

Cance WG, Wells SA. Multiple endocrine neoplasia type IIa. *Curr Probl Surg* 22:1, 1985.

Lairmore TC, Ball DW, Baylin SB, Wells SA. Management of pheochromocytomas in patients with multiple endocrine neoplasia type 2 syndromes. *Ann Surg* 217:595, 1993.

Sabiston DC Jr (ed). *Textbook of Surgery: The Biological Basis of Modern Surgical Practice* (14th ed). Philadelphia: Saunders, 1991.

Adrenal Tumors

Douglas S. Tyler

The diagnosis and treatment of adrenal tumors require a sound fundamental knowledge of adrenal endocrine physiology. The clinical manifestations of hyperaldosteronism, hypercortisolism, and pheochromocytoma result from hypersecretion of adrenal endocrine products. Biochemical diagnosis and radiographic localization are required prior to surgical intervention. Adrenocortical carcinoma, a rare tumor that is potentially curable by surgery, must be differentiated from the more common metastatic tumors and computed tomography (CT)–detected "incidentalomas" of the adrenal glands, which rarely require surgical intervention.

Primary Hyperaldosteronism

Primary hyperaldosteronism is the clinical syndrome that results from hypersecretion of aldosterone. This condition is due to adrenal hyperplasia in about 40% of cases and to adrenal adenoma about 60% of the time. Other rare causes of primary aldosteronism include glucocorticoid-suppressible hyperaldosteronism, adrenocortical carcinoma, and aldosterone-secreting ovarian tumors. Primary hyperaldosteronism is responsible for approximately 0.5-1.0% of all cases of hypertension and roughly 5–10% of surgically correctable cases of hypertension.

CLINICAL MANIFESTATIONS

The main problem in diagnosing primary hyperaldosteronism is that the symptoms are usually mild and nonspecific. The most common symptoms are headache, fatigue, polydypsia, polyuria, and nocturia. Hypertension is almost always present but is frequently mild, with diastolic blood pressures below 120 mm Hg in over 70% of cases.

DIAGNOSIS

Patients suspected of having primary hyperaldosteronism should undergo a thorough evaluation. Initial laboratory findings that support the diagnosis, especially in patients not currently receiving diuretic therapy, include an elevated urine chloride level and hypokalemia accompanied by metabolic alkalosis. Initially, all nonessential medications should be stopped for at least 2 weeks. Estrogens and spironolactone should be discontinued for at least 6 weeks. Patients should then be placed on a salt-loading diet (10–12 g NaCl/day). During salt loading urine should be collected over 24 hours and measurements made of aldosterone, sodium, and potassium. Serum levels of aldosterone and electrolytes and plasma renin activity should also be measured. Patients with primary hyperaldosteronism do not have suppressed aldo-

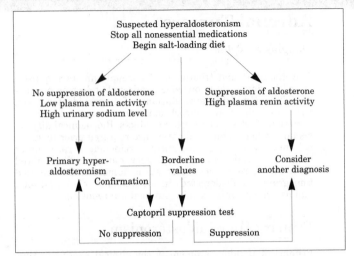

Fig. 14-1. Algorithm for patients with suspected primary hyperaldosteronism.

sterone production during the salt loading, but rather continue to have urinary aldosterone levels that are usually higher than 14 mg per day, a urinary potassium level higher than 25 mEq per day, and low plasma renin activity. Potassium supplementation should also be given during the period of salt loading because severe hypokalemia (K<3mEq) can inhibit aldosterone production in some patients. Other useful tests used to diagnose hyperaldosteronism include the Lasix stimulation test and the IV saline loading test.

If there is any doubt about the diagnosis, a captopril suppression test should be performed. The patient takes 25 mg of captopril PO in the morning; 2 hours later, plasma aldosterone levels and plasma renin activity are measured. Patients with essential hypertension should have a drop in their plasma aldosterone level and a rise in their plasma renin activity. In contrast, patients with primary hyperaldosteronism will show no change in their plasma aldosterone levels or their plasma renin activity. Our approach to patients suspected of having primary hyperaldosteronism is shown in Fig. 14-1.

Imaging studies of the adrenals with high-resolution thin-slice CT scans or magnetic resonance imaging (MRI) can identify lesions 7–10 mm or larger. The presence of a mass in association with the laboratory diagnosis of primary hyperaldosteronism is diagnostic of an adenoma. Patients who have negative or equivocal findings on CT scans or MRI may benefit from iodocholesterol (NP-59) scanning or adrenal venous sampling. The iodocholesterol scan will demonstrate symmetric uptake by both adrenals in patients with hyperplasia but uptake only within the tumor in a patient with an adenoma. Adrenal venous sampling, although not frequently needed, is the most sensitive method of differentiating hyperplasia from an adenoma.

TREATMENT

The treatment of primary hyperaldosteronism depends on the cause. Adrenal hyperplasia is best managed medically using the aldosterone antagonist spironolactone. Most patients can achieve adequate control of their blood pressure with this medicine alone or in conjunction with other anti-hypertensives. When a benign adenoma is diagnosed, the appropriate therapy consists of surgical resection. Preoperatively, patients should be placed on spironolactone and given potassium supplements to help normalize their fluid and electrolyte levels over a 3- to 4-week period.

A posterior flank incision is the preferred approach when excising an aldosterone-secreting adenoma. Adrenalectomy performed in this way is associated with minimal morbidity and mortality. The early results from surgical resection of an adenoma are good, with 95% of patients becoming normotensive and eukalemic. However, within 3 years 20–30% of the patients develop recurrent hypertension. The etiology of the hypertension is not clear, but it is usually not associated with hypokalemia.

Approximately 2% or less of adrenocortical carcinomas cause isolated hyperaldosteronism. In this rare situation, an anterior approach to surgical exploration should be taken to facilitate resectability and allow assessment for metastatic disease.

Hypercortisolism

Cushing's syndrome refers to the state of hypercortisolism that can result from a number of different pathologic processes (Table 14-1). Cortisol regulation involves feedback loops on the pituitary gland and hypothalamus. Approximately 70% of the cases of hypercortisolism are secondary to hypersecretion of adrenocorticotropic hormone (ACTH) from the pituitary gland, a condition called *Cushing's disease*. Most of the time a small pituitary adenoma is found to be the cause. Hypersecretion of cortisol from the adrenal glands accounts for approximately 10–20% of cases of Cushing's syndrome. The underlying cause is an adrenal adenoma 50–60% of the time and an adrenocortical carcinoma 20–25% of the time. Bilateral adrenal hyperplasia accounts for the remaining 20–30% of cases. Although the etiology of autonomously functioning bilateral adrenal hyperplasia is unclear, several reports suggest that some cases may be due to an aberrant sensitivity of the adrenal glands to gastric inhibitory polypeptide, which is released in response to eating.

Ectopic secretion of ACTH, referred to as *ectopic ACTH syndrome*, causes about 15% of cases of Cushing's syndrome. Ectopic ACTH syndrome is usually caused by malignant

Table 14-1. Causes of Cushing's syndrome

Cushing's disease (due to pituitary adenoma)
    Associated with diffuse adrenal hyperplasia
    Associated with micronodular hyperplasia
    Associated with macronodular hyperplasia
Ectopic adrenocorticotropin syndrome
Ectopic corticotropin-releasing factor syndrome
Adrenal tumors
    Single adenoma
    Multiple adenomas
    Carcinoma
Primary adrenocortical hyperplasia
Exogenous steroids

tumors, with carcinoma of the lung, carcinoma of the pancreas, carcinoid tumors, and malignant thymoma accounting for 80% of such cases. Ectopic secretion of corticotropin-releasing factor is exceedingly rare but has been reported in a few cases.

CLINICAL MANIFESTATIONS

Weight gain is the most common feature of hypercortisolism and occurs predominantly in the truncal area. Centripetal obesity combined with muscle wasting in the extremities, fat deposition in the head and neck region, and a dorsal kyphosis secondary to osteoporosis gives the patient a very characteristic habitus. Hypertension, striae, and virilization in females are three other common findings.

DIAGNOSIS

The work-up for Cushing's syndrome should be aimed first at establishing the diagnosis and then at determining the etiology. To establish the diagnosis, a state of hypercortisolism must be documented. The adult adrenal glands secrete on average 10–30 mg of cortisol each day. The secretion follows a diurnal variation: Cortisol levels tend to be high early in the morning and low in the evening. The variability of plasma cortisol levels requires that morning (8 A.M.) plasma cortisol levels be used as part of an overnight low-dose dexamethasone suppression test as screening for Cushing's syndrome.

To determine the etiology of the elevated cortisol level, plasma ACTH levels must be checked. ACTH secretion also follows a diurnal variation preceding that of cortisol by 1–2 hours. Suppressed levels of ACTH are seen in patients with adrenal adenomas, adenocortical carcinomas, or autonomously functioning adrenal hyperplasia. In such cases, autonomous secretion of cortisol by the pathologic process in the adrenal gland inhibits ACTH release by the pituitary. Patients with Cushing's disease—that is, a pituitary adenoma secreting ACTH—usually have plasma ACTH levels that are elevated or within the upper limits of normal. When there is an ectopic source of ACTH secretion, the plasma ACTH level is usually markedly elevated.

A number of other tests are sometimes used to help establish the diagnosis of Cushing's syndrome as well as to distinguish between pituitary, adrenal, and ectopic etiologies. The dexamethasone suppression test is the most widely used. The overnight dexamethasone suppression test requires the patient to take 1 mg of dexamethasone at 11:00 P.M.; the plasma cortisol level is measured at 8:00 A.M. the following morning. In a person without Cushing's syndrome, cortisol release will be suppressed, with plasma cortisol levels lower than 5 mg/dl. In contrast, 98% of patients with Cushing's syndrome will have plasma cortisol levels that remain above 5 mg/dl.

To confirm the presence of Cushing's syndrome, the low-dose and high-dose dexamethasone suppression test can be performed. For this test, urine is collected over 24 hours for 6 consecutive days for measurement of free cortisol and 17-hydroxycorticosteroid (17-OHCS). During the first 2 days no dexamethasone is taken, and urinary cortisol is measured to establish baseline values. During the third and fourth days, the patient takes 0.5 mg of dexamethasone every 6 hours. Hypercortisolism is confirmed if urinary cortisol levels do not decline below 20 mg/g creatinine/day and/or if urinary 17-OHCS levels stay above 2 mg/g creatinine/day. On the fifth and sixth days, the patient takes 2 mg of dexamethasone every 6 hours. Individuals who have Cushing's disease usually show a reduction in their urinary cortisol levels to 50% of the baseline obtained on days 1 and 2. The cortisol levels of patients with an ectopic ACTH syndrome or autonomously functioning adrenal pathology (neoplasm or hyperplasia) do not fall below 50% of the baseline.

The metyrapone test is also occasionally used to differentiate between the various etiologies of Cushing's syndrome. Metyrapone inhibits the enzyme 11b-hydroxylase, which converts 11-deoxycortisol to cortisol as well as converting 11-deoxycorticosterone to corticosterone and aldosterone. The inhibition of cortisol production in the normal adrenal gland by metyrapone is sensed in the pituitary gland and results in increased production of ACTH. The ACTH stimulates the adrenal cortex to produce cortisol precursors that can then be detected in either the blood or urine. A decline in urinary and serum cortisol levels also occurs. On the day before the test begins, patients collect a baseline 24-hour urine sample and have blood drawn for baseline plasma cortisol and 11-deoxycortisol measurements. The patient then takes 30 mg/kg of metyrapone at midnight. Eight hours later the patient has plasma cortisol and 11-deoxycortisol levels rechecked. In addition, the patient collects another 24-hour urine sample. The pituitary gland of patients with Cushing's disease senses the decreased levels of cortisol; ACTH release is increased, which results in elevated serum deoxycortisol and urinary 17-OHCS levels accompanied by decreased serum cortisol levels. The pituitary gland of patients with

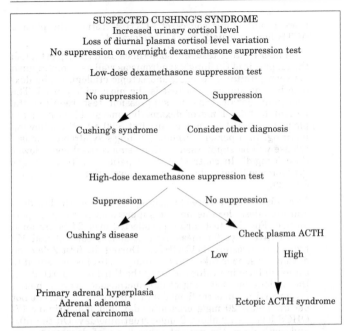

SUSPECTED CUSHING'S SYNDROME
Increased urinary cortisol level
Loss of diurnal plasma cortisol level variation
No suppression on overnight dexamethasone suppression test

Low-dose dexamethasone suppression test

No suppression   Suppression

Cushing's syndrome   Consider other diagnosis

High-dose dexamethasone suppression test

Suppression   No suppression

Cushing's disease   Check plasma ACTH

Low   High

Primary adrenal hyperplasia
Adrenal adenoma   Ectopic ACTH syndrome
Adrenal carcinoma

Fig 14-2. Work-up for suspected Cushing's syndrome. (ACTH = adreno-corticotropic hormone.)

ectopic ACTH syndrome or autonomously functioning adrenal tissue is chronically suppressed and does not respond to changes in cortisol levels. Therefore serum deoxycortisol and urinary 17-OHCS levels remain unchanged from the baseline values.

An overview of our approach to patients suspected of having Cushing's syndrome is shown in Fig. 14-2. Initial screening involves 24-hour urine collections for measurement of free cortisol levels and measurement of morning and evening plasma cortisol levels to determine whether the hormone has a diurnal variation. An overnight dexamethasone suppression test is then performed in patients with either elevated urinary cortisol levels or loss of their diurnal variation in cortisol secretion. Patients with suppressed cortisol levels do not have Cushing's syndrome. Patients without suppressed cortisol levels receive a low-dose, high-dose dexamethasone test and/or a metyrapone test. Patients whose cortisol levels are suppressed after the low-dose, high-dose dexamethasone test or who are metyrapone responsive have Cushing's disease and should have a CT scan of the head, with special focus on the pituitary region. In patients whose cortisol levels are not suppressed after the low-dose, high-dose dexamethasone test or who are metyrapone unresponsive, we check the plasma ACTH level. High ACTH levels indicate ectopic ACTH syndrome. These patients should have a CT scan of

Table 14-2. Perioperative steroid coverage and replacement

Day	Steroid dose
Major procedure	
Preop	Hydrocortisone, 100 mg IV q6h beginning at midnight on the evening prior to surgery
1 postop	Hydrocortisone, 100 mg IV q6h
2[a] postop	Hydrocortisone, 80 mg IV q6h
3 postop	Hydrocortisone, 60 mg IV q6h
4 postop	Hydrocortisone, 40 mg IV q6h
5 postop	Hydrocortisone, 20 mg IV q6h
6[b–d] postop	Hydrocortisone, 10 mg IV q6h
Minor procedure	
Preoperatively	Hydrocortisone, 100 mg IV (single dose)
Evening after surgery	Hydrocortisone, 20 mg IV (single dose)

[a]Patients can be put on an oral equivalent of hydrocortisone (usually prednisone) at any time once they are tolerating oral intake.
Patients who have a postoperative complication require additional steroid coverage
[b]After 6 days the patient can be placed back on his or her preoperative steroid therapy.
[c]Patients with forms of Cushing's syndrome that lead to suppression of native adrenal tissue (adrenal adenoma, adrenal carcinoma) may require a prolonged period before completely weaning off steroids from a baseline dose of 40 mg/day.
[d]Patients who undergo bilateral adrenalectomy require lifelong glucocorticoid and mineralocorticoid replacement in the form of cortisol acetate (25 mg PO every morning and 12.5 mg PO every evening) and fluorohydrocortisone (0.1 mg PO every morning) after steroid weaning completed (postoperative day 7).

the chest and abdomen in an attempt to identify the underlying malignancy. Patients with low plasma ACTH levels have adrenal pathology as the etiology of their Cushing's syndrome. An abdominal CT scan will help separate an adrenal neoplasm from primary adrenal hyperplasia. Radioisotope imaging of the adrenals with labeled iodocholesterol can help distinguish primary adrenal hyperplasia, which should demonstrate bilateral uptake, from a cortisol-secreting adenoma, which leads to suppression of the contralateral gland and thus uptake only by the adenoma. Adrenocortical carcinomas usually do not take up radiolabeled iodocholesterol.

TREATMENT

The appropriate management of Cushing's syndrome depends on the underlying etiology. Patients with Cushing's disease should undergo transphenoidal resection of their pituitary adenoma when it is believed to be resectable. Remission of symptoms is seen in more than 80% of patients with a single adenoma but is less likely in the presence of extrasellar extension, macronodular disease of the pituitary, or pituitary corticotropic hyperplasia. Bilateral adrenalectomy is rarely performed and should be reserved for patients who fail to respond to hypophysectomy. If bilateral adrenalectomy is performed, patients require not only perioperative steroid coverage (Tables 14-2 and 14-3) but also lifelong

Table 14-3. Comparison of steroid preparations

Steroid	Half-life (hours)	Glucocorticoid activity (relative to cortisone)	Mineralocorticoid activity (relative to cortisone)
Cortisol	8–12	1	1
Cortisone	8–12	0.8	0.8
Prednisone	12–36	4	0.8
Prednisolone	12–36	4	0.8
Methylprednisolone	12–36	5	0.5
Triaminolone	12–36	5	0
Betamethasone	36–72	10	0
Dexamethasone	36–72	25	0

replacement of both glucocorticoids and mineralocorticoids. Some groups have advocated heterotopic autotransplantation of adrenal tissue after bilateral adrenalectomy as a way to minimize steroid utilization and prevent Nelson's syndrome. When this procedure is performed, approximately 4 g of each gland is sliced into 1- to 2-mm sections and placed into a muscle pocket in the paraspinous or rectus abdominis muscle.

Patients with a neoplasm of the adrenal gland, whether adenoma or carcinoma, should undergo resection of the involved side. Although almost all adenomas can be resected, adrenocortical carcinomas that secrete cortisol are resectable in only 25–35% of patients. Chemotherapy has been disappointing in patients with unresectable disease. Symptomatic relief of the hypercortisol state can be achieved with various agents, including aminoglutethimide, metyrapone, mitotane, or ketoconazole.

Patients with autonomously functioning bilateral adrenal hyperplasia require bilateral adrenalectomy with or without heterotopic autotransplantation. To date medical therapy has not been effective for this condition.

Finally, patients with ectopic ACTH syndrome should have the underlying malignant lesion resected if possible. Bilateral adrenalectomy should be reserved for the small group of patients whose primary tumor is unresectable and whose symptoms of cortisol excess cannot be controlled medically.

Pheochromocytoma

In large series of hypertensive patients, approximately 0.1–0.2% of patients are found to have pheochromocytomas. These neuroectodermal tumors arise from chromaffin cells in the adrenal medulla. About 10% of the time, pheochromocytomas can be found in both adrenal glands, with multiple tumors being present in some cases. Ten percent of pheochromocytomas can be found in extra-adrenal sites, where they are more appropriately called *paragangliomas* because of their close association with ganglia of the sympathetic nervous system. The most common extra-adrenal sites include the organ of Zuckerkandl (located between the inferior mesenteric artery and the aortic bifurcation), the urinary bladder, the thorax, and the renal hilum.

Histologic evidence of malignancy in pheochromocytomas can be demonstrated approximately 10% of the time; malignancy is more commonly seen with extra-adrenal lesions than with those arising in the adrenal glands. Documenting malignancy can be difficult because invasion of adjacent organs or metastatic disease must be present. Furthermore, both benign and malignant lesions may show tumor penetration of the gland's capsule, invasion of veins draining the gland, cellular pleomorphism, mitoses, and atypical nuclei. Familial pheochromocytomas account for about 10% of cases and are usually benign. The familial syndromes associated with pheochromocytomas include multiple endocrine neoplasia types IIa and IIb, in which bilateral tumors are common, as well as the neuroectodermal dysplasias consisting of neurofibromatosis, tuberous sclerosis, Sturge-Weber syndrome, and von Hippel-Lindau disease, in which pheochromocytoma is usually unilateral. Patients with these syndromes require close follow-up and periodic screening for pheochromocytoma, especially before any planned surgical procedure.

CLINICAL MANIFESTATIONS

The clinical manifestations of pheochromocytoma can be varied and at times quite dramatic. Hypertension, sustained or paroxysmal, is the most common clinical finding. Paroxysmal elevations in blood pressure can vary markedly in frequency and duration. A number of things can stimulate increases in blood pressure, ranging from heavy physical exertion to eating foods high in tyramine. Other common symptoms include excessive sweating, palpitations, tremulousness, anxiety, and chest pain. Most symptoms appear secondary to the excess catecholamine secretion by the tumors. Patients with functioning tumors are rarely asymptomatic, and nonfunctioning tumors are extremely rare.

DIAGNOSIS

The diagnosis of pheochromocytoma is made by documenting the excess secretion of catecholamines. Twenty-four–hour urine collections should be tested for free catecholamines (dopamine, epinephrine, and norepinephrine) and their metabolites (normetanephrine, metanephrine, vanillylmandelic acid). Elevated levels of catecholamines or their metabolites are seen in more than 90% of patients with pheochromocytoma. Plasma levels of free catecholamines are also usually elevated. However, because plasma values frequently overlap those seen in essential hypertension, the urinary measurements are accepted as being more sensitive. The adrenal glands and the organ of Zuckerkandl produce the enzyme phenylethanolamine-N-methyl-transferase, which converts norepinephrine to epinephrine. Pheochromocytomas that arise elsewhere do not contain this enzyme and thus do not produce much, if any, epinephrine. As a result, extra-adrenal pheochromocytomas secrete predominantly dopamine and norepinephrine.

When the urinary values of catecholamines show only borderline elevation the clonidine suppression test, a provocative test, helps differentiate pheochromocytoma from other causes of hypertension. Clonidine should suppress the centrally mediated release of catecholamines in all patients except those with pheochromocytomas, in whom the tumors usually function autonomously. Plasma catecholamine levels are measured 3 hours after giving a PO dose of clonidine (0.3 mg). A pheochromocytoma can be ruled out in patients in whom the plasma catecholamine level is lower than 500 pg/ml at 3 hours.

Once the diagnosis of pheochromocytoma is made, localization studies can be carried out. CT can detect 95% of adrenal masses larger than 6–8 mm and is usually performed first because it can also identify extra-adrenal intra-abdominal pheochromocytomas. An MRI may also be useful because T2-weighted images can clearly identify chromaffin tissue and because MRI gives an adrenal mass to liver ratio of greater than 3. This ratio is much higher than would be seen for adenomas or adenocarcinomas of the adrenal. ^{131}I-Metaiodobenzylguanidine (MIBG) scanning is another imaging procedure that is helpful in localizing extra-adrenal, metastatic, and/or bilateral pheochromocytomas. The radiolabeled amine is selectively picked up by chromaffin tissue and can identify the majority of pheochromocytomas, regardless of their location. Using these techniques, it is rare to have a patient whose pheochromocytoma cannot be localized preoperatively. In such rare instances, arteriography and/or venous sampling may be useful.

TREATMENT

After diagnosis and localization of the pheochromocytoma, careful preoperative preparation is required to prevent a cardiovascular crisis during surgery due to excess catecholamine secretion. The main focus of the preoperative preparation is adequate alpha-adrenergic blockade and complete restoration of fluid and electrolyte balances. Phenoxybenzamine is the alpha-adrenergic blocking agent of choice and is usually begun at a dose of 10 mg twice a day. The dosage is gradually increased over a 1- to 3-week period until adequate blockade is reached. The total dosage used should not exceed 1 mg/kg/day. Alpha-methyltyrosine, a competitive blocker of tyrosine conversion to dihydroxyphenylalanine, is another drug that can be used alone or together with phenoxybenzamine to inhibit catecholamine synthesis by 50–80%. Use of a beta-adrenergic blocking agent is somewhat controversial. Proponents of beta blockade feel that it helps prevent tachycardia and other arrhythmias. When used, a dose of 10 mg of propranolol given PO three times a day is recommended for 3 days preoperatively. Dosages as high as 50 mg four times a day may be necessary if there is persistent tachycardia (heart rate >140 beats/minute). The beta blocker should not be given unless alpha blockade has been established; otherwise, the beta blocker would inhibit epinephrine-induced vasodilation, leading to more significant hypertension and left heart strain. In addition to requiring pharmacologic preparation, patients with pheochromocytoma may require correction of fluid volume depletion as well as any concurrent electrolyte imbalances.

The perioperative management of patients with pheochromocytoma can be difficult. Rarely is the alpha-adrenergic blockade complete. The anesthesiologist should be prepared to treat a hypertensive crisis with sodium nitroprusside and tachyarrhythmias with either a beta blocker or lidocaine. Central venous access and right heart catheterization should be obtained preoperatively. The surgical exploration should be done through an anterior approach (bilateral subcostal incision) so that both glands can be evaluated and the abdomen examined for metastatic disease. The surgeon should try to manipulate the tumor as little as possible and to ligate the tumor's venous outflow via the adrenal vein as early in the procedure as possible.

Postoperatively, patients need to be monitored in an intensive care unit for 24 hours so they can be observed for arrhythmias and for hypotension secondary to a compensatory vasodilation that can occur once the excess catecholamine secretion has been stopped. Sometimes hypertension can remain a problem postoperatively, especially in those patients who had sustained hypertension preoperatively.

The best currently available palliation for unresectable or metastatic disease is alpha blockade with phenoxybenzamine. Alpha-methyltyrosine can also be used, with good palliation. The most commonly used chemotherapy regimens for pheochromocytoma are high-dose streptozocin and a combination of cyclophosphamide, vincristine, and dacarbazine. The overall response rates with these regimens is approximately 50%. Radiation has been effective only for bony metastases. More recently, there has been a some enthusiasm for treating metastatic lesions with a therapeutic dose of ^{131}I-MIBG. Unfortunately, a high percentage of metastatic pheochromocytomas do not take up ^{131}I-MIBG; therefore the response rate, as manifested by a reduction in urinary catecholamines, is only about 50%. Objective responses as determined by imaging studies are seen even less frequently.

The 5-year survival rate for patients with malignant pheochromocytoma is approximately 43% as compared with a 97% 5-year survival rate for benign lesions.

Adrenocortical Carcinoma

Adrenocortical carcinoma is a rare malignancy with approximately 150–200 new cases reported each year in the United States. There is a bimodal age distribution, with incidence peaking in young children and then again between 40 to 50 years of age.

CLINICAL MANIFESTATIONS

Patients with adrenocortical carcinoma usually present with vague abdominal symptoms secondary to an enlarging retroperitoneal mass or with clinical manifestations of overproduction of one or more steroid hormones. Most of these tumors are functional as measured by biochemical parameters. Fifty percent secrete cortisol, producing Cushing's syndrome. The work-up and management of patients with Cushing's syndrome are described in that section in this chapter. Another 10–20% of adrenocortical carcinomas produce various steroid hormones, causing varying degrees of virilization in females, feminization in males, and/or hypertension.

DIAGNOSIS

The work-up of these patients involves a careful biochemical screening including a 24-hour urine collection to measure levels of cortisol, aldosterone, catecholamines, metanephrine, vanillylmandelic acid, 17-OHCS, and 17-keto-steroids. The results serve mainly to guide perioperative replacement therapy as well as to rule out pheochromocytoma.

High-resolution abdominal CT and MRI are the best ways to obtain images of the adrenal glands. CT can usually identify lesions as small as 7 mm. MRI may be especially helpful not only in identifying tumor extension up the inferior vena cava but also in differentiating between various lesions based on the adrenal to liver ratio on T2-weighted images. Adenomas usually have ratios of 0.7–1.4; malignant lesions, whether primary or metastatic to the adrenal gland, have ratios of 1.4–3.0; and pheochromocytomas usually have ratios greater than 3.0. Chest radiography is helpful in ruling out pulmonary metastasis. Adrenal arteriography and venography are usually reserved for selected patients who have large lesions that may distort the usual anatomy in the region of the tumor. The current staging system for adrenocortical carcinomas is shown in Tables 14-4 and 14-5.

TREATMENT

Surgery is the treatment of choice for adrenocortical carcinomas. Approximately 50% of the tumors are localized to the adrenal gland at the time of initial exploration. Radical en bloc resection that includes adjacent organs, if necessary, provides the only chance for long-term cure. Unfortunately,

Table 14-4. Staging for adrenocortical carcinoma

Tumor size	
T1	Tumor <5 cm, no invasion
T2	Tumor >5 cm, no invasion
T3	Tumor outside adrenal in fat
T4	Tumor invading adjacent organs
Lymph node status	
N0	No positive lymph nodes
N1	Positive lymph nodes
Metastases	
M0	No distant metastases
M1	Distant metastases

Table 14-5. Staging criteria and median survival for adreno-cortical carcinoma

Stage	Criteria	Median survival (years)
I	T1 N0 M0	5
II	T2 N0 M0	5
III	T1–2 N1 M0; T3 N0 M0	2.3
IV	Any T, any N M1; T3–4 N1 M0	1

85% of patients develop metastatic disease. The 5-year survival rate for all patients approaches only 20–25%.

Common sites of recurrence include lungs, lymph nodes, liver, peritoneum, and bone. Resection of recurrent disease, including pulmonary metastases, can prolong survival for about 1 year and control the symptoms related to excess hormone production. Therefore after a curative resection, patients need to be monitored closely with monthly urinary steroid profiles as well as frequent abdominal CT and chest radiography. Adjuvant therapy for adrenocortical carcinoma has had minimal impact, if any, on disease progression.

Radiation can provide palliation for bone metastases and recurrent, unresectable abdominal tumors; however, it has failed to prolong survival. No chemotherapeutic agent or combination of agents has been shown to be consistently effective against unresectable disease. Mitotane has been one of the most commomly used chemotherapy agents against this neoplasm because of its ability to palliate the endocrine effects of the tumor. This drug is an isomer of DDT and not only inhibits steroid production but also leads to atrophy of adrenocortical cells. Mitotane is associated with a number of side effects in the gastrointestinal and neuromuscular systems. In addition, the drug appears to have a narrow therapeutic range and requires close monitoring of serum levels.

Incidentalomas

With the widespread use of abdominal CT, asymptomatic adrenal lesions are being discovered with increasing frequency. These lesions, termed *incidentalomas*, are seen in 0.6–1.3% of routinely performed abdominal imaging studies and up to 9% in autopsy series. Although most of these lesions are benign adenomas, many can cause problems either by being hormonally active or by becoming an invasive malignancy.

All patients with incidentalomas should have measurement of serum electrolyte levels and a 24-hour urine collection to determine levels of vanillylmandelic acid, metanephrine, catecholamines, cortisol, aldosterone, 17-OHCS, and 17-ketosteroids. Any hormonally active lesion, regardless of size, should be resected.

If the incidentaloma is nonfunctioning, the risk of its being malignant seems to be related to its size. Lesions larger than 100 g, which corresponds to a diameter of approximately 6 cm, should be resected because as many as 35% are malignant. Although observation is generally recommended for lesions smaller than 3.5 cm in diameter, the management of tumors between 3.5 and 6 cm is more controversial. MRI appears to be useful in helping determine which lesions less than 6 cm should be removed. By using the adrenal mass to liver ratio on T2-weighted images, one can separate adenomas, which have a ratio of less than 1.4, from malignant lesions (primary or metastatic), which have a ratio greater than 1.4. Any suspicious lesion should be resected. A lesion that is followed rather than resected needs to be reimaged at 3, 6, and 12 months to determine whether it is growing and, if so, at what rate. Figure 14-3 provides an overview of our approach to patients with incidentalomas.

Metastatic Lesions

The metastasis of tumors to the adrenal glands is relatively common. Based on autopsy studies, 42% of lung tumors, 16% of stomach tumors, 58% of breast tumors, 50% of malignant melanomas, and a high percentage of renal and prostate tumors have metastasized to the adrenals at the time of death. Only rarely are problems related to the metastases, such as adrenal insufficiency, encountered because more than 90% of the gland must be replaced before clinically detectable alterations in gland function are appreciated. When adrenal insufficiency does occur, it is usually in the setting of grossly enlarged adrenal glands as detected by CT.

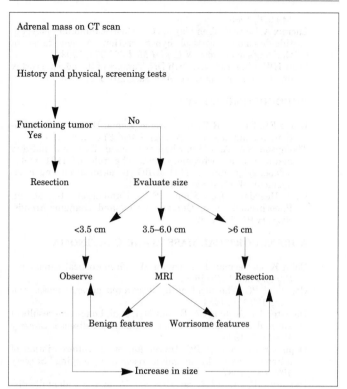

Fig. 14-3. Algorithm for the work-up and treatment of an adrenal incidentaloma.

Selected References

PRIMARY HYPERALDOSTERONISM

Bravo EL, Tarazi RC, Dustan HP, et al. The changing clinical spectrum of primary aldosteronism. *Am J Med* 74:641, 1983.

Grant CS, Carpenter P, van Heerden JA, et al. Primary aldosteronism: Clinical management. *Arch Surg* 119:585, 1984.

Young WF, Klee GC. Primary aldosteronism. *Endocrinol Metab Clin North Am* 17:367, 1988.

HYPERCORTISOLISM

Brunicardi FC, Rosman PM, Lesser KL, et al. Current status of adrenalectomy for Cushing's disease. *Surgery* 98:1127, 1985.

Carpenter PC. Cushing's syndrome: Update of diagnosis and management. *Mayo Clin Proc* 61:49, 1986.

Jex RK, van Heerden JA, Carpenter PC, et al. Ectopic ACTH syndrome: Diagnostic and therapeutic aspects. *Am J Surg*

149:276, 1985.

Lacroix A, Bolte E, Tremblay J, et al. Gastric inhibitory polypeptide-dependent cortisol hypersecretion: A new cause of Cushing's syndrome. *N Engl J Med* 327:974, 1992.

Scott HW, Abumrad NN, Orth DN. Tumors of the adrenal cortex and Cushing's syndrome. *Ann Surg* 201:586, 1985.

PHEOCHROMOCYTOMA

Bravo EL, Gifford RW. Pheochromocytoma: Diagnosis, localization, and management. *N Engl J Med* 311:1298, 1984.

Thompson NW, Allo MD, Shapiro B, et al. Extra-adrenal and metastatic pheochromocytoma: The role of I131 metaiodobenzylguanidine (I131-MIBG) in localization and management. *World J Surg* 8:605, 1984.

van Heerden JA, Sheps SG, Hamberger B, et al. Pheochromocytoma: Current status and changing trends. *Surgery* 91:367, 1982.

ADRENOCORTICAL MASSES AND CARCINOMA

Cohn K, Gottesman L, Brennan M. Adrenocortical carcinoma. *Surgery* 100:1170, 1986.

Copeland PC. The incidentally discovered adrenal mass. *Ann Surg* 199:116, 1984.

Demeter JG, De Jong SA, Brooks MH, et al. Long-term results of adrenal autotransplantation in Cushing's disease. *Surgery* 108:1117, 1990.

Doppman JL, Reinig JW, Dwyer AJ, et al. Differentiation of adrenal masses by magnetic resonance imaging. *Surgery* 102:1018, 1987.

Herrera MF, Grant CS, van Heerden JA, et al. Incidentally discovered adrenal tumors: An institutional perspective. *Surgery* 110:1014, 1991.

Luton JP, Cerdas S, Billaud L, et al. Clinical features of adrenocortical carcinoma, prognostic factors, and the effect of mitotane therapy. *N Engl J Med* 322:1195, 1990.

Ross NS, Aron DC. Hormonal evaluation of the patient with an incidentally discovered adrenal mass. *N Engl J Med* 323:1401, 1990.

Carcinoma of the Thyroid and Parathyroid Glands

Elizabeth A. Blair and George Barnes, Jr.

Thyroid Cancer

EPIDEMIOLOGY

Thyroid cancer constitutes approximately 1% of all human malignancies, with an estimated incidence in the United States of 13,000 cases in 1994. The majority of these cases—over 75%—occur in women. Carcinoma of the thyroid is considered an indolent disease, with many deaths occurring from other causes. An estimated 1,000–1,200 patients die annually of this disease, with 65% of the deaths in women. Overall, thyroid cancer is the most common endocrine malignancy, representing 90% of the cases.

The prevalence of thyroid nodules increases linearly with age, with spontaneous nodules occurring at a rate of 0.08% per year beginning early in life and extending into the eighth decade. Clinically apparent nodules are present in 4–7% of the adult population, occurring more commonly in women and increasing with age.

Few risk factors have been confirmed for thyroid carcinoma, with the exception of radiation exposure. A history of ionizing radiation is an accepted major risk factor for thyroid malignancy, usually the papillary type. Approximately 9% of thyroid cancers are associated with prior radiation exposure. The risk of cancer from radiation increases linearly with doses from 6.5 cGy to a peak of 2,000 cGy, flattening at higher doses and causing thyroid ablation. The radiation-exposed patient is more likely to have multifocal disease. Radiation exposure in childhood is also associated with an increased risk of benign thyroid nodules, estimated to be 20–30%, compared to the incidence in the general population of 4%. The incidence of cancer in a cold nodule is 10–20% in the general population; however, radiation increases that risk to 30–50%. The role of racial and genetic factors, diet, iodine consumption, and iodine deficiency in the etiology of thyroid carcinoma is ill defined except for medullary carcinoma. Patients with multiple endocrine neoplasia syndrome type II (MEN-II) are genetically at risk for medullary carcinoma and with familial cases, represent 20% of all medullary cases (see Chapter 13).

The presence of a point mutation in the *ras* oncogene has been identified in 40–50% of follicular carcinomas of the thyroid. In addition, a similar percentage of benign follicular adenomas have the same *ras* mutation, suggesting that this mutation is important in the etiology of these tumors.

PATHOLOGY

The majority of malignant tumors of the thyroid gland are of glandular epithelial origin, with the remaining types arising from parafollicular C cells or from nonepithelial stromal elements. The World Health Organization classification of malignant epithelial thyroid tumors is as follows: papillary carcinoma, follicular carcinoma, medullary carcinoma, anaplastic (undifferentiated) carcinoma, and lymphoma. More than 90% of thyroid carcinomas are of the well-differentiated histologic variety: papillary and follicular.

Papillary carcinoma is a well-differentiated form of thyroid carcinoma and is also the most common type, representing 60–70% of all cases. Multifocality is a prominent feature of this pathologic type and has been documented in up to 80% of patients with papillary cancer. Papillary carcinoma occurs as an irregular solid or cystic mass that arises from follicular epithelium. It is nonencapsulated but sharply circumscribed. Microscopically, the hallmark is papillary fronds of epithelium. Rounded calcific deposits (psammoma bodies) can be found in 50% of lesions. Since papillary carcinomas are not encapsulated and invade regional lymphatics, cervical lymph node metastases are common. Papillary carcinoma is the predominant type found in patients with a history of prior radiation exposure. There is no evidence that tumors associated with radiation exposure are unusual or more aggressive than the naturally occurring variety, and they should be managed according to general treatment principles. Overall these patients have a good prognosis, and 80% of them will survive 10 years.

Follicular carcinoma is the second most common malignancy of the thyroid and is considered a well-differentiated tumor, comprising 15–20% of thyroid cancers. It is often difficult to histologically confirm the diagnosis of follicular carcinoma due to its similarity to benign follicular adenomas. Follicular carcinoma is usually encapsulated and consists of highly cellular follicles; most are single, solid, and noncystic without central necrosis. This pathologic type is the most common found in association with endemic goiter. Hematogenous metastases are more common with follicular carcinoma than with papillary carcinoma, and the prognosis is somewhat poorer. Approximately 60% of patients will survive 10 years after treatment for follicular carcinoma.

Hürthle cell neoplasms are thought to be variants of follicular carcinoma within the thyroid, yet are distinct pathologic entities. They represent 5% of thyroid carcinomas. The histopathologic diagnosis of malignancy, as in follicular carcinoma, is difficult to make without the presence of vascular or capsular invasion. The incidence of lymph node metastases is slightly higher in Hürthle cell carcinomas than in follicular carcinomas. The ability of Hürthle cell carcinomas to absorb radioactive iodine is significantly lower than that of follicular carcinomas.

Medullary carcinomas arise from calcitonin-secreting parafollicular C cells of the thyroid gland. These lesions represent 5% of all thyroid cancers, with 20% of patients exhibiting an autosomal dominant inheritance pattern. The sporadic form usually occurs unilaterally, while familial forms are bilateral or are associated with C cell hyperplasia in the contralateral lobe. In inherited forms, the bilateral or multicentric C cell hyperplasia precedes and later undergoes transformation to medullary thyroid carcinoma. Histologically medullary carcinoma is an ill-defined, nonencapsulated, invasive mass. It is composed of columns of epithelial cells and dense stroma that stains for amyloid and collagen. Calcitonin may be identified by immunohistochemical stains. These lesions are slow growing but metastasize by both lymphatic and hematogenous routes. Regional metastases occur early in the course of the disease, usually before the primary reaches 2 cm in size and are present in 50% of patients at the time of diagnosis. Cervical and upper mediastinal lymph nodes are the usual sites involved. Overall 10-year survival rates are 90% with disease confined to the thyroid, 70% with cervical metastases, and 20% with distant metastases. Prognosis for medullary thyroid carcinoma falls between that of anaplastic tumors and well-differentiated tumors. Poor prognostic factors include age greater than 50 years, metastases at the time of diagnosis, and MEN-IIb. Seventy percent of the patients with MEN-IIb have metastasis at the time of diagnosis; less than 5% survive 5 years.

Anaplastic carcinoma is undifferentiated and represented by small cells of variable characteristics. These are rapidly growing tumors, usually greater than 6 cm in size and often inoperable. Anaplastic thyroid carcinoma is aggressive and lethal. These tumors invade local structures and metastasize locally and distantly. At the time of diagnosis, 25% are invading the trachea, 90% have regional metastases, and 50% have distant metastases to the lung. Although rare, it is considered one of the deadliest malignancies. Treatment seldom results in cure, with a mean survival of 6 months and a 5-year survival rate of 7%.

Lymphomas are also small-cell tumors that enlarge rapidly. Lymphomas may be primary or secondary. In patients with disseminated lymphoma, 20% involve the thyroid at autopsy. Histologically, non-Hodgkin's, histiocytic lymphoma is the most common form of primary thyroid lymphoma. Thyroid lymphoma is rare, occurring with a peak onset in the seventh decade and a 6:1 female preponderance. Prognosis is related to the extent of disease at the time of diagnosis. When lymphoma is confined to the thyroid gland, the 5-year survival rate is 75–85% with radiation therapy. Survival at 5 years decreases to 35% with regional metastases and 5% with disseminated disease.

DIAGNOSIS

The majority of patients with thyroid cancer will have no specific symptoms. A change in the size of a thyroid nodule or pain from hemorrhage into a nodule may occasionally bring the patient to the physician. Hoarseness, dysphagia, dyspnea or hemoptysis are symptoms resulting from invasion of surrounding anatomic structures and are rare in well-differentiated thyroid carcinomas.

A thorough physical examination is the most important initial diagnostic step. The presence of a single or dominant nodule, usually over 1 cm in diameter with a hard consistency and fixation, is characteristic of cancer. Not infrequently, especially in children, the initial manifestation of thyroid carcinoma is a palpable cervical lymph node. The presence of discrete 1- to 2-cm lymph nodes in conjunction with a thyroid nodule suggests malignancy. Palpable adenopathy is most often found along the middle and lower portions of the jugular vein but may be located lateral to the sternocleidomastoid muscle in the lower portion of the posterior cervical triangle. Physical findings of concern are vocal cord paralysis, fixation of the thyroid nodule, and tracheal deviation or invasion. Cervical spine flexibility should be assessed to ensure that the necessary hyperextension of the neck can be achieved for adequate operative exposure. Laryngeal function should be evaluated with either indirect mirror or flexible fiberoptic examination.

A variety of diagnostic tests are available to help distinguish benign from malignant disease. The most desirable and cost-effective strategy uses the minimum number of studies to distinguish lesions that require surgical intervention from those that do not. The ultimate goal is to avoid operating on benign lesions whenever possible. Figure 15-1 broadly outlines how we evaluate and treat the thyroid nodule or mass.

The fine-needle aspiration (FNA) and interpretation of cytology by an experienced pathologist is probably the single most useful procedure. This test is safe and cost effective, and when performed by an experienced cytopathologist, accuracy in the diagnosis of thyroid cancer is greater than 90%. The accuracy is greatest for lesions between 1 and 4 cm, since smaller lesions are difficult to sample and larger lesions have an increased sampling error due to the large area of the lesion. Lesions are generally classified as negative, positive, or suspicious for malignancy. Distinguishing a follicular adenoma from a follicular carcinoma is not possible with an FNA biopsy since pathologic examination demonstrating capsular or vascular invasion is required. In general, the results obtained by FNA are used to help plan further management of the patient, but the individual clinical situation should be the most important consideration.

Ultrasonography of the thyroid is an accurate method for establishing the consistency of the nodule (solid or cystic), multicentricity, and presence of lymph node enlargement. Ultrasound can detect lesions as small as 1 mm; however, the percentage of these small lesions that are malignant is unknown. Unfortunately, interpretation depends on the experience of the imaging expert, and currently no specific

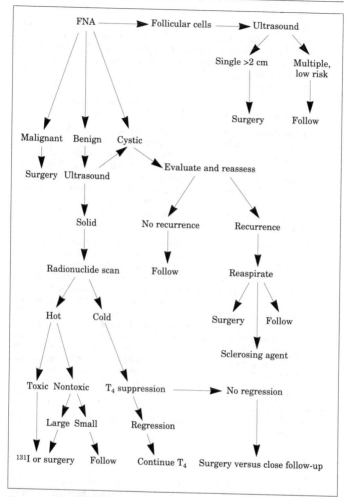

Fig. 15-1. Steps involved in the work-up of a thyroid nodule at M. D. Anderson. (FNA = fine-needle aspiration.)

sonographic criteria can distinguish benign from malignant nodules. Solid lesions have a 15–20% risk of malignancy, while the risk in cystic lesions greater than 4 cm is 15% and is considered minimal in smaller cystic lesions. In addition, ultrasound-assisted FNA is useful when the tumor is difficult to palpate or in a deep location.

Radionucleotide scintigraphy (^{99}Tc-pertechnetate, iodine ^{125}I or ^{131}I) was previously used as the first diagnostic step in evaluating palpable thyroid masses. Since most thyroid carcinomas and many benign nodules will appear cold on scan, the main limitation of this imaging modality is its inability to distinguish between benign and malignant lesions. Approximately 16% of cold nodules, 9% of warm, and 4% of hot lesions will harbor a malignancy. Although a cold lesion has the greatest probability of being malignant, the presence of a hot lesion on thyroid scan does not exclude malignancy.

A chest roentgenogram is important to evaluate for pulmonary metastases and identify tracheal deviation.

Other diagnostic imaging studies are seldom needed for evaluation of a patient with a thyroid nodule. Computerized tomography (CT) and magnetic resonance imaging (MRI) are useful in large or recurrent cancers suspected of invasion into the surrounding soft tissue. When indicated by the history and physical findings, CT or MRI of the neck and upper mediastinum may be used to delineate extrathyroidal extension or to determine the presence of significant cervical and/or mediastinal metastases.

Preoperative laboratory assessment should include thyroid function testing and a serum calcium measurement. Thyroid function studies do not help in making the diagnosis of cancer, but the presence of hypothyroidism or hyperthyroidism in a patient with a thyroid nodule is important, particularly when considering general anesthesia. Parathyroid function should be assessed by measuring calcium level, as the incidence of parathyroid adenomas and other hyperfunctioning anomalies of the parathyroid gland are more frequent in the presence of thyroid nodules or carcinoma. Thyroid antibody tests are important when thyroiditis is a consideration. Serum calcitonin measurements are only indicated when a family history of medullary carcinoma is present or an MEN syndrome is likely. Serum thyroglobulin levels are useful mainly for follow-up studies following treatment of differentiated thyroid carcinoma and are not a part of the diagnostic evaluation.

TREATMENT

Controversy continues over what to do in the presence of a thyroid nodule, the extent of resection necessary in cases of papillary and follicular cancer, the role of postresection thyroid hormone suppression, and the appropriate use of postoperative therapeutic radioactive [131]I.

Staging and Prognosis

Since well-differentiated thyroid cancer is associated with a favorable prognosis, many authors have attempted to tailor their surgical approach to the prognosis of the disease. Prognostic groupings have been defined for differentiated thyroid carcinoma based on age and gender of the patient and on findings at the time of surgery. Two widely used prognostic schemes are recognized by the acronyms AGES and AMES. The letters stand for *age* at the time of diagnosis,

Table 15-1. AJCC TNM classification of thyroid gland carcinoma

Primary tumor (T)	
T1	Diameter <3 cm
T2	Diameter >3 cm
T3	Multifocal tumor
T4	Fixation or invasion
Nodal involvement (N)	
Nx	Nodes cannot be assessed
N0	No clinically or pathologically positive nodes
N1	Clinically or pathologically positive nodes
Metastases (M)	
Mx	Not assessed
M0	No known metastases
M1	Distant metastases present

metastasis to distant sites, *extent (size)* of the primary tumor, and histologic *grade* of the tumor.

At the University of Texas M. D. Anderson Cancer Center, we define three risk groups: high, medium, and low. The high-risk group is comprised of men over 40 years of age and women over 50 years of age with follicular carcinoma. These patients have a relapse rate of 40% and a 36% death rate from their cancer. The low-risk group refers to differentiated carcinoma in men less than 40 years of age and women under the age of 50 with any histology. Their recurrence rate is 11% and death rate is 4%. Children and adolescents fall into the low-risk category and have an excellent prognosis. The intermediate risk group includes males over the age of 40 and women over 50 with papillary carcinoma. The recurrence rate for this group is 29%, with a death rate of 21%.

In general, the prognosis for papillary thyroid carcinoma is influenced by age, gender, extent of disease, and volume of the primary tumor. Over 50% of patients will have metastases to the regional lymphatics, and 10% will develop hematogenous metastases. Overall, these patients have a good prognosis, and 80% of them will survive 10 years. The prognostic significance of lymph node metastases continues to be debated; in patients with papillary cancer who are less than 40 years of age, the significance is considered negligible. The minimal effect of lymph node metastases on prognosis is reflected in the American Joint Committee on Cancer (AJCC) staging system (Tables 15-1 and 15-2). In this system, papillary carcinoma has stage I and stage II, which differ only by the presence or absence of distant disease. It is only for patients over 45 years of age that lymph node metastases are factored into the staging prognosis. The diminished importance of lymph node metastases is based on data suggesting that microscopic metastases are present in up to 80% of lymph nodes examined, yet only 10% of patients develop clinically significant disease. In addition, if long-term survival is examined in patients under 40 years, the presence of positive nodes is not a significant negative prognostic factor in papillary carcinoma. Survival for thyroid carcinoma according to stage is shown in Table 15-3.

Table 15-2. AJCC staging of thyroid gland cancer

Histologic type	Stage	<45 years of age	>45 years of age
Papillary	Stage I	Any T, any N, M0	Any T, N0 M0, T1 N1 M0
	Stage II	Any T, any N, M1	T2–4, N1, M0
	Stage III	None	None
	Stage IV	None	Any T, any N, M1
Follicular	Stage I	Any T, any N, M0	Any T, any N, M0
	Stage II	Any T, any N, M1	T2–4, N0, M0
	Stage III	None	Any T, N1, M0
	Stage IV	None	Any T, any N, M1
Medullary	Stage I	None	None
	Stage II	Any T, any N, M0	None
	Stage III	None	Any T, any M, M1
	Stage IV	Any T, any N, M1	Any T, any N, M1
Undiffer- entiated	Stage I	None	None
	Stage II	None	None
	Stage III	None	None
	Stage IV	Any T, any N, M1	Any T, any N, M1

Table 15-3. Ten-year survival rates for thyroid carcinoma by stage

Stage	10-year survival (%)
I	95
II	50–95
III	15–50
IV	<15

The prognosis of follicular carcinoma is somewhat poorer than with papillary carcinoma. Approximately 60% of patients will survive 10 years after treatment for follicular carcinoma. Additionally, hematogenous metastases are more common in follicular carcinoma.

Surgical Resection

Surgical resection is the principal treatment used in thyroid cancer. Accepted surgical management varies from a thyroid lobectomy and isthmusectomy to a total thyroidectomy and modified neck dissection (Table 15-4).

Thyroidectomy is indicated in the management of a patient with a thyroid nodule in the following circumstances:

1. Palpable thyroid abnormality or cold nodule in a patient with a history of irradiation to the neck.

2. Palpable nodule in a patient under 20 years of age or a solid, single nodule in a patient over 60 years of age.

3. FNA suggestive or indicative of thyroid malignancy.

4. A thyroid mass with physical findings suggestive of malignant disease (fixed to surrounding structures, vocal cord paralysis, etc.).

Table 15-4. Recommended treatment of thyroid cancer

Lesion	Treatment
Papillary	
<1.5 cm	Lobectomy and isthmusectomy
>1.5 cm	Total thyroidectomy
Follicular	Total thyroidectomy
Hürthle	
Benign	Lobectomy and isthmusectomy
Malignant	Total thyroidectomy
Medullary	Total thyroidectomy and central neck dissection

5. Proof of cervical metastasis or a thyroid mass with cervical lymph node enlargement.

6. Histologically or cytologically proven metastatic thyroid carcinoma.

7. All solitary cold nodules or dominant nodules in a multinodular gland that fail to respond to suppressive hormonal therapy.

The management of well-differentiated thyroid cancer is controversial. Proponents of total thyroidectomy argue that (1) this operation can be performed safely with a 2% incidence of permanent recurrent nerve injury or permanent hypoparathyroidism; (2) there is a risk of persistent or recurrent cancer in the residual thyroid after lesser surgery; and (3) residual thyroid tissue left after less than total thyroidectomy hampers detection of metastases by radioiodine scans and thyroglobulin. Advocates of more conservative procedures such as thyroid lobectomy and isthmusectomy or near-total thyroidectomy argue that (1) there is a decreased risk of recurrent laryngeal nerve and parathyroid gland injury with conservative surgery; (2) it is rare for a total thyroidectomy to remove all the thyroid gland; (3) occult foci of papillary carcinoma left behind with conservative surgery are rarely of clinical significance; (4) clinically significant recurrences after conservative surgery can be safely managed by re-operation; and (5) there are no data to show a survival benefit for total thyroidectomy over thyroid lobectomy for well-differentiated lesions.

Lobectomy with isthmusectomy is an appropriate treatment for a small papillary cancer less than 1.5 cm in diameter and in patients at low risk of death from thyroid cancer (i.e., men younger than 40 years, women younger than 50, no metastasis, low-grade tumor). Data from Mazzaferri et al. have shown excellent survival in this group of patients treated with less than a total resection. An incidental microscopic carcinoma found at the time of thyroidectomy for other reasons does not require further treatment.

At M. D. Anderson we perform a total or near-total thyroidectomy for all papillary cancers larger than 1.5 cm, those associated with a history of previous radiation, gross disease in both lobes, and all follicular cancers. This approach is used for papillary carcinoma because of its multifocal nature, and local control is improved. In follicular cancer, removal of all thyroid tissue facilitates postoperative radionuclide scanning and allows for adjuvant ^{131}I treatment of distant metastases.

Although total thyroidectomy is our treatment of choice for follicular carcinoma and Hürthle cell carcinoma, the diagnosis may not be ascertained by frozen-section examination at the time of surgery. Patients with a minimally invasive, small (<1 cm) follicular tumor or a single, well-encapsulated, benign Hürthle cell neoplasm may be treated by thyroid lobectomy and isthmusectomy. All other patients should undergo a total thyroidectomy. When the diagnosis of follicular carcinoma is confirmed postoperatively, a completion thyroidectomy should be performed in high-risk patients (i.e., men older than 40 years, women older than 50, lesions >1 cm, patients with distant metastasis).

In medullary carcinoma, all patients should undergo a total thyroidectomy combined with a central paratracheal neck dissection to remove all disease. This procedure is important because medullary tumors do not concentrate radioiodine, the disease is multifocal, metastases occur early, and nonsurgical treatments are noneffective. Identifying C cell hyperplasia in the contralateral lobe indicates a familial case and the need for family screening.

Anaplastic carcinoma is an aggressive lesion that is rarely resectable at presentation. The diagnosis is usually made by core needle biopsy. Treatment consists of combination radiotherapy and chemotherapy. Resectable lesions are treated by total thyroidectomy and wide local excision of adjacent soft tissues. Resected patients are treated with postoperative adjuvant chemotherapy and radiotherapy.

Surgical Technique

Surgical resection of a possible thyroid cancer requires meticulous dissection of the ipsilateral thyroid compartment, identification and preservation of the recurrent laryngeal nerve, and complete resection of the affected lobe and thyroid isthmus. Identification of the ipsilateral parathyroid glands should be attempted, but preservation may be impossible if there is extensive invasion by cancer or clinical metastases in the paratracheal area. If the diagnosis of cancer is confirmed by frozen-section histologic examination of the specimen, total thyroidectomy is completed by resecting the opposite lobe, taking special care to identify and spare parathyroid glands and their blood supply. Once the thyroid gland is removed, the posterior surface is carefully inspected for any possible parathyroid tissue. If the parathyroid is identified, a portion is sent for frozen-section examination, with the remnant kept in physiologic solution (Tissuesol or Ringer's solution). If parathyroid tissue is confirmed, the preserved portion is minced and implanted in a small pocket created in the sternocleidomastoid muscle.

In addition to thyroidectomy, we recommend a compartmental lymph node dissection. Dissection of the lymphoareolar tissue in this area is the best way to avoid reexploration for future recurrence.

The surgical procedure may be carried out under local or general anesthesia. The approach to the thyroid gland itself is through a transverse incision, from 1.5 to 6.0 inches in length, approximately 1–2 finger breadths above the clavicles. The subplatysmal flaps are elevated superiorly to the level of the thyroid notch and inferiorly to the suprasternal notch. Separation of the fascia between the strap muscles and the sternocleidomastoid muscles is done to facilitate exposure of the gland and allow inspection of the lower jugular lymph nodes. The strap muscles are separated in the midline and can be divided on the side of the primary tumor if necessary. Portions of the strap muscles adherent to the gland are resected with the specimen. The thyroid compartment may be approached laterally along the anterior border of the sternocleidomastoid muscle or medially through the midline raphe of the strap muscles.

Palpable adenopathy or clinical suspicion of lymphatic metastasis in the high-risk patient requires that a neck dissection be performed. In these cases, all areolar and lymphatic tissue along the internal jugular vein and carotid vessels from the subdigastric area down to the supraclavicular fossa is resected. The middle thyroid veins are divided during this portion of the procedure. The dissection is continued medially, allowing for identification and dissection of the recurrent laryngeal nerve. All lymphoareolar tissue in the thyroid compartment and upper mediastinum to the level of the innominate vein is accessible through a collar incision. This tissue contains the lymph nodes of the central compartment and is dissected medially and superiorly in continuity with the specimen. A nonrecurrent laryngeal nerve on the right side may be recognized as it originates high from the vagus nerve. Nonrecurrent laryngeal nerves may be found in proximity to the superior thyroid vessels or the inferior thyroid artery.

The thyroid vessels are identified and ligated close to the gland. The superior pole vessels are individually transected with a small curved or right angle hemostat. The superior laryngeal nerve should be identified between the thyroid vessels as it crosses the constrictor muscle and enters the cricothyroid muscle. Caution is warranted as the position of the superior nerve in relation to the vascular pedicle may vary.

Dissection of the gland is continued inferiorly on the posterior aspect of the gland, incising the fascia that secures the gland (visceral and suspensory ligament). The recurrent laryngeal nerve, if not previously located, is identified in the paratracheal groove inferior to the gland and is dissected superiorly. The inferior artery is identified and its branches are individually ligated as they enter the thyroid gland, taking care not to injure the recurrent nerve. The anatomic relationship of the nerve and the inferior artery is extremely variable. Also, the nerve may divide into several branches at the level of the inferior thyroid artery. All nerve branches should be preserved in the course of the dissection. Careful dissection is continued up to where the nerve enters the larynx. All parathyroid-like tissue should be respected and left attached to individual vascular pedicles. Surgical loupes are often helpful for this part of the dissection.

Any extrathyroidal extension of carcinoma into surrounding tissues needs to be clearly delineated. Judicious resection of the invaded structure should be accomplished, including resection of laryngeal nerves, tracheal rings, or portions of the larynx, to ensure complete surgical extirpation. Local invasion of tissues surrounding the thyroid, though rare, is a source of significant morbidity and mortality. Uncontrolled local recurrence is a major cause of mortality from thyroid cancer, making local control a key issue in these patients. Fortunately, locally invasive thyroid carcinoma can often be resected with a much narrower margin than other carcinomas that arise in tissues surrounding the thyroid.

Dissection of the opposite lobe, when indicated, proceeds similarly to the dissection of the involved lobe. The most delicate and important part of the dissection of the opposite lobe consists of the identification and preservation of the recurrent laryngeal nerve and the parathyroid glands and their blood supply. Often a small portion of thyroid tissue may have to be spared (subtotal resection) to preserve the vascular pedicle to the parathyroid tissue. Meticulous dissection of the parathyroid glands and their vascular supply, and autotransplantation of devascularized parathyroid tissue are important techniques that have contributed to a lower incidence of permanent hypoparathyroidism.

At the completion of the procedure, hemostasis is obtained and the wound is irrigated with normal saline. One or two drains are placed for vacuum aspiration.

Neck Dissection

The necessity and extent of neck dissection for follicular and papillary carcinomas is another subject of controversy. Follicular carcinoma rarely metastasizes to the regional lymph nodes, while papillary carcinoma frequently spreads to regional nodes. Neck dissection is obviously indicated for palpable adenopathy. Elective neck dissections have not conclusively been proved to be more effective than observation and therapeutic dissection. Careful intraoperative assessment of the regional nodes and sampling or dissection of the central compartment lymph nodes is advisable, however, during surgical resection of papillary carcinomas to avoid the necessity of later repeat dissection for recurrent disease.

When neck dissection for differentiated thyroid carcinoma is indicated, all the nodal groups at highest risk for metastasis should be included. The so-called central or interjugular tracheal compartment contains the first echelon of lymph nodes for the thyroid gland. The nodes along the jugular vein from the subdigastric area to the root of the neck are important metastatic sites. Another route of lymphatic spread for thyroid cancer is along the inferior thyroid artery as it courses behind the common carotid artery and to the lower portion of the posterior triangle of the neck. The classic radical neck dissection, with removal of internal jugular vein, sternocleidomastoid muscle, and accessory nerve, is seldom necessary. Most often, a comprehensive modified neck dissection sparing the above structures is the appropriate cancer operation for metastatic thyroid cancer. A central, bilateral neck dissection, clearing all lymphatic tissue from hyoid bone to the brachiocephalic vein and between the carotid arteries, is considered standard therapy in medullary carcinoma, with a formal modified dissection reserved for patients with positive nodes.

Adjuvant Therapy

Postoperative thyroid-stimulating hormone (TSH) suppression with thyroid hormone for well-differentiated cancers has been shown in retrospective studies to decrease local recurrence rates as compared to surgery alone; however, no controlled clinical trials are available to support this approach. Our philosophy is to treat patients postoperatively with thyroid hormone.

The use of therapeutic ablation of remnant thyroid tissue after thyroidectomy is well established, though criteria for the use of postoperative radioactive iodine vary from institution to institution. Our practice after total thyroidectomy for follicular or papillary carcinoma of the thyroid is to delay thyroid hormone replacement for 4–6 weeks to maximize iodine uptake during scanning. Most patients will develop some symptoms of hypothyroidism, though few suffer distress. A tracer dose of radioactive iodine is then administered and a whole-body scan is performed. This allows scintigraphic staging of disease and may show the presence and extent of metastases that are minimally recognizable by conventional techniques. Approximately 60–80% of well-differentiated tumors take up radioiodine.

Radioactive ^{131}I at therapeutic levels (usually 100 mCi) is indicated for patients with papillary or follicular carcinomas who are less than 20 or older than 40 years of age, patients 20–40 years of age with papillary or follicular carcinomas and either known residual tumor or metastasis, and patients with recurrent cancer. Occasionally, patients with unresectable cancer are treated with radioactive iodine. Adjuvant treatment with ^{131}I and external beam radiotherapy is useful for control of close or microscopically involved margins. Long-term survival and palliation are frequently possible for patients who have extensive extrathyroidal spread and soft-tissue invasion due to differentiated thyroid carcinoma.

External beam radiotherapy (55 Gy in 5.0–5.5 weeks) is an accepted adjuvant treatment for patients with recurrent or locally invasive differentiated carcinoma who do not capture iodine. The use of this treatment in the adjuvant setting to control microscopic foci of differentiated carcinoma reduces the incidence of regional recurrence. In addition, external beam radiotherapy is an accepted treatment modality for nonresectable disease and for palliation of painful distant metastasis, especially in the bone.

After surgery and subsequent ^{131}I ablation therapy, all patients receive hormonal replacement treatment (levothyroxin sodium) at a dose of 100–200 µg/day. The dose varies among patients and needs to be adjusted to suppress the TSH to low or undetectable levels. The dose typically requires modification 3–4 months after completion of treatment.

Adjuvant therapy for other types of thyroid cancers such as Hürthle cell, medullary, and anaplastic carcinoma is less effective. The problem with Hürthle cell and medullary carcinomas is their lack of consistent uptake of radioactive iodine. In addition, they arise from a tissue that does not contain TSH receptors, and thus they are not sensitive to suppression.

Overall cytotoxic chemotherapy has not been very effective in the treatment of thyroid carcinomas. However, radiation therapy combined with doxorubicin has been used in patients with anaplastic carcinomas with some response.

SURVEILLANCE

A coordinated plan of follow-up for thyroid carcinomas must consider the varied presentations possible for recurrent disease. Most patients are seen every 6 months for 1–2 years postoperatively and then yearly. Follow-up visits typically include measuring the serum thyroglobulin level and a chest x-ray. This protocol may vary depending on the risk group of the patient and special circumstances. When indicated, a repeat ^{131}I scan is done after temporary (4–6 weeks) deletion of hormonal replacement. Subsequent therapeutic doses of radioactive iodine may be administered.

Over 50% of patients with papillary carcinomas of the thyroid who die of their disease, die with central neck disease, while most of the recurrences of follicular carcinomas occur distantly. Patients with papillary carcinoma of the thyroid have a high (40%) incidence of lymph node metastases. The most common sites of distant metastases for thyroid cancers are lungs, bone, soft tissues, brain, liver, and adrenal glands. Lung metastases more commonly occur in young patients, whereas bone metastases occur more commonly in older patients. Thyroglobulin values normally range between 2.5 and 28.0 ng/ml but drop after thyroidectomy or ablation and serve as a sensitive indicator of recurrent or persistent disease.

Follow-up for medullary carcinoma differs in that no scanning or thyroglobulin measurements are used. Instead, calcitonin is used to follow these patients. Similarly, Hürthle cell, anaplastic carcinoma, and lymphoma cannot be followed by thyroid scanning and require regular physical exam and x-ray studies for follow-up.

Parathyroid Carcinoma

EPIDEMIOLOGY

Carcinoma of the parathyroid gland is a rare lesion. Its incidence as a cause of hyperparathyroidism varies from 0.5 to 4.0%. The incidence is equally divided between men and women and usually is diagnosed in the fifth decade. The rarity of this tumor has limited the accumulation of natural history data and etiologic factors that might cause it. Associations with familial hyperparathyroidism or MEN-I syndrome have been described. External irradiation has also been reported in association with parathyroid carcinoma.

The natural history of parathyroid carcinoma is one of a slow-growing, persistent, locally recurrent tumor. The local recurrence rate has been estimated to range from 36 to 69%, and overall survival is less than 50%. The major cause of death is hypercalcemia. Distant metastases tend to occur late, with lung, liver, bone, and pancreas being frequent sites.

CLINICAL PRESENTATION

The clinical presentation of patients with parathyroid carcinoma is usually severe hyperparathyroidism. The serum calcium level in carcinoma patients averages more than 14 mg/dl, compared to lower levels of 10 or 11 mg/dl seen with benign causes of hyperparathyroidism. As a result, renal (60%) and skeletal (50%) involvement in parathyroid carcinoma is significantly increased compared to benign causes of primary hyperparathyroidism, where renal and skeletal disease occur in 48% and 20% of patients, respectively. The presence of a palpable neck mass in a patient with hyperparathyroidism should raise the suspicion of parathyroid carcinoma.

DIAGNOSIS

Preoperative localization studies are also useful in parathyroid carcinoma. Real-time ultrasound of the neck is an effective localization study. Malignancy is suggested by signs of gross invasion and marked irregularity of the tumor margins.

Unless the tumor is clinically virulent, differentiation of benign from malignant remains difficult. The findings of invasion of surrounding structures, metastases, or recurrenct tumor point to malignancy. The histologic criteria for a diagnosis of parathyroid malignancy are (1) fibrous capsule and/or fibrous trabeculae, (2) a trabecular or rosette-like cellular architecture, (3) the presence of mitotic figures, and (4) capsular or vascular invasion.

TREATMENT

Surgery is the most effective therapy for carcinoma of the parathyroid glands. Parathyroid cancer has a propensity for local recurrence and rarely metastases to regional nodes. Therefore resection should be performed as an en bloc procedure. En bloc in this case usually requires a thyroid lobectomy and excision of paratracheal alveolar tissue, local lymph nodes, and the thymic tongue. A neck dissection is not necessary at the time of the initial procedure unless clinically positive lymph node metastases are demonstrated.

METASTATIC DISEASE

Localization of metastatic foci is important if treatment of recurrent parathyroid cancer is planned. Thallium chloride scintiscanning is useful for locating cervical or upper mediastinal recurrence. CT scan is effective for identification and localization of mediastinal or pulmonary metastases. Venous catheterization and selective venous sampling are helpful in situations where noninvasive studies fail to show recurrent tumors.

The principal cause of death and the most difficult problem in the long-term management of patients with carcinoma of the parathyroid gland is hypercalcemia. Surgical excision of recurrent carcinoma offers the best palliation. There are no effective chemotherapeutic agents that inhibit tumor growth or affect the secretion of parathyroid hormone in parathyroid carcinoma, and as a result medical management is used only to control hypercalcemia. See Chapter 19 for a discussion of the management of hypercalcemia.

Selected References

Anderson BJ, Samaan NA, Vessilopoulou-Sellin R, et al. Parathyroid carcinoma: Features and difficulties in diagnosis and management. *Surgery* 94:906, 1983.

Boring CC, Squires TS, Tong T. Cancer statistics, 1993. *CA* 43:7, 1993.

Cady B, Rossi R. An expanded view of risk: January 29, 1994 group definition in differentiated thyroid carcinoma. *Surgery* 104:947, 1988.

Clark OH, Duh QY. Thyroid cancer. *Med Clin North Am* 75:21, 1991.

Devine RM, Edis AJ, Banks PM. Primary lymphoma of the thyroid: A review of the Mayo Clinic experience through 1978.

World J Surg 5: 33, 1981.

Duh QY, Sancho JJ, Greenspan FS, et al. Medullary thyroid carcinoma: The need for early diagnosis and total thyroidectomy. *Arch Surg* 124:1206, 1989.

Harness JK, Thompson NW, McLeod MK, et al. Follicular carcinoma of the thyroid gland: Trends and treatment. *Surgery* 96:972, 1984.

Hay ID, Grant CS, Taylor WF, et al. Ipsilateral lobectomy versus bilateral lobar resection in papillary thyroid carcinoma: A retrospective analysis of surgical outcome using a novel prognostic scoring system. *Surgery* 102:1089, 1987.

Hedinger C, Williams ED, Sorbin LH. The WHO histological classification of thyroid tumors: A commentary on the second edition. *Cancer* 63:908, 1989.

Kenady DE, McGrath PC, Schwartz RW. Treatment of thyroid malignancies. *Curr Opin Oncol* 3:128, 1991.

Krubsack AJ, Wilson SD, Lawson TL, et al. Prospective comparison of radionucleotide, computed tomographic, sonographic, and magnetic resonance localization of parathyroid tumors. *Surgery* 106: 639, 1989.

Mazzaferri EL, Young RL. Papillary thyroid carcinoma: A 10-year follow-up report of the impact of therapy in 576 patients. *Am J Med* 70:511, 1981.

McHenry C, Jarosz H, Davis M, et al. Selective postoperative radioactive iodine treatment of thyroid carcinoma. *Surgery* 106:956, 1989.

McLeod MK, Thompson NW. Hürthe cell neoplasm of the thyroid. *Otolaryngol Clin North Am.* 23:441, 1990.

Nel CJC, van Heerden JA, Goellner JR, et al. Anaplastic carcinoma of the thyroid: A clinicopathologic study of 82 cases. *Mayo Clin Proc* 60:51, 1985.

Niederle B, Roka R, Schemper M, et al. Surgical treatment of distant metastases in differentiated thyroid cancer: Indication and results. *Surgery* 100:1088, 1986.

Norton JA. Reoperative parathyroid surgery: Indication, intraoperative decision-making and results. *Prog Surg* 18:133, 1986.

Norton JA, Doppman JL, Jensen RT. Cancer of the Endocrine System. In VT DeVita, S Hallman, SA Rosenberg (eds), *Cancer: Principle and Practice of Oncology.* Philadelphia: Lippincott, 1989.

Obara T, Fujimoto Y. Diagnosis and treatment of patients with parathyroid carcinoma: An update and review. *World J Surg* 15:738, 1991.

Merino MJ, Boice JD, Ron E, et al. Thryoid cancer: A lethal endocrine neoplasm. *Ann Intern Med* 115:133, 1991.

Rosen IB, Sutcliffe SB, Gospodarowicz MK, et al. The role of surgery in the management of thyroid lymphoma. *Surgery* 104:1095, 1988.

Samaan NA, Schultz PN, Hickey RC, et al. The results of various modalities of treatment of well differentiated thyroid carcinoma: A retrospective review of 1599 Patients. *J Clin Endocrinol Metab* 75:714, 1992.

Sandelin K, Thompson NW, Bondeson L. Metastatic parathyroid carcinoma: Dilemmas in management. *Surgery* 110: 978, 1991.

Shortell CK, Andrus CH, Phillips CE, et al. Carcinoma of the parathyroid gland: A 30-year experience. *Surgery* 110:704, 1991.

Thomas CG. Role of thyroid-stimulating hormone suppression in the management of thyroid cancer. *Semin Surg Oncol* 7:115, 1991.

Wynne AG, van Heerden JA, Carney JA, et al. Parathyroid carcinoma: Clinical and pathological features in 43 patients. *Medicine* 71:197, 1992.

Hematologic Malignancies and Splenic Tumors

James A. Reilly, Jr.

Leukemia and lymphoma account for 6–8% of adult cancers and about 8% of the deaths from malignancy in the United States. In children younger than 15 years, leukemias are the most common malignancies, with non-Hodgkin's lymphoma fourth in frequency.

Leukemia and lymphoma patients are usually referred to a surgeon with a specific request: diagnostic biopsy, vascular access, staging laparotomy, or therapeutic splenectomy. Surgeons must be familiar with this group of disorders, both to perform the operation appropriately and to know the procedure's probability of success and risks. At times a major procedure is unlikely to achieve the desired result, or the patient's limited life expectancy makes such an operation unwise.

The Leukemias

The chronic proliferative diseases appear to be a spectrum of disorders ranging in increasing severity from polycythemia vera and essential thrombocythemia to myeloid metaplasia to chronic myelogenous leukemia (CML). A few patients with polycythemia vera and essential thrombocythemia and a larger percentage of patients with myeloid metaplasia will ultimately develop leukemia.

POLYCYTHEMIA VERA AND ESSENTIAL THROMBOCYTHEMIA

Polycythemia vera is associated with an autonomous expansion of the red blood cell mass and volume with a variable effect on white blood cells (WBCs) and platelets, whereas essential thrombocythemia is characterized by an increase in the megakaryocyte lineage, with a greatly increased platelet count and a variable effect on erythrocytes and WBCs. In both diseases there is an increased risk of thrombosis and, paradoxically, of hemorrhage. Three-fourths of patients with polycythemia vera will have palpable splenomegaly, and about half will have hepatic enlargement. Phlebotomy, low-dose chemotherapy, or a combination of these modalities is the primary treatment for patients with polycythemia vera and essential thrombocythemia. Because of the risk of hemorrhage, any operation should be avoided in these patients until the polycythemia is under control.

While splenectomy has little or no role in the management of most patients with polycythemia vera or essential thrombocythemia, a small number of patients develop a condition similar to myeloid metaplasia and require splenectomy. The operative risks are greater and the survival is poorer in this group than in patients with myeloid metaplasia. Patients with polycythemia vera and essential thombocythemia should be treated with aggressive nonoperative therapy and offered splenectomy only when pain, anemia, and thrombocytopenia are refractory to other treatment. Splenectomy does not increase the survival rate, but it may improve the quality of life.

MYELOID METAPLASIA

Myeloid metaplasia is characterized by fibrosis of the bone marrow and extramedullary hematopoiesis, chiefly in the spleen, liver, and lymph nodes. As the spleen enlarges, the hematopoietic function it serves may be overwhelmed by destructive hypersplenism (excessive destruction of one or more of the blood components, usually by an autoimmune mechanism).

Although some patients are asymptomatic, most present with fatigue, anorexia and weight loss, or symptomatic splenomegaly. Leukocytosis and thrombocytosis may be present; other hematologic abnormalities such as diminished WBC and platelet counts may result from passive splenic sequestration or active destruction. Active splenic destruction may be humorally mediated (related to specific antibody recognition) or cell mediated (probably by activated macrophages). Peripheral blood smears often demonstrate large platelets, nucleated red cells, anisocytosis, and immature myeloid elements. The diagnosis is made by bone marrow biopsy. In about 5% of cases myeloid metaplasia will progress to CML or acute myeloblastic leukemia.

Initial management may include transfusions, steroids, androgens, cytotoxic chemotherapy, and splenic irradiation. If these measures are not effective in treating the complications of hypersplenism, a splenectomy may be indicated. Splenectomy does not prolong survival but may improve the quality of life. The response rate for anemia varies from 75 to 95% following splenectomy. The morbidity of splenectomy ranges from 35 to 75% and the mortality rate from 5 to 18%.

At the University of Texas M. D. Anderson Cancer Center, patients who have myeloid metaplasia with myelofibrosis are advised to undergo splenectomy under the following conditions: (1) for severe anemia due to hypersplenism when medical management is unsuccessful; (2) for chronically symptomatic splenomegaly; or (3) for the development of worsening congestive heart failure caused by a shunt effect through the spleen. Adequate bone marrow activity must be verified before splenectomy is contemplated. If the spleen is the major site of hematopoiesis, splenectomy may result in severe pancytopenia. A bone marrow biopsy and nuclear medicine bone marrow scan may define the hematopoietic productivity of the marrow cavity.

CHRONIC MYELOGENOUS LEUKEMIA

CML, also known as chronic granulocytic leukemia, involves a clonal proliferation of myeloid stem cells. About 90% of patients will have a translocation of chromosomes 9 and 22; this translocation is called the *Philadelphia chromosome*. The Philadelphia chromosome may be followed clinically to help assess response to therapy.

CML has both a chronic benign phase and a phase of acute blastic transformation. Most patients present with symptoms of the chronic phase, which include fatigue, weakness, night sweats, low-grade fever, and abdominal pain. Splenomegaly may be an isolated finding during physical examination. The WBC count and the platelet count may be elevated; however, the platelets may not function normally. Hypersplenism may result in anemia or thrombocytopenia. Patients with the chronic phase of CML should be evaluated every 3–6 months. The median duration of the chronic phase is about 45 months, but some patients may live up to 20 years with this condition. CML will progress from the chronic benign phase to the acute leukemic transformation phase in about 80% of patients.

The acute or accelerated stage of CML may be heralded by progressive fatigue, high fevers, increasingly symptomatic splenomegaly, anemia, thrombocytopenia, basophilia, and bone or joint pain. In addition to the Philadelphia chromosome, other deletions and translocations may be detected. The WBC count may markedly increase and may not be readily controlled by medical means. Increased splenic destruction of blood components may be manifested by more frequent infections or bleeding episodes. Average survival is approximately 6 months, and during this period, the disease may become resistant to chemotherapy. Blast crisis is heralded by large numbers of these immature cells in the circulation, with a decrease in other cellular components; this is usually a preterminal event.

Currently, CML patients are treated with either standard chemotherapy or interferon-alpha (IFN-α) when they become symptomatic in the chronic phase of the malignancy. Splenectomy is generally used as palliation for either painful splenomegaly or refractory anemia. For CML patients whose disease becomes resistant to IFN-α, a splenectomy may improve response to this therapy. Removal of an enlarged spleen prior to bone marrow transplantation may improve survival either by eliminating a focus of disease or by decreasing transfusion requirements. However, splenectomy has not been proved necessary in all CML patients undergoing transplantation. Symptoms due to splenomegaly will likely be improved by splenectomy, but the response is variable when splenectomy is performed to correct dyscrasias. Splenectomy does not delay blast transformation, and its effect on survival is controversial. Because patients in the accelerated phase of the disease may have a limited survival period, splenectomy in that group should be avoided except in patients undergoing bone marrow transplantation.

Table 16-1. Rai staging of chronic lymphocytic leukemia

Stage	Criteria
0	Lymphocytosis (WBCs >15,000/μl with >40% lymphocytes in the bone marrow)
I	Lymphocytosis with lymphadenopathy
II	Lymphocytosis with enlarged liver or spleen (lymphadenopathy not necessarily present)
III	Lymphocytosis with anemia. Anemia may be due to hemolysis or to decreased production (lymphadenopathy or hepatosplenomegaly need not be present)
IV	Lymphocytosis with thrombocytopenia (platelet count <100,000/μl) anemia, and lymphadenopathy

WBC = white blood cell.

CHRONIC LYMPHOCYTIC LEUKEMIA

Chronic lymphocytic leukemia (CLL) is the most common leukemia in the Western hemisphere. It is typified by an accumulation of long-lived, mature-appearing but functionally inactive B cells. The median age of onset is in the seventh decade, and the incidence continues to increase beyond that age.

CLL patients may present with enlarged, painless lymph nodes, weakness, weight loss, and anorexia. As the disease progresses, they may develop more pronounced lymphadenopathy and splenomegaly. There may be a decrease in red blood cell count due to either bone marrow infiltration with leukemic cells or a Coombs-positive hemolytic anemia. About 20% of patients will develop a second malignancy, most commonly lung cancer, melanoma, or sarcoma. CLL may have either an indolent or an aggressive course, with patient survival ranging from 1 to 20 years. CLL patients have a progressive loss of immune function, and infection is the most common cause of death.

Previously, treatment was withheld in the early stages until signs of progression occurred. Currently, at M. D. Anderson, treatment is still not generally started in the Rai stage 0 patients (lymphocytosis only), but chemotherapy is used to treat other early-stage patients (Rai stage I or II) with poor prognostic signs and all patients with Rai stage III or IV disease (Table 16-1). Fludarabine is used in conjunction with granulocyte-macrophage colony stimulating factor (GM-CSF). Splenectomy may be recommended for patients refractory to fludarabine or for patients with symptomatic splenomegaly or hypersplenism if perioperative risk factors are low.

HAIRY CELL LEUKEMIA

Hairy cell leukemia (HCL) is a monoclonal lymphoproliferative disorder of mature B cells. It comprises only 2–5% of all leukemias, and there is a 3:1 male predominance. The pathognomonic hairy cells are named for their cytoplasmic projections; they may be found in both the bone marrow and the peripheral circulation.

Patients with HCL may complain of weakness and fatigue. Splenomegaly is almost universally present. About 10% of patients with HCL will have such mild symptoms that they never require treatment. The majority of patients will require therapy for neutropenia, splenomegaly, hypersplenism, or bone marrow failure. Infection related to neutropenia is the most common cause of death.

Early efforts to use chemotherapy to treat HCL were unsuccessful because the degree of associated myelosuppression was not tolerable. Splenectomy became the treatment of choice and was associated with increased survival. Since that time, more effective chemotherapeutic agents have become available. At M. D. Anderson splenectomy is not used in the routine management of patients with HCL. Instead, they are treated with IFN-α, deoxycoformycin, or chlorodeoxyadenosine. The overall response rate to IFN-α is between 80 and 90%. If relapse occurs, chlorodeoxyadenosine is usually effective in regaining control of the disease.

ACUTE LYMPHOCYTIC AND MYELOGENOUS LEUKEMIA

Except in cases of splenic rupture, splenectomy has no role in the management of patients with acute lymphocytic or acute myelogenous leukemia during induction chemotherapy or during relapse. In rare cases, patients in complete remission require splenectomy because of persistent fungal granulomas of the spleen.

SPLENIC RUPTURE IN LEUKEMIA

Splenic rupture is a rare event in leukemic patients and is almost always associated with some form of trauma. There is no increased risk with any particular type of leukemia, but patients with splenomegaly may be more susceptible to splenic trauma. The reported incidence of rupture from four series was 0.72%. Leukemic patients make up only 3.5% of those with spontaneous splenic rupture.

Signs and symptoms include abdominal tenderness and rigidity, shifting dullness, and tachycardia. The chest radiograph may demonstrate an elevated hemidiaphragm or a pleural effusion. A high index of suspicion is necessary in evaluating patients with splenomegaly and abdominal pain since the precipitating event may have been so minor as to not be remembered.

Survival rates vary with the rapidity of diagnosis and of performance of splenectomy. Patients who survive splenectomy following rupture have a life expectancy similar to that of other patients with the same type of leukemia.

The Lymphomas

HODGKIN'S DISEASE

The prognosis of patients with Hodgkin's disease (HD) has improved dramatically over the past 20 years. This advancement is due to increased knowledge of the biology of the disease and more effective use of radiotherapy and multiagent chemotherapy. The role of staging laparotomy continues to evolve as nonoperative staging becomes increasingly accurate and as subsets of patients are identified who are unlikely to benefit from the information laparotomy provides.

HD is characterized by the presence of multinucleated Reed-Sternberg (RS) cells or one of their variants. As opposed to non-Hodgkin's lymphoma, in which a monoclonal population of malignant lymphocytes usually predominates, in HD the malignant cells are a minority population outnumbered by inflammatory cells.

HD patients typically present with nontender lymphadenopathy. The cervical nodes are most commonly involved; other regions, including axillary, inguinal, mediastinal, and retroperitoneal nodes, are less frequently affected at presentation. The presence or absence of B symptoms should be elucidated from the patient's history. B symptoms include any one of the following: unexplained fever with temperature over 38°C, night sweats significant enough to require changing bed clothes, or weight loss of more than 10% of body weight over 6 months. Although classic for HD, the Pel-Ebstein fever, with progressively shortening intervals between fevers, is a relatively rare phenomenon.

The physical examination should include an evaluation of all lymph node–bearing areas, including Waldeyer's tonsillar ring, and palpation for liver or splenic enlargement. Initial work-up should include a complete blood count with differential count, liver function tests, and a chest radiograph. A bone marrow biopsy is useful to determine the extent of the disease. Excisional biopsy of the largest node that is likely to provide the diagnosis should be performed. Careful selection of the biopsy site is important because some areas, particularly the inguinal region, frequently contain nondiagnostic inflammatory nodes.

Other clinical staging tools include computed tomography (CT), nuclear medicine scans, and bipedal lymphangiography. CT is used to detect mediastinal and abdominal lymphatic enlargement; however, nodes containing HD often are not enlarged. Gallium scans have been useful in detecting mediastinal and peripheral nodal disease. Bipedal lymphangiography may detect changes in femoral, inguinal, external iliac, and retroperitoneal nodes. Use of lymphangiography has improved the staging of HD because this procedure identifies lymphatic enlargement as well as changes in the architecture of normal-sized nodes caused by neoplastic involvement.

Table 16-2. Ann Arbor staging system for Hodgkin's disease

Stage	Criteria
I	Involvement of a single lymph node region (I) or a single extralymphatic organ or site (IE)
II	Involvement of two or more lymph node regions on the same side of the diaphragm (II) or of an extralymphatic organ and its adjoining lymph node site (IIE)
III	Involvement of lymph node sites on both sides of the diaphragm (III) or localized involvement of an extra-lymphatic site (IIIE), spleen (IIIS), or both (IIISE)
IV	Diffuse or disseminated involvement of one or more extralymphatic organs with or without associated lymph node involvement
A	Asymptomatic
B	Fever, night sweats, or weight loss of more than 10%

The prognosis of patients with HD depends on the histologic subtype and stage of disease at presentation. The Rye modification of the Lukes-Butler classification of HD identifies four histologic subtypes: lymphocyte predominant, nodular sclerosis, mixed cellularity, and lymphocyte depleted. These subtypes are determined by the specific variant of RS cell, the ratio of these cells to the normal population, and the degree of sclerosis. The nodular sclerosis subtype has the best prognosis, followed by lymphocyte predominant, mixed cellularity, and finally lymphocyte depleted.

The Ann Arbor staging system (Table 16-2) is used for staging HD based on the extent of disease. Clinical staging includes all data from the history and physical examination and nonoperative diagnostic studies. Pathologic staging includes additional information obtained from a staging laparotomy. The Ann Arbor stages are subclassified to reflect lymphatic disease and involvement of extranodal areas designated by *E* for involvement of an extralymphatic site (i.e., stomach or small intestine) or *S* for splenic involvement. Disease is further subclassified according to the presence or absence of systemic symptoms of the disease.

Increasing knowledge of the effect of patient characteristics, histologic subtype, and stage of disease have allowed more individualized treatment of patients, with dramatic improvements in survival. Staging laparotomy was first introduced to define disease extent in all presentations of HD. Subsequently, investigators performed staging by laparotomy to determine which patients had early-stage disease that could be treated by local irradiation and which had extensive disease requiring systemic therapy. Previously, up to 40% of patients who underwent staging laparotomy had a change in their clinical stage. Both improvements in the accuracy of radiologic diagnostic procedures and more intensive use of chemotherapeutic and radiation treatments earlier in the course of the disease have decreased the number of patients who require staging laparotomy.

Currently at M. D. Anderson nonoperative staging and prognostic factors are used to guide therapy in about 80% of patients. Certain subsets of patients have been identified who almost never require staging laparotomy. An example is females with lymphocyte-predominant histology and stage IA disease. This group can be effectively treated with mantle radiotherapy (axilla, neck, and mediastinum) because they almost never have disease below the diaphragm. Patients who will require chemotherapy with or without radiation because of extensive disease or poor prognostic factors also will not benefit from the information gained by a staging laparotomy. Conversely, other patients may benefit from the procedure if a negative staging laparotomy allowed treatment with radiation therapy alone. This group includes those without B symptoms, who have no hilar disease, and whose mediastinal involvement is less than one-third of the chest diameter. Most centers have eliminated staging laparotomy in pediatric patients with HD.

Components of a Staging Laparotomy

For staging laparotomy of HD, the abdomen is entered through a midline incision from the xyphoid process to below the umbilicus. A thorough exploration is performed to identify palpable abnormalities. This includes bimanual palpation of the liver, examination of the bowel and mesentery, and exploration of the major nodal groups. Lymph nodes containing disease are often normal in size. The areas most likely to contain disease include the spleen and the splenic, celiac, and portal lymph nodes.

Splenectomy and liver biopsies are performed early in the procedure so that ample time is available to ensure hemostasis. The spleen should routinely be removed because it may contain nonpalpable disease. In children, some surgeons advocate performing a partial splenectomy to prevent a lifetime risk of asplenic sepsis. Splenic nodes, along with the distal 3 cm of the splenic artery and vein, should be removed in continuity with the spleen. The ends of the splenic vessels are marked with titanium clips to guide future radiotherapy should it be necessary.

A wedge biopsy is obtained from one or both lobes of the liver, and a deeper biopsy with a Tru-cut core needle is done on both lobes. Additional wedge biopsies should be done on any grossly abnormal areas of the liver.

As each nodal group is dissected, it is sent as a separate specimen in sterile saline to the pathologist, and the area is marked with titanium clips. The gastrohepatic ligament is incised, and lymph nodes along the hepatic artery leading to the celiac axis are removed. The sentinel node at the junction of the portal vein with the duodenum, along with any other nodes along the porta hepatis, are excised. The transverse colon is retracted superiorly, and the small bowel is reflected to the patient's right to visualize the aorta. The retroperitoneum is incised over the aorta from the left renal vein down to the iliac bifurcation. The nodes between the aorta and the inferior mesenteric vein are excised. Nodes along the iliac vessels and within the mesentery seldom contain disease, but they should be sampled and submitted for review. Any lymph nodes that appeared abnormal on the lymphangiogram should also be removed.

If a bone marrow biopsy has not been performed preoperatively, it should be obtained from the iliac crest while the patient is under general anesthesia. Oophoropexy was once routinely performed in females of reproductive age, but currently its use is limited to patients with suspected iliac nodal involvement. Some surgeons recommend performing appendectomy during the staging procedure.

The morbidity rate is generally less than 10%, and deaths related to staging laparotomy are rare. Complications include wound problems, atelectasis, pneumonia, pulmonary embolus, and infection. Any complications that delay the initiation of needed systemic therapy or radiotherapy are potentially serious. Long-term complications include small-bowel adhesions and asplenic sepsis.

NON-HODGKIN'S LYMPHOMA

Patients in the United States with non-Hodgkin's lymphoma (NHL) characteristically have a monoclonal proliferation of lymphocytes, with 80% of cases being of B cell derivation and the remainder originating from T cells. The diagnosis of various subsets of B cell NHL depends on the identification of histopathologic markers using monoclonal antibodies and of cellular morphology; criteria assessed are a diffuse versus follicular (nodular) pattern of lymph node involvement, small versus large cell type, and cleaved versus noncleaved nuclear morphology. With this information, the lymphoma can be categorized according to the Working Formulation, which is a modification of the Lukes and Collins schema. Although an in-depth discussion of this classification system is beyond the scope of this chapter, the Working Formulation has simplified our understanding of the behaviors of these subtypes by placing them into one of three categories, depending on whether patients have a low, intermediate, or high risk of death due to the disease. The T cell NHLs are much more difficult to identify precisely and to place into prognostic groups.

The majority of NHL patients present with superficial adenopathy, most commonly in the cervical lymph nodes. These nodes are generally enlarged and not tender. The Ann Arbor system (see Table 16-2) is used to stage these patients, but it is less helpful in NHL than in HD because over half of

NHL patients present with stage III or IV disease and about 20% present with B symptoms.

Because NHLs do not spread in the orderly manner that HD does, the surgeon is generally asked to see NHL patients to perform a diagnostic biopsy, to establish vascular access for chemotherapy, or to treat complications of therapy. Staging laparotomy is not indicated in these patients. Splenectomy is necessary, though rarely, for hypersplenism, massive splenomegaly, or a persistent splenic focus of disease, usually in those with low-grade lymphomas. Although primary splenic lymphoma is unusual, splenectomy may be beneficial for patients with isolated splenic disease. This diagnosis is often made only after splenectomy is performed for hypersplenism or splenomegaly. If the lymphoma is localized to the spleen, the prognosis is similar to that of other stage I patients.

Diagnostic Biopsy for Lymphoma

When lymphoma is suspected, proper planning and execution of the biopsy are crucial to enable the pathologist to make a diagnosis. Since preservation of the architecture aids in histologic diagnosis, efforts should be made to avoid traction or cautery. The largest node found on physical examination should be biopsied. If several nodal areas are enlarged, biopsy of the cervical area is preferred to biopsy of an axillary node, which in turn is superior to biopsy of nodes from the inguinal region. In suspected extranodal disease or in the case of matted nodes, it is important to excise as generous an amount of tissue as possible. Communication with the pathologist is important to guarantee that adequate tissue is sent and that it is delivered in an acceptable fashion. In general, the specimen is sent fresh, in saline, or wrapped in a saline-soaked sponge. It is important that the specimen be sent directly to the pathologist and that there is an indication that the diagnosis of lymphoma is suspected. Needle biopsies rarely provide an adequate amount of tissue, although they may be helpful in ruling out a carcinoma or sarcoma or in suspected relapse of lymphoma when a tissue diagnosis is needed before treatment.

Miscellaneous Splenic Tumors

SPLENIC CYSTS

A splenic cyst may be confused with a neoplastic process when detected as a palpable abnormality or an unexpected radiologic finding. Patients often present with vague symptoms, possibly due to cyst enlargement. Although parasitic cysts are extremely rare in the United States, they are more common outside this country. Parasitic cysts are most commonly due to an echinococcal infection. Nonparasitic cysts make up 75% of splenic cysts in the United States and are classified as primary if they have a true cellular lining or secondary if they lack this layer. Primary splenic cysts may be congenital, due to an embryologic remnant, or neoplastic. The neoplastic cysts include epidermoid cysts, dermoid cysts, lymphangiomas, and cavernous hemangiomas. Secondary cysts are the more common type of nonparasitic cyst and are thought to be the result of splenic injury and resultant hematoma.

Splenic cysts rarely require treatment unless they become infected, hemorrhage, or perforate. Treatment may consist of a partial or total splenectomy; marsupialization or drainage procedures should be avoided.

INFLAMMATORY PSEUDOTUMOR

Inflammatory pseudotumor, also known as plasma cell granuloma, has histologic features of inflammation and mesenchymal repair. Such masses can be found in various locations in the body, including the respiratory system, gastrointestinal tract, orbit, and lymph nodes. When a pseudotumor is detected in the spleen, it may be mistaken for lymphoma. Pseudotumors are thought to occur at sites of previous trauma or infection. Unfortunately, the definitive diagnosis can be made only after excision.

NONLYMPHOID TUMORS

The spleen is involved with various benign and malignant nonlymphoid tumors. Benign vascular tumors include hemangioma, lymphangioma, and hemangioendothelioma. Lipoma and angiomyolipoma are also encountered. Angiosarcoma of the spleen confers a poor prognosis; this tumor has been associated with exposure to thorium dioxide, vinyl chloride, and arsenic. Kaposi's sarcoma may be found as an isolated process in the spleen. Other splenic sarcomas, including malignant fibrous histiocytoma, fibrosarcoma, and leiomyosarcoma, are extremely rare.

SPLENIC METASTASIS

Considering the large percentage of the total blood flow that supplies the spleen, it is a surprisingly rare site for metastasis. In autopsy series of cancer patients, the finding of metastasis involving the spleen ranges from 1.6 to 30%. Splenic metastasis is rarely a clinically relevant problem. Melanoma, breast, and lung cancer are the most frequently detected metastases. Splenomegaly is an unusual finding with solitary metastasis. Several small series have reported the use of splenectomy for an isolated splenic metastasis. Resection with curative intent is rarely possible with splenic metastasis, but splenectomy may be necessary for complications such as perforation, splenic vein thrombosis, and growth into adjacent viscera.

Splenectomy

SPLENECTOMY FOR HYPERSPLENISM

Anemia, neutropenia, and thrombocytopenia may occur for a number of reasons in patients with hematologic malignancies. Because only patients with excessive destruction of a blood component will benefit from a splenectomy, a careful work-up should be done to identify the etiology of the process. Patients with hypersplenism may present with a normal-sized spleen, and others may have massive splenomegaly without hypersplenism.

Infusion of the patient's or normal donor platelets tagged with ^{111}indium is helpful in determining whether the spleen is the site of destruction. Patients with an acquired hemolytic anemia generally have a positive Coombs' test, and the detection of the warm antibody is a good indication that splenectomy will be beneficial. Although chromium-labeled red blood cell scans may be useful in demonstrating decreases in red blood cell survival, they are not as helpful in identifying the site of sequestration. In cases of suspected splenic sequestration, a bone marrow biopsy is important to determine whether adequate precursor cells are available or whether the patient depends on the hematopoietic activity of the spleen.

Splenectomy in patients with CML has been associated with severe bleeding problems. These may be related to impaired clot formation caused by proteases and serases produced by granulocytes. CML patients with severe leukocytosis should receive chemotherapy in an attempt to decrease the WBC count to approximately 20,000 cells/μl. Experience at M. D. Anderson suggests that splenectomy is best avoided in CML patients whose WBC counts cannot be controlled with chemotherapy. Splenectomy should also be avoided in CML patients who have had splenic irradiation.

Bleeding and infection are the greatest perioperative risks. Qualitative platelet function should be evaluated rather than relying on a platelet count. The template bleeding time is currently the most widely available laboratory value for identifying adequacy of platelet function. The patient's current and recent medications should be carefully reviewed to identify any drugs that may impair coagulation. Because of potential bleeding problems associated with certain antibiotics, prophylactic coverage must be carefully chosen to avoid increasing the risk of hemorrhage.

Although splenectomy may be performed through either a midline or a subcostal approach, the midline incision is preferred when coagulation defects, thrombocytopenia, or splenomegaly is present. After the splenic pedicle is clamped, thrombocytopenic patients are transfused with fresh single-donor platelets to achieve a platelet count of over 60,000 cells/μl. Careful hemostasis at the conclusion of the procedure is mandatory. Postoperatively, patients should be monitored closely during the first 48 hours for signs of bleeding.

A blood count with differential and platelet counts should be obtained every 6 hours for the first 24 hours after the operation. Decreasing platelet and blood counts, despite adequate replacement, suggest an ongoing bleeding process.

SPLENECTOMY FOR THE MASSIVELY ENLARGED SPLEEN

Indications for splenectomy in patients with massively enlarged spleens include debilitating symptoms of splenomegaly, excessive destruction of blood components, and concerns of possible splenic rupture. These patients often complain of chronic severe upper abdominal and back pain, impaired respiration, and early satiety. Hypersplenism may be present. Depending on the size of the spleen and the body habitus, the patient may be judged to be at increased risk of splenic trauma.

Preoperatively, it is important to check quantitative and qualitative platelet function values and coagulation studies because hemorrhage is the major complication of splenectomy in this group. Portal venous contrast studies should be performed in patients with possible portal hypertension. In splenic vein thrombosis, splenectomy is appropriate, but otherwise it may deprive a patient with portal hypertension of the option of a splenorenal shunt.

Adequate blood products must be available preoperatively. The blood of these patients may be difficult to crossmatch because of numerous past transfusions, and fresh single-donor platelets may be required. Patients should undergo routine bowel preparation, and prophylactic antibiotics should be given.

A midline, rather than subcostal, incision is preferred because the rectus muscles are not severed, which limits bleeding. With increasing size, the spleen becomes more of a midline structure and lends itself to this approach. Prior to mobilization of the spleen, its vessels should be isolated. The gastrocolic omentum is divided, the lesser sac is entered, and the splenic artery is identified along the posterior-superior surface of the pancreas. The artery is doubly ligated but left intact. The splenic vein is not disturbed yet. The spleen may decrease 20–30% in size at this point and allow platelet transfusion without consumption. The splenic flexure of the colon is mobilized, the splenic ligaments are divided, and the spleen is delivered from the splenic fossa. The normally avascular splenic ligaments often contain small vessels in the presence of hematologic malignancies. Dense adhesions between the spleen and the diaphragm may complicate mobilization, and when dissection is particularly difficult, it is better to resect part of the diaphragm with the spleen than to risk hypertrophy of splenic remnants. Such adhesions are formed in areas of splenic infarction and are the most frequent sites of postoperative bleeding in this group of patients. After the spleen is mobilized, the artery and vein are suture ligated and divided. Liver biopsy may be indicated if involvement by lymphoma is suspected. If an injury to the pancreatic tail is recognized, it should be repaired and drained appropriately. Achieving hemostasis in the splenic bed is crucial and may require suture ligation, cautery, platelet transfusions, and thrombostatic agents. Drains do not reliably warn of postoperative hemorrhage or prevent infection, and except in cases of pancreatic injury, they are not routinely used. Postoperatively, patients should be closely monitored for signs of bleeding or infection.

Prophylaxis for Asplenic Sepsis

Patients with hematologic malignancies who undergo splenectomy are at greater risk for asplenic sepsis than are those who have the procedure for other indications. Some hematologic malignancy patients, especially those with CML and CLL, are at increased risk for sepsis even before splenectomy. The risk of overwhelming postsplenectomy infection (OPSI) is greatest for children. The expected death rate from OPSI in children is 1 in every 300–350 patient-years, and in adults it is 1 in every 800–1,000 patient-years. For all patients, the risk is greatest for the first few years following splenectomy, but deaths attributed to OPSI have occurred 30 or more years after splenectomy.

Following splenectomy, there is loss of the opsonins tuftsin and properdin, a decrease in immunoglobulin M production, impaired phagocytosis, and altered cellular immunity. Poorly opsonized bacteria are best cleared by the spleen, and following the spleen's removal patients are particularly susceptible to the encapsulated bacteria.

Vaccination can decrease the risk of postsplenectomy pneumococcal infection. The 23-valent form of the pneumococcal vaccine should be used. The vaccine is most effective when given several weeks preoperatively. Nevertheless, despite the diminished immunity obtained if the vaccine is given after splenectomy, adequate protection is still achieved in most patients. In patients who are not immunized preoperatively there is no benefit from delaying the immunization for several weeks after surgery, so these patients should be vaccinated without delay. Leukemic patients may not be able to develop antibodies in response to pneumococcal vaccine, but it may still be worthwhile to vaccinate this group. Booster immunizations with the pneumococcal vaccine have no proven benefit. Certain subsets of patients are at increased risk of infection with *Haemophilus influenzae* and *Neisseria meningitidis* and should receive the appropriate vaccinations.

Long-term use of prophylactic oral antibiotics is often recommended in the pediatric population or in patients who may have difficulty reaching a physician. Penicillin is commonly prescribed to these patients, but the benefit of this practice has never been proved.

Selected References

Boring CC, Squires TS, Tong T. Cancer statistics, 1993. *CA* 43:7, 1993.

Brenner B, Nagler A, Tatarsky I, et al. Splenectomy in agnogenic myeloid metaplasia and postpolycythemic myeloid metaplasia. *Arch Intern Med* 148:2501, 1988.

Canady MR, Welling RE, Strobel SL. Splenic rupture in leukemia. *J Surg Oncol* 41:194, 1989.

Dawes LG, Malangoni MA. Cystic masses of the spleen. *Am Surg* 52:333, 1986.

Edwards MJ, Balch CM. Surgical aspects of lymphoma. *Adv Surg* 22:225, 1989.

Farrar WB, Kim JA. Biopsy techniques to establish diagnosis and type of malignant lymphoma. *Surg Oncol Clin North Am* 2:159, 1993.

Feldman EJ, Arlin ZA. Modern management of chronic myelogenous leukemia (CML). *Cancer Invest* 6:737, 1988.

Flexner JM, Stein RS, Greer JP. Outline of treatment of lymphoma based on hematologic and clinical stage with expected end results. *Surg Oncol Clin North Am* 2:283, 1993.

Hagemeister FB, Fuller LM, Martin RG. Staging Laparotomy: Findings and Applications to Treatment Decisions. In L Fuller (ed), *Hodgkin's Disease and Non-Hodgkin's Lymphoma in Adults and Children*. New York: Raven, 1988.

Harris NL. The pathology of lymphomas: A practical approach to diagnosis and classification. *Surg Oncol Clin of North Am* 2:167, 1993.

Hubbard SM, Longo DL. Treatment-related morbidity in patients with lymphoma. *Curr Opin Oncol* 3:852, 1991.

Johnson HA, Deterling RA. Massive splenomegaly. *Surg Gynecol Obstet* 168:131, 1989.

Klein B, Stein M, Kuten A, et al. Splenomegaly and solitary spleen metastasis in solid tumors. *Cancer* 60:100, 1987.

Kluin-Nelemans HC, Noordijk EM. Staging of patients with Hodgkin's disease: What should be done? *Leukemia* 4:132, 1991.

Kurzrock R, Talpaz M, Gutterman JU. Hairy cell leukaemia: Review of treatment. *Br J Haematol* 79(Suppl 1):17, 1991.

McBride CM, Hester JP. Chronic myelogenous leukemia: Management of splenectomy in a high-risk population. *Cancer* 39:653, 1977.

Morgenstern L, Rosenberg J, Geller SA. Tumors of the spleen. *World J Surg* 9:468, 1985.

Mower WR, Hawkins JA, Nelson EW. Postsplenectomy infection in patients with chronic leukemia. *Am J Surg* 152:583, 1986.

Pollock R, Hohn D. Splenectomy. In MS Roh, FC Ames (eds), *Advanced Oncologic Surgery*. New York: Mosby-Wolfe, 1994.

Shaw JHF, Print CG. Postsplenectomy sepsis. *Br J Surg* 76:1074, 1989.

Styrt B. Infection associated with asplenia: Risks, mechanisms, and prevention. *Am J Med* 88:33N, 1990.

Wiernik PH, Rader M, Becker NH, et al. Inflammatory pseudotumor of spleen. *Cancer* 66:597, 1990.

Genitourinary Cancer

Mark G. Delworth and Colin P. N. Dinney

Genitourinary cancers account for 16% of malignancies in humans. Prostate cancer is now the most common malignancy in American males. As the incidence of genitourinary cancers continues to increase, a clear understanding of the diagnosis and treatment of these diseases is essential. In this chapter, we review the current management of prostate, bladder, renal, and testicular neoplasms.

Prostate Cancer

EPIDEMIOLOGY AND ETIOLOGY

Prostate cancer is the most common malignancy of men. From 1973 to 1988, the incidence of prostate cancer increased by an estimated 2.8% per year to a rate of 102 cases per 100,000 males in 1988. The incidence continues to climb and is higher for blacks than whites. Prostate cancer rarely occurs before age 50 years; incidence increases through the ninth decade of life. Some of this increased incidence may be attributed to the increase in prostate cancer screening using prostate-specific antigen (PSA) and transrectal ultrasound (TRUS). Carcinoma of the prostate is the second leading cause of solid cancer mortality in men, with rates of 47 per 100,000 black males and 23 per 100,000 white males. Thirty percent of men older than 50 years with no clinical evidence of prostate cancer will have a focus of cancer within the prostate on autopsy.

Many factors have been proposed as associated with the development of prostate cancer. The presence of an intact hypothalamic-pituitary-gonadal axis and advanced age are the most universally accepted risk factors. The relatively low rate of prostate cancer in the Orient is thought to be partially due to low-fat diets. It is unclear whether the increased mortality of prostate cancer in blacks is due to unique racial biologic factors or differences in health care delivery. Other factors that have been implicated (but not proved to play a role) in the development of prostate cancer include increased physical activity, increased sexual activity, cadmium exposure, increased zinc intake, and estrogen intake.

Evidence has shown that a man with one, two, or three first-degree relatives affected with prostate cancer has a two times, five times, or 11 times increased risk, respectively, for the development of prostate cancer. A Mendelian pattern of autosomal dominant transmission of prostate cancer accounts for 43% of disease occurring before age 55 years and 9% of all prostate cancers occurring by age 85 years.

ANATOMY

The normal prostate weighs 15–20 g and is divided into three major glandular zones. The *peripheral zone* constitutes 70% of the prostate and is the area palpated during digital rectal examination (DRE). The area around the ejaculatory ducts is called the *central zone* and accounts for 25% of the gland. The *transitional zone* makes up the 5% of the prostate gland around the urethra. In a pathologic review of 104 prostates from patients who underwent radical prostatectomy, 68% of the cancers were located in the peripheral zone, 24% in the transitional zone, and only 8% in the central zone. Almost all stage A (nonpalpable) cancers in that study were found in the transitional zone, the area most susceptible to benign prostatic hyperplasia.

SCREENING

Although there are good screening methods for prostate cancer, controversy surrounds the concept of screening for this disease. First, there is no consensus as to the optimal management of early-stage disease. Second, the cost of a national screening effort for all men over age 50 years would be high and possibly not cost effective.

DIAGNOSIS

Patients with low-volume clinically localized prostate cancer are typically asymptomatic; abnormalities are detected by DRE or elevated serum PSA level. Advanced prostate cancer can be asymptomatic; present as local symptoms of urinary hesitancy, frequency, and urgency; or present as systemic symptoms of weight loss, fatigue, and bone pain.

Prostatic acid phosphatase (PAP) levels were widely used in the past as markers of prostate cancer; however, their use has been supplanted by PSA. PAP remains useful in the detection of metastatic disease and is a part of the staging system for prostate cancer, although it exhibits greater specificity but less sensitivity than PSA in the detection of metastatic disease.

PSA is a serine protease produced by the epithelium of the prostate. PSA is not specific for prostate cancer and can be elevated in such benign conditions of the prostate as prostatitis, prostatic infarction, and prostatic hyperplasia. Transurethral resection of the prostate (TURP) and prostatic needle biopsy have been shown to increase significantly the serum PSA level above baseline for up to 8 weeks. DRE, cystoscopy, and TRUS do not alter serum PSA to a clinically significant degree. Only 4% of men with a PSA <4 ng/ml will have prostate cancer detectable by biopsy, while 58% with a PSA >10 ng/ml will have prostate cancer. A palpable abnormality on DRE is associated with a 36% incidence of prostate cancer compared to a 5% incidence of prostate cancer in patients with a normal DRE.

TRUS is performed using real-time imaging with a 7-MHz transducer, which allows both transverse and sagittal imaging of the prostate. Prostate cancer typically appears as a hypoechoic region within the prostate. TRUS can also be used to measure the dimensions of the prostate to calculate the glandular volume.

Lymphatic metastases can be detected by computed tomography (CT), lymphangiography, and magnetic resonance imaging (MRI). However, the only reliable method for staging pelvic lymph nodes is a staging pelvic lymphadenectomy.

Radionuclide bone scan remains the most sensitive test to detect skeletal metastases. However, Chybowski et al. reviewed the medical records of 521 patients and found that only one patient with a PSA level below 20 ng/ml had evidence of skeletal metastasis. Therefore based on these data, radionuclide bone scans may not be necessary for staging prostate cancer patients who have a low serum PSA level and no skeletal symptoms. When bone metastases are present, 80% are osteoblastic, 15% are mixed osteoblastic-osteolytic, and 5% are osteolytic. A chest radiograph is performed to detect the presence of pulmonary metastases.

The diagnosis of prostate cancer is made by the histologic finding of prostate cancer in a prostatic biopsy, in a prostatic needle aspiration, or in tissue obtained from prostatectomy for benign disease. Adenocarcinoma is the predominant cell type of prostate cancer and is the only type discussed in this chapter.

GRADING AND STAGING

The University of Texas M. D. Anderson Cancer Center grading system is based on the percentage of glandular formation by the tumor cells. Grade 1 carcinoma has greater than 75% gland formation; grade 2 has 51–75%; grade 3 has 26–50%; and grade 4 has less than 25% gland formation. The M. D. Anderson grading system has been shown to correlate with survival. The Gleason grading system is the other major grading system and recognizes five histologic patterns of prostate cancer. The scores of the predominant and secondary patterns are added to yield a range of tumor grades from 2 to 10.

The biologic behavior of the tumor can be further categorized by stage, which accounts for tumor volume and location. Prostate cancer typically spreads to the pelvic lymph nodes, bone, and lungs. The Organ Systems Coordinating Center and Hopkins (modified Jewett) staging systems are shown in Table 17-1.

MANAGEMENT OF LOCAL DISEASE

In 1987 the National Cancer Institute published a consensus statement on the treatment of early-stage prostate cancer. They concluded: "Radical prostatectomy and radiation thera-

Table 17-1. Staging systems for prostate cancer

	Hopkins	OSCC
Primary tumor		
Anatomic relationship indefinable		TX
Digitally unrecognizable cancer		TA
<5% total surgical specimen, low or medium grade	A1	TA1
>5% total surgical specimen, any grade	A2	TA2
TA, but not A1 or A2		TAX
Digitally palpable cancer, organ-confined	B	TB
< half of one lobe, regardless of location	B1	TB1
> half lobe but <1 lobe	B1	TB2
>1 lobe or bilaterally palpable cancer	B2	TB3
Palpable cancer extending beyond prostate	C	TC
Extension beyond margin unilaterally		TC1
Extension beyond margin bilaterally		TC2
Extension into bladder, rectum, levator muscles, or pelvic side walls		TC3
Nodal status		
No regional lymph node metastases		N0
Microscopic regional lymph node metastasis, proven histologically	D1	N1
Gross regional lymph node metastases	D1	N2
Extraregional lymph node metastases		N3
Minimal requirements have not been met		NX
Distant metastases		
No evidence of metastases		M0
Elevated acid phosphatase only	D0	M1
Visceral and/or bone metastases	D2	M2
Minimal requirements not met		MX

OSCC = Organ Systems Coordinating Center.

py are clearly effective forms of treatment in the attempt to cure tumors limited to the prostate for appropriately selected patients. . . . What remains unclear is the relative merit of each in producing lifelong freedom from cancer recurrence. . . . Properly designed and completed randomized trials that evaluate both disease control and quality of life after modern radiation therapy compared with radical prostatectomy are essential."

Surgery

The surgical excision of prostate cancer by complete removal of the prostate, seminal vesicles, and ampullae of the vasa deferentia was first performed in the early 1900s. This procedure, known as a *radical prostatectomy*, can be performed using a perineal or retropubic approach.

Gibbons et al. reviewed their experience of total prostatectomy in 215 patients and found that overall and disease-free survival rates, respectively, were 94% and 86% at 5 years, 75% and 67% at 10 years, and 55% and 48% at 15 years. Morbidity has decreased significantly over the past several decades. Leandri et al. reported on 620 patients and found a 6.9% early complication rate, 1.3% late complication rate, and 0.2% mortality rate. Sexual potency was maintained in 71% in whom a nerve-sparing technique was used, and 5% experienced stress incontinence after 1 year.

Radiotherapy

External beam radiotherapy has been used for the definitive treatment of localized and regionally extensive prostatic ade-nocarcinoma. At M. D. Anderson, 60–70 Gy was given to 114 patients with localized prostate cancer as primary therapy. The 5- and 10-year uncorrected survival rates are compara-ble to radical surgery (89% and 68%, respectively). In this series there was no difference in survival between patients with stages A and B disease. Skeletal metastases were the major site of relapse. Serious complications developed in only 1.8% of treated patients. At M. D. Anderson we currently rec-ommend radical prostatectomy for the treatment of early-stage prostate cancer. Primary radiotherapy is reserved for patients with significant comorbid medical illnesses.

Stage C Disease

Stage C prostate cancer involves areas outside the prostatic capsule, such as fat, seminal vesicles, levator muscles, or other adjacent structures. This stage of prostate cancer is associated with a 53% incidence of lymph node metastases and a decreased overall survival rate. At M. D. Anderson, stage C disease is treated with primary radiotherapy with 5-, 10-, and 15-year uncorrected actuarial survival rates of 72%, 47%, and 17%, respectively. The local control rate in our expe-rience with stage C disease is 75% at 15 years of follow-up.

Treatment modalities, other than radiotherapy, used for stage C disease include radical prostatectomy, TURP, and hormonal therapy. Tumor grade, stage, bulk of tumor, and seminal vesicle involvement in stage C disease are associat-ed with the interval between radical prostatectomy and dis-ease progression. The actuarial 5-year survival rate for patients with stage C disease who have undergone TURP in stage C disease is 64%, making TURP an option for patients with short life expectancies, such as the very elderly and those with serious coexisting medical problems. Currently, several groups are investigating the use of hormonal thera-py in an attempt to downstage B2/C tumors before extirpa-tive surgery.

Stage D Disease

Approximately 20% of patients present with stage D1 prostate cancer, and 75% of these patients will develop bone metastases. As with other stages of prostate cancer, there appears to be a great deal of variability within D1 disease. Barzell et al. found that patients with low-volume nodal disease had a 71% 5-year metastasis-free survival with treatment. However, a similar population of patients followed for 10 years had a 14% disease-free survival rate. The optimal treatment for D1 disease is controversial. Observation, hormonal treatment, radiation, cytoreductive surgery, and combinations of these have been used with various degrees of success. For patients with low-volume nodal disease, cytoreductive surgery combined with hormonal treatment appears to yield the best 5-year disease-free survival rate: 65–95%.

Stage D2 represents systemic disease. Patients have a median survival of 30 months, with an estimated 5-year survival rate of 20%. The treatment of metastatic prostate cancer is androgen ablation therapy. The hypothalamus produces luteinizing hormone–releasing hormone (LHRH) and corticotropin-releasing factor (CRF), which stimulate the anterior pituitary to release adrenocorticotropic hormone (ACTH) and luteinizing hormone (LH). LH stimulates testosterone production by the testes, and ACTH stimulates the adrenals to produce androstenedione and dehydroepiandrosterone, precursors of testosterone and dihydrotestosterone (DHT). Although the testes are the major source of testosterone, the adrenals can supply up to 20% of the DHT found in the prostate.

Early androgen ablation therapy consisted of either estrogen supplementation or bilateral orchiectomy. More recently, LHRH agonists have been developed that chronically stimulate the pituitary, resulting in a decrease in LH release. This, in turn, leads to castrate levels of testosterone production by the testes. Flutamide, an antiandrogen, works by blocking uptake or binding of androgen in target tissues.

Bilateral orchiectomy, estrogens, and LHRH agonists appear to have equal efficacy when used as monotherapy for metastatic prostate cancer. Total androgen ablation with an LHRH agonist plus an antiandrogen may be more effective than any form of monotherapy. Despite effective initial therapy, the eventual emergence of androgen-insensitive tumor cells leads to the demise of the patient.

Bladder Cancer

EPIDEMIOLOGY AND ETIOLOGY

Bladder cancer is the second most common genitourinary malignancy. It is the fourth most common cancer in males and the eleventh most common cancer in females. The incidence is lowest in black females (6 per 100,000) and highest in white males (33 per 100,000). White males also have the highest mortality rate—6 deaths per 100,000.

The etiology of urothelial cancers, of which bladder cancer is the most common, is well established. Cigarette smoking has been linked to 30–40% of all cases of bladder cancer. The chemicals 1-naphthylamine, 2-naphthylamine, benzidine, and 4-aminobiphenyl have been shown to promote urothelial carcinogenesis. Workers in the textile, leather, aluminum refining, rubber, and chemical industries who are exposed to high levels of these chemicals have an increased incidence of bladder cancer. Other chemicals that have been linked to urothelial cancer are MBUCCA (plastics industry), phenacetin, and the antineoplastic agents cyclophosphamide and chlornaphazine. In addition, recurrent bladder infections, as well as infections with the parasite *Schistosoma haematobium* , have been associated with squamous cell carcinoma of the bladder.

PATHOLOGY

The urinary bladder is a hollow viscus that functions in both the storage and evacuation of urine. Histologically, the bladder is composed of mucosa, lamina propria, muscularis, and serosa (limited to the dome). Localized bladder cancer is classified as *superficial disease*, which is limited to the mucosa and lamina propria, or *invasive disease*, which extends into the muscularis and beyond. About 70% of newly diagnosed bladder cancer is superficial, while the remaining 30% is invasive or metastatic. Once a bladder cancer extends through the basal layer of the mucosa, it may invade blood vessels and lymphatics, thereby providing a route of metastasis. Carcinoma in situ, an aggressive form of superficial disease, is composed of anaplastic cells limited to the mucosal layer.

The World Health Organization (WHO) classifies epithelial tumors of the bladder into four histologic types: transitional cell carcinoma (TCC) (91%), squamous cell carcinoma (7%), adenocarcinoma (2%), and undifferentiated carcinoma (<1%). However, up to 20% of TCCs contain areas of squamous differentiation, and up to 7% contain areas of adenomatous differentiation. The remainder of this section discusses TCC.

CLINICAL PRESENTATION

Eighty percent of all patients who present with bladder carcinoma have gross or microscopic hematuria, typically painless and intermittent. About 20% of patients complain of symptoms of vesical irritability, including urinary frequency, urgency, and dysuria. Other symptoms include pelvic pain, flank pain (from ureteral obstruction), and lower extremity edema. Patients with systemic disease may present with anemia, weight loss, and bone pain.

DIAGNOSIS

A patient who presents with hematuria or other symptoms of bladder cancer should undergo a thorough urologic evaluation consisting of a history, physical examination, urinalysis, intravenous urogram, and cystoscopic examination of the urinary bladder with barbotage of urine for cytologic examination. The most useful of these steps is the examination of the bladder using a rigid or flexible cystoscope. Papillary and sessile tumors are easily visualized through the cystoscope; carcinoma in situ, however, can appear as normal mucosa. Fewer than 60% of bladder tumors can be seen on an intravenous urogram, but this examination will also identify other abnormalities that may be present in the genitourinary tract. Results of barbatoge of urine can be expected to be positive in 10% of patients with grade 1 tumors, 50% of patients with grade 2 tumors, and up to 90% of patients with grade 3 tumors or carcinoma in situ. Flow cytometric examination of urine can detect hyperdiploid cell lines with a high degree of sensitivity. Quantitative fluorescent image analysis, a relatively new method of detection that combines quantification of DNA and morphometric analysis, is reported to be both sensitive (76%) and specific (94%).

GRADING AND STAGING

The WHO uses a grading system based on the cytologic features of the tumor. Grade 1 represents a well-differentiated tumor; grade 2, a moderately differentiated tumor; and grade 3, a poorly differentiated bladder cancer.

Once a bladder tumor is diagnosed, the urologist must accurately stage the tumor. The initial transurethral resection of the bladder tumor (TURBT) will determine the histologic depth of invasion of the tumor as well as the presence or absence of dysplasia or carcinoma in situ. A bimanual examination should be performed at the time of resection to determine whether a mass is present and, if so, whether it is fixed or mobile.

Further work-up for detecting metastasis consists of a CT scan, liver function tests, a chest radiograph, and a bone scan (if the alkaline phosphatase level is elevated or the patient's symptoms suggest systemic disease). The Jewett-Strong-Marshall and International Union Against Cancer (TNM) staging systems are listed in Table 17-2.

MANAGEMENT

Superficial Bladder Cancer

The majority of bladder cancers present as superficial disease. Approximately 70% of these superficial cancers are papillary, 10% are nodular, and 20% are mixed. After the initial treatment of superficial bladder cancer, the cancer can be cured, can recur with the same stage and grade, or can recur with progression of stage or grade. Risk factors associated with both disease recurrence and progression include a high tumor grade, lamina propria invasion, dysplasia else-

Table 17-2. Staging systems for bladder cancer

	Jewett-Strong-Marshall stage	TNM stage	
		Clinical	Pathologic
No tumor in specimen	O	T0	Po
Carcinoma in situ	O	Tis	Pis
Noninvasive papillary tumor	O	TA	PA
Lamina propria invasion	A	T1	P1
Superficial muscle invasion	B1	T2	P2
Deep muscle invasion	B2	T3A	P3
Invasion of perivesical fat	C	T3B	P3
Invasion of contiguous organ	D1	T4	P4
Regional lymph node metastases	D1		
Single homolateral node			N1
Bilateral regional or contralateral nodes			N2
Fixed regional nodes			N3
Juxtaregional lymph node metastases	D2		N4
Distant metastases	D2	M1	M1

where in the bladder, positive urinary cytology findings, and tumor diameter larger than 5 cm.

Initial treatment of superficial bladder cancer focuses on eradication of the existing disease and prophylaxis against disease recurrence or progression. TURBT has been the standard treatment for existing stage TA and T1 tumors as well as visible stage Tis tumors. Other treatment modalities for the eradication of superficial disease include laser fulguration and photodynamic therapy. The advantage of transurethral resection over the other modalities is that it provides tissue for histologic examination.

Patients with high-grade TA or T1 lesions, multiple tumors, recurrent tumors, tumors associated with Tis, aneuploid tumors, tumors larger than 5 cm, and persistently positive cytology findings may be candidates for adjuvant intravesical therapy. Intravesical agents can be used as therapeutic, adjuvant, or prophylactic treatment for bladder cancer. Thiotepa, mitomycin C, doxorubicin, and etoglucid are the chemotherapeutic agents used most frequently. Bacillus Calmette-Guérin (BCG), a live attenuated tuberculosis organism, has become the most widely used intravesical agent in superficial bladder cancer. BCG enhances the patient's own immune response against the tumor, providing resistance to disease recurrence and progression. Although specific dose scheduling varies, most treatment regimens include intravesical treatment weekly for a period of 4–8 weeks, followed by an optional series of maintenance treatments administered over many months.

Invasive Bladder Cancer

Tumors that have penetrated the muscularis propria are considered invasive. There are several options for treatment of patients with invasive tumors. A small subset of patients may be eligible for bladder-sparing therapy. With aggressive transurethral re-resection of invasive bladder tumors, a 67% survival rate can be obtained for those retaining their bladder (median follow-up was 5 years). Patients with a muscle invasive tumor that is primary and solitary, does not have surrounding urothelial atypia, and allows for a 2-cm surgical margin may be candidates for partial cystectomy. At M. D. Anderson, data have shown that approximately 5% of patients are actually suitable for bladder-sparing surgery; 5-year survival rates have been comparable to those achieved with radical cystectomy.

Primary external beam radiotherapy has been used to treat invasive bladder cancer. Treatment protocols advocate doses of 65–70 Gy. Five-year survival rates range from 21 to 52% for stage B2 and 18 to 30% for stage C. Local recurrence occurs in 50–70% of these patients. Stage T4 lesions fare worse, with 5-year survival rates consistently below 10%. Thus, external beam radiotherapy may be useful in patients who do not wish to have surgery or for whom radical surgery is medically contraindicated; however, the survival rate for radiotherapy is below that for radical surgery.

Radical cystectomy with pelvic lymphadenectomy is performed with the intent to remove all localized and lymphatic disease present. At M. D. Anderson, the 5-year actuarial survival rate for patients with invasive bladder carcinoma after radical cystectomy alone is 79% for stage B, 46% for stage C, 54% for stage D with nodal spread, and 32% for stage D with visceral metastases. The local recurrence rate is 7% and the operative mortality rate 1.1%. Fourteen percent of patients undergoing cystectomy with lymphadenectomy are found to have unsuspected metastases to the pelvic lymph nodes. The majority of these cases involve one or two nodes limited to an area below the bifurcation of the common iliac arteries and medial to the external iliac artery.

Once a patient undergoes cystectomy, the ureters must be diverted into an alternate drainage system. The most common urinary diversion used today is the cutaneous ureteroileal diversion popularized by Bricker in the 1950s. This form of urinary diversion involves the anastomosis of each ureter to the proximal end of an isolated piece of ileum; the distal end is brought out as a cutaneous stoma for drainage into a urinary appliance.

Metastatic Disease

Cisplatin appears to be the single agent with the greatest activity against TCC of the bladder; however, single-agent therapy response rates are only in the range of 10–30%. The highest response rates documented to date have been with regimens that include cisplatin, methotrexate, vinblastine, and doxorubicin (M-VAC). In the M. D. Anderson trial of M-VAC, a complete response rate of 35% and a partial response rate of 30% were observed. Other trials have documented similar response rates, with median survival of approximately 1 year. Many groups have proposed the use of M-VAC in both a neoadjuvant and adjuvant setting. Data from prospective randomized trials are needed to clarify the role M-VAC should play in each of these areas.

Renal Cancer

EPIDEMIOLOGY AND ETIOLOGY

Tumors of the renal and perirenal tissues comprise 2–3% of all adult visceral tumors. Renal cell carcinoma (RCC) represents 85% of all renal parenchymal tumors and is the only renal tumor discussed in this chapter. In 1994, an estimated 27,600 people will be diagnosed with renal cancer and 11,300 people will die of this disease. Males are affected twice as often as females. RCC most frequently occurs in the fifth to sixth decade of life.

In contrast with the known causes of bladder cancer, the etiology of RCC is unknown. It has been speculated that smoking, industrial contamination, asbestos, petroleum by-products, and viruses may play roles in the development of RCC. RCC may occur either sporadically or genetically as part of von Hippel-Lindau disease, which is characterized by cerebellar hemangioblastoma, retinal angiomata, bilateral RCC, and islet cell tumors of the pancreas. Both disease types have a common genetic mechanism that includes loss of a region of chromosome 3. RCC is also associated with polycystic kidney disease, "horseshoe kidneys," and acquired renal cystic disease.

PATHOLOGY

The majority of RCCs have their origin in the proximal tubular cell of the kidney. The tumor is multicentric in up to 7% of cases. Local extension of the tumor is limited by the renal capsule and Gerota's fascia surrounding the kidney. The predominant cell type is clear cell, but granular and spindle-shaped cells also may be present. The tumor cells are typically rich in glycogen and lipid, giving the tumor a clear cell appearance microscopically and a characteristic yellow appearance grossly.

CLINICAL PRESENTATION

RCC has often been called "the internist's tumor" because of its subtle presentation. Gross or microscopic hematuria, the most common presenting symptom, is present in more than half of patients with RCC. The classic triad of hematuria, abdominal mass, and flank pain occurs in about 19% of patients. Paraneoplastic syndromes occur in 10–40% of cases and consist of pyrexia, anemia, erythrocytosis, hypercalcemia, liver dysfunction (Stauffer's syndrome), and hypertension. Other symptoms can include bone pain and central nervous system abnormalities, as up to 30% of patients present with bone and brain metastases.

DIAGNOSIS

The work-up of a patient with the above symptoms should include a history, physical examination, complete blood count, serum chemistry panel, urinalysis, urine culture, and IV urogram. Typically, the IV urogram will show a renal mass (if present), which can be categorized as solid, cystic, or indeterminate. Cystic masses should undergo renal ultrasound, which will confirm the characteristics of a simple renal cyst (through transmission, smooth wall, posterior enhancement). A patient with a solid or indeterminate mass or complex cyst should have a contrast-enhanced CT scan. In most cases, the CT scan will define the nature of the mass. A renal angiogram can be used to demonstrate hypervascularity, which is present in 90% of RCCs, as well as provide useful information for planning an operative procedure, especially when a partial nephrectomy is considered. If any of the studies obtained suggests involvement of the renal vein or vena cava, an abdominal ultrasound, color Doppler, or MRI study should be obtained to assess the extent of the tumor thrombus. In contrast to the management of other renal tumors, a surgeon may perform a radical nephrectomy for RCC without preoperative histologic diagnosis of the tumor.

If a mass suggests RCC, a metastatic work-up consisting of a chest radiograph, CT scan (if not already obtained), and liver function tests should be performed. The most common sites of metastases of RCC in decreasing order are the lung, bone, and regional lymph nodes. If the patient does not have an elevated alkaline phosphatase level or skeletal pain, a bone scan is usually not required. A CT scan of the brain can be performed if there is any suspicion of brain metastases; however, this is not done routinely.

GRADING AND STAGING

There is no universal grading system for RCC. Patients with the sarcomatoid variant seem to fare slightly worse than those with the granular or clear cell type, and it is generally agreed that the sarcomatoid cell type is found in more aggressive tumors.

The Robson and TNM staging systems, the most commonly used in the United States, are shown in Table 17-3.

MANAGEMENT

Localized Renal Cell Carcinoma

Surgical excision is the only effective treatment of localized RCC. In a radical nephrectomy, the kidney, ipsilateral adrenal, and surrounding Gerota's fascia are all resected en

Table 17-3. Staging systems for renal cell cancer

	Robson	TNM
Tumor confined by renal capsule	I	
Small tumor, minimal calyceal distortion		T1
Large tumor, calyceal deformity		T2
Tumor extension to perirenal fat or ipsilateral adrenal, confined by Gerota's fascia	II	T3a
Renal vein involvement	IIIa	T3b
Renal vein and vena caval involvement below the diaphragm	IIIa	T3c
Vena caval involvement above the diaphragm	IIIa	T4b
Lymphatic involvement	IIIb	
Single homolateral regional node		N1
Multiple regional, contralateral, or bilateral nodes		N2
Fixed regional nodes		N3
Juxtaregional nodes involved		N4
Combination of IIIa and IIIb	IIIc	
Spread to contiguous organs except ipsilateral adrenal	IVa	T4a
Distant metastases	IVb	M1

bloc. Although no randomized study has proved its benefit over simple nephrectomy, radical nephrectomy has the theoretic advantage of removing the lymphatics within the perinephric fat. Up to 20% of patients have evidence of regional lymphatic metastases without distant disease. The 5-year survival rates for patients with positive lymph nodes range from 8 to 35%. Extended lymphadenectomy has never been proved to be of benefit in patients who undergo radical nephrectomy, and many surgeons prefer to do a limited node dissection, which has limited morbidity, for prognostic information.

The surgical approach to radical nephrectomy is determined by the size and location of the tumor as well as the surgeon's preference. A modified flank, midline, or subcostal (chevron) incision can be used. Large upper-pole tumors may be approached through a thoracoabdominal incision for greater exposure. Since the incidence of ipsilateral adrenal metastasis in lower-pole tumors is rare, it is acceptable not to remove the adrenal at the time of nephrectomy for a lower-pole lesion.

Approximately 15–20% of RCCs invade the renal vein, and 8–15% invade the vena cava. Involvement of RCC in the renal vein usually does not pose a significant problem. Vena caval involvement, however, may require additional extensive procedures. Vena caval thrombi have been divided by many authors into three groups. Type 1 thrombi (50%) are completely infrahepatic, type 2 (40%) are intrahepatic, and type 3 (10%) extend up into the right atrium of the heart. In cases with vena caval involvement it is imperative that the surgeon be familiar with techniques of vascular surgery, and consideration should be given to consulting with a cardiothoracic surgeon, especially for type 3 thrombi.

There are situations in which radical nephrectomy may not be the best option for the patient. For example, in cases of bilateral tumor involvement, renal insufficiency, a solitary kidney, or von Hippel-Lindau disease, a parenchyma-sparing procedure may be indicated. In this procedure, the renal artery is temporarily occluded, the kidney cooled down, and partial nephrectomy or wedge resection performed. Frozen sections of the surgical margins are typically analyzed to ensure adequacy of resection. After restoration of arterial blood flow, the renal capsule is closed or, alternatively, omentum or perirenal fat is sutured to the defect to promote healing. Five-year survival rates after partial nephrectomy for patients with stage I and II disease are approximately 70% and 60%, respectively.

Advanced Renal Cell Carcinoma

Approximately 10% of patients present with locally advanced disease that has invaded adjacent structures. In general, the 3-year survival rate for these patients after surgery is less than 10%. Nephrectomy in this situation is done to improve the quality of life for symptomatic patients rather than to prolong survival. Recently, however, nephrectomy has also been performed in the presence of metastatic disease to satisfy clinical protocols that require removal of the primary lesion.

Distant metastatic disease can be categorized as a solitary metastasis or bulky metastatic disease. Several studies have shown improved 3-year survival rates, ranging from 20 to 60%, after radical nephrectomy with removal of a solitary metastasis. Solitary lung metastases appear to be associated with better survival rates than metastases to other organ sites.

Cytotoxic chemotherapy is ineffective in RCC; the highest objective response rate for single-agent therapy is only 16%. Thus, medical treatment for metastatic RCC has focused on the use of immunotherapy. The combination of alpha-interferon (IFN-α) and interleukin-2 (IL-2) has yielded response rates of 21–50% in various trials. In addition, it has been shown that both IFN-α and IL-2 can be given subcutaneously on an outpatient basis with side effects that are well tolerated. Currently, it is unclear whether nephrectomy will augment this response.

Testicular Cancer

EPIDEMIOLOGY AND ETIOLOGY

Malignant tumors of the testis are rare. It is estimated that 6,800 cases of testis cancer will be diagnosed in 1994, but only 325 men will die of this disease. Ninety-five percent of these tumors are of germ cell origin. Although testis tumors can occur at any age, specific tumor types tend to occur at different ages. Choriocarcinomas tend to occur between 24 and 28 years of age, embryonal carcinomas from 26 to 34 years of age, seminomas from 32 to 42 years of age, and lymphomas and spermatocytic seminomas after the age of 50 years.

The most well-known etiologic factor in the development of testis cancer is cryptorchidism. Between 3 and 11% of all cases of testis cancer occur in cryptorchid testes. Although trauma to the testis has been linked to testis cancer, there is no evidence of a definite relationship.

CLINICAL PRESENTATION

Testicular cancer typically presents as a painless testicular enlargement. Advanced disease can present as back pain, flank pain, or systemic symptoms. The differential diagnosis includes varicocele, hydrocele, hematoma, epididymitis, orchitis, and inguinal hernia.

DIAGNOSIS

Although the diagnosis is usually evident at physical examination to an experienced clinician, scrotal ultrasound can be useful in establishing the diagnosis. Any solid testicular mass is considered a testicular tumor until proved otherwise. Once a testicular tumor is suspected, the patient's levels of the tumor markers alpha-fetoprotein (AFP) and human chorionic gonadotropin (HCG) should be tested. Following this, he should undergo a radical (inguinal) orchiectomy. There is no role for fine-needle aspiration or Tru-cut biopsy in the work-up of this disease.

After radical orchiectomy, a CT scan of the chest, abdomen, and pelvis should be performed. If they were initially elevated, tumor markers should be reanalyzed following orchiectomy, after allowing the appropriate time for each marker to return to baseline.

STAGING

The M. D. Anderson staging system for testicular cancer is outlined in Table 17-4. In terms of biologic behavior and therapy, testicular tumors can be categorized as seminomatous or nonseminomatous germ cell tumors (NSGCT). Seminomas are radiosensitive and chemosensitive tumors that undergo lymphatic spread in an orderly fashion. In contrast, NSGCT are less radiosensitive and have a higher metastatic rate than seminomas.

MANAGEMENT

Seminomatous Germ Cell Tumors

Stage I and IIA seminomas are typically treated with radiotherapy to the ipsilateral iliac and periaortic areas up to the

Table 17-4. M. D. Anderson Cancer Center staging systems for testicular cancer

	Stage
Seminoma	
Confined to testicle	I
Retroperitoneal disease only, mass <10 cm	IIA
Retroperitoneal disease only, mass >10 cm	IIB
Supradiaphragmatic nodal disease	IIIA
Visceral disease	IIIB
Nonseminomatous germ cell tumor	
Confined to testicle	I
Negative clinical, positive surgical RPLND or elevated markers postorchiectomy	IIA
RPLND mass <2 cm	IIB
RPLND mass <5 cm	IIC
RPLND mass <10 cm	IID
Supraclavicular nodal disease	IIIA
Elevated marker(s) post-RPLND dissection	IIIB1
Pulmonary disease (minimal or advanced)	IIIB2
Advanced abdominal disease (mass >10 cm)	IIIB3
Visceral disease other than lung	IIIB4
β-hCG >50,000 IU, ±IIIB2, –IIIB4	IIIB5

RPLND = retroperitoneal lymph node dissection; β-hCG = human chorionic gonadotropin (beta subunit).

level of the diaphragm after radical orchiectomy. Using radiotherapy, the cure rate for stage I disease approaches 100%. Although 10–15% of patients with stage IIA disease have relapses, over half of these respond successfully to salvage therapy, yielding a survival rate of 95% for patients with stage IIa disease.

Stage IIB or III disease is usually treated with cisplatin- or carboplatin-based chemotherapy. Surgery is generally reserved for lymphatic disease that does not respond to chemotherapy or radiotherapy. Using this approach, 5-year disease-free survival rates of 86% and 92% have been obtained for patients with stages IIB and III disease, respectively.

Nonseminomatous Germ Cell Tumors

The optimal therapy for stage I disease is controversial; options include surveillance, retroperitoneal lymph node dissection (RPLND), and primary systemic chemotherapy. Overall, about 20–30% of stage I patients who undergo surveillance relapse. Wishnow et al. at M. D. Anderson Cancer Center found that patients with vascular invasion in their tumor, AFP levels greater than 80 ng/ml, or more than 80% embryonal elements in their tumor were at high risk for relapse. Twenty to thirty percent of patients who undergo RPLND are upstaged to stage II, allowing rational use of adjuvant chemotherapy. In addition, RPLND offers excellent local control for stage I tumors. After treatment with RPLND (and chemotherapy, if needed), survival rates are 99% for stage I and 95% for those upstaged to stage IIA.

The recurrence rate after RPLND for stage IIA disease is less than 20%. Thus, both RPLND and primary systemic chemotherapy have been used to treat low-volume retroperitoneal disease. Survival rates of 97% or better have been associated with both forms of therapy.

Because of the high recurrence rates associated with RPLND for stage IIB and III NSGCTs, primary systemic chemotherapy is the treatment of choice for this disease. RPLND is used to remove any residual disease that may be present after primary chemotherapy and to determine the need for further therapy. Recent experience with chemotherapy for advanced NSGCT at M. D. Anderson has shown survival rates of 96% and 76% for low- and high-volume stage III disease, respectively.

Since a majority of NCGCTs produce either AFP or β-hCG, these markers are helpful in monitoring the patient for treatment response and recurrent disease.

Despite the relatively early age of onset of testis cancer, this disease remains one of the most curable cancers in humans.

Selected References

PROSTATE CANCER

Barzell W, Bean MA, Hilaris BS, Whitmore WF Jr. Prostatic adenocarcinoma: Relationship of grade and local extent to the pattern of metastases. *J Urol* 118:278, 1977.

Brawn PN, Ayala AG, von Eschenbach AC, et al. Histologic grading study of prostate adenocarcinoma: The development of a new system and comparison of other methods—a preliminary study. *Cancer* 49:525, 1982.

Chybowski, FM, Keller JJ, Bergstralh EJ, Oesterling JE. Predicting radionuclide bone scan findings in patients with newly diagnosed untreated prostate cancer: Prostate specific antigen is superior to all other clinical parameters. J Urol 145:313, 1991.

Cooner WH, Mosley BR, Rutherford JR, et al. Prostate cancer detection in a clinical urological practice by ultrasonography, digital rectal examination and prostate specific antigen. *J Urol* 143:1146, 1990.

Crawford ED, Nabors WL. Total androgen ablation: American experience. *Urol Clin North Am* 18:55, 1991.

Gibbons RP, Correa RJ Jr, Brannen GE, et al. Total prostatectomy for localized prostate cancer. *J Urol* 131:73, 1984.

Kazlowski JM, Grayhack JT. Carcinoma of the Prostate. In JY Gillenwater, JT Grayhack, SS Howards, et al. (eds), *Adult and Pediatric Urology*. Chicago: Year Book, 1987.

McNeal JE, Redwine EA, Freiha FS, et al. Zonal distribution of prostatic adenocarcinoma. *Am J Surg Pathol* 12:897, 1988.

National Institutes of Health. Consensus development conference on the management of clinically localized prostate cancer (1987: Bethesda, MD). NCI monograph no. 7, NIH publication no. 88-3005. Washington, DC: U.S. Government Printing Office. Pp. 3–6, 1988.

Scardino PT, Frankel JM, Wheeler TM, et al. The prognostic significance of post-irradiation biopsy results in patients with prostate cancer. *J Urol* 135:510, 1986.

Stamey TA, McNeal JE. Adenocarcinoma of the Prostate. In PC Walsh, AB Retik, TA Stamey, et al (eds), *Campbell's Urology* (6th ed). Philadelphia: Saunders, 1992.

Wynder EL, Mabuchi K, Whitmore WF. Epidemiology of cancer of the prostate. *Cancer* 28:344, 1971.

Zagars GK, von Eschenbach AC, Johnson DE, et al. The role of radiation therapy in stages A2 and B adenocarcinoma of the prostate. *Int J Radiat Oncol Biol Phys* 14:701, 1988.

BLADDER CANCER

Catalona WJ. Bladder Cancer. In JY Gillenwater, JT Grayhack, SS Howards, et al (eds), *Adult and Pediatric Urology*. Chicago: Year Book, 1987.

Cummings KB, Barone JG, Ward WS. Diagnosis and staging of bladder cancer. *Urol Clin North Am* 19:429, 1992.

Heney NM, Ahmad S, Flanagan MJ, et al. Superficial bladder cancer: Progression and recurrence. *J Urol* 130:1083, 1983.

Lamm DL. Long term results of intravesical therapy for superficial bladder cancer. *Urol Clin North Am* 19:573, 1992.

Logothetis CJ, Dexeus FH, Finn L, et al. A prospective randomized trial comparing MVAC and CISCA chemotherapy for patients with metastatic urothelial tumors. *J Clin Oncol* 8:1050, 1990.

RENAL CANCER

Couillard DR, deVere White RW. Surgery of renal cell carcinoma. *Urol Clin North Am* 20:263, 1993.

Williams RD. Renal, Perirenal, and Ureteral Neoplasms. In JY Gillenwater, JT Grayhack, SS Howards, et al (eds), *Adult and Pediatric Urology*. Chicago: Year Book, 1987.

Wirth MP. Immunotherapy for metastatic renal cell carcinoma. *Urol Clin North Am* 20:283, 1993.

TESTIS CANCER

Logothetis CJ. The case for relevant staging of germ cell tumors. *Cancer* 65:709, 1990.

Sternberg CN. Role of primary chemotherapy in stage I and low-volume stage II nonseminomatous germ-cell testis tumors. *Urol Clin North Am* 20:93, 1993.

Wishnow KI, Johnson DE, Swanson DA, et al. Identifying patients with low-risk clinical stage I nonseminomatous testicular tumors who should be treated by surveillance. *Urology* 34:339, 1989.

Gynecologic Oncology

Alton V. Hallum, III, Robert L. Coleman,
and Judy Wolf

The surgical oncologist and gynecologic oncologist share a common territory—the abdomen. Familiarity with all disease processes affecting the abdominal cavity is necessary. Unfortunately, the subspecialization of medicine not only challenges physicians to keep pace with advances in their own practice, it also makes learning about trends in other fields a herculean task. This chapter discusses the basics of gynecologic oncology so that these disease processes are considered when examining patients and appropriate management occurs when one encounters these neoplasms unexpectedly. Emphasis is placed on diagnosis, staging, and surgical management.

Ovarian Cancer

EPITHELIAL OVARIAN CANCER

Epidemiology and Etiology

Carcinoma of the ovary is the fourth most common cause of death from cancer in women, accounting for 5% of all cancer-related deaths. Approximately one-fourth of all gynecologic malignancies are of ovarian origin, and 47% of all gynecologic cancer-related deaths are due to ovarian cancer. This is primarily because the disease frequently is not diagnosed until an advanced stage: Almost 60 percent of patients will have stage III or stage IV disease at presentation. The lifetime risk of developing ovarian cancer is approximately 1 in 70. Incidence increases with age and peaks in the eighth decade of life.

The majority (85–90%) of ovarian cancers are epithelial in origin. The other classes of ovarian neoplasms—sex cord–stromal tumors and germ cell tumors—are rare.

Risk Factors

Three hereditary patterns have been linked to epithelial ovarian cancer, although they account for only 3–5% of ovarian cancer cases. Site-specific ovarian cancer, familial breast and ovarian cancer, and Lynch type II syndrome (nonpolyposis colon cancer, endometrial cancer, and ovarian cancer) make up the known hereditary conditions. All three are transmitted as autosomal dominant traits with variable penetrance. The age of onset for patients with hereditary forms of ovarian cancer is usually the fifth decade of life or earlier, while nonhereditary forms usually occur in the sixth decade or later. These patients have an increased incidence of bilateral ovarian tumors as well as multiple primary sites of cancer. The presence of two first-degree relatives with ovarian cancer is a marker of high risk for familial ovarian cancer.

Screening

Unfortunately, there is no effective screening program for ovarian cancer. Most epithelial ovarian neoplasms are sporadic in nature and are associated with no predisposing risk factors. Ovarian cancer has no preclinical phase, and early-stage cancers are usually discovered incidentally. Presently available screening techniques are not sufficiently sensitive or specific when used alone. When the tests are used in combination, sensitivity and specificity improve but not enough to justify general use, as screening becomes very expensive when the yield is relatively low.

Clinical Presentation and Diagnostic Work-Up

Symptoms noted most frequently at the time of diagnosis are usually related to disseminated disease: abdominal discomfort and pain, abdominal distention, early satiety, dyspepsia, constipation, dysuria, and urinary frequency. These symptoms may be due to the presence of bulky tumor or ascites but can also occur with other neoplasms of the abdominal viscera or with metastatic disease to the abdomen. Because symptoms are nonspecific, there is frequently a delay in the diagnosis of ovarian cancer.

Early-stage ovarian cancer is usually discovered as an asymptomatic adnexal mass on routine pelvic examination. The majority of such adnexal masses are benign, especially in premenopausal women. When a pelvic mass is encountered in a woman of reproductive age, repeat pelvic examination or ultrasonography should be performed in approximately 6 weeks to determine whether spontaneous regression of the mass has occurred, as often happens when the mass is a corpus luteum or functioning cyst. The presence of solid elements, irregular borders, internal papillary projections, multiple septae, and/or bilateral tumors on ultrasound examination increases the probability that an ovarian mass is malignant.

When ovarian cancer is suspected, the work-up should begin with a complete history and physical examination, including pelvic examination and Papanicolaou (Pap) smear. Pelvic ultrasound is frequently used to determine the relationship of the mass to the other pelvic viscera, as well as to evaluate abnormalities of the uterine corpus, endometrial thickness, and the presence of ascites, hydroureter, and hydronephrosis. Computed tomography (CT) or magnetic resonance imaging (MRI) is also done to evaluate the presence of extraovarian disease. The most common sites for bulky metastases include the omentum, peritoneal surfaces, bowel mesentery, sigmoid colon, and retroperitoneal lymph nodes. Other radiographic studies to consider in the preoperative evaluation include chest radiograph, IV pyelogram, and barium enema x-ray study. A barium enema study is especially helpful in postmenopausal women because the signs and symptoms of ovarian cancer and colorectal carcinoma can be similar. Proctosigmoidoscopy may be useful if colon cancer cannot be ruled out. A mammogram should also be considered to exclude the possibility of metastatic breast cancer, which can occasionally present as bilateral ovarian metastases.

Routine blood tests should include a serum CA-125 determination. Eighty to 85% of patients with epithelial ovarian cancer will have an elevated CA-125 level (serum level >35 units/ml), whereas fewer than 1% of nonpregnant healthy women will have a CA-125 that high. This marker is most frequently elevated in patients with serous neoplasms, although elevations can be seen with mucinous adenocarcinoma.

In premenopausal women, other nonmalignant conditions can cause elevations in CA-125: pregnancy, endometriosis, pelvic inflammatory disease, and ovulation. Other malignancies also can cause an elevation in the CA-125 level, so this marker should not be considered specific for ovarian cancer. In patients with preoperatively elevated marker levels, CA-125 can also be used to monitor response to adjuvant chemotherapy.

Surgical Staging

Ovarian cancer is staged by laparotomy. Laparotomy allows quantification of the extent of disease and, when no gross extraovarian disease is evident, permits a detailed search for microscopic disease to be performed. In patients with extensive disease, laparotomy allows debulking of the tumor mass, which improves clinical outcome. The International Federation of Gynecology and Obstetrics (FIGO) surgical staging system is outlined in Table 18-1.

Traditionally, a midline incision is used to evaluate an adnexal or pelvic mass that may be an ovarian cancer. After the abdomen is entered, cytologic washings are obtained from the pelvis, paracolic gutters, and right hemidiaphragm. These washings are especially important when the cancer appears confined to the ovary. The volume of ascites should be noted and a sample submitted for cytologic examination. If there is no evidence of extraovarian spread, resection of the adnexal mass should be performed with particular care taken not to rupture the ovarian capsule. The spilling of malignant cells into the peritoneal cavity may adversely affect the patient and is an indication for upstaging of the disease (see Table 18-1). Frozen-section evaluation of the adnexal mass will guide further management. If an ovarian malignancy is diagnosed and is apparently confined to the ovary, a meticulous search of all peritoneal surfaces should be performed. Omentectomy should be performed and random peritoneal biopsies should be taken from the pelvis, paracolic gutter, and diaphragm. Any adhesions should also be submitted for pathologic examination. Pelvic and para-aortic lymph node sampling should then be performed. This aggressive search for microscopic disease often will lead to a change in the clinical stage of disease. Approximately 30% of

Table 18-1. FIGO (1986) staging system for ovarian cancer

Stage	Characteristics
I	Growth limited to the ovaries
IA	Growth limited to one ovary; no ascites; no tumor on the external surfaces; capsule intact
IB	Growth limited to both ovaries; no ascites; no tumor on the external surfaces; capsule intact
IC	Tumor either stage IA or stage IB but with tumor on the surface of one or both ovaries, or with capsule ruptured, or with ascites containing malignant cells or with positive peritoneal washings
II	Growth involving one or both ovaries on pelvic extension
IIA	Extension or metastases to the uterus or tubes
IIB	Extension to other pelvic tissues
IIC	Tumor either stage IIA or IIB with tumor on the surface of one or both ovaries, or with capsule(s) ruptured, or with ascites containing malignant cells or with positive peritoneal washings
III	Tumor involving one or both ovaries with peritoneal implants outside the pelvis or positive retroperitoneal or inguinal nodes; superficial liver metastases equals stage III; tumor is limited to the true pelvis but with histologically verified malignant extension to small bowel or omentum
IIIA	Tumor grossly limited to the true pelvis with negative nodes but with histologically confirmed microscopic seeding of abdominal peritoneal surfaces
IIIB	Tumor of one or both ovaries; histologically confirmed implants of abdominal peritoneal surfaces, none exceeding 2 cm in diameter; nodes negative
IIIC	Abdominal implants greater than 2 cm in diameter or positive retroperitoneal or inguinal nodes
IV	Growth involving one or both ovaries with distant metastases; if pleural effusion is present, there must be positive cytologic test results to allot a case to stage IV; parenchymal liver metastases equals stage IV

patients will be upstaged, with three-fourths of these patients having stage III disease.

Ovarian cancer tends to metastasize within the abdomen, with spread over peritoneal surfaces. Therefore after the extent of spread is documented, efforts are directed at maximally resecting all gross disease. Optimal cytoreductive surgery—less than 2 cm of residual disease—depends on the skill and determination of the surgeon. Several series have shown that this degree of cytoreductive surgery could be accomplished with an average success rate of 35% and a range of 17–87%.

Survival strongly correlates with volume of residual disease after cytoreductive surgery. Griffiths performed linear regression analysis on 102 patients with stage II and III ovarian cancer. The median survival of patients with no

Table 18-2. Survival by stage in epithelial ovarian cancer

Stage	5-year survival
I	Up to 80%
II	Up to 60%
III	15%
IV	5%

gross residual disease was 39 months, while patients with residual tumor larger than 1.45 cm in greatest diameter had a median survival of 12.7 months. Incomplete debulking with implants greater than 1.5 cm in diameter affords no survival advantage. Several subsequent studies corroborated the impact of residual disease on survival.

Cytoreductive surgery remains the foundation of therapy for advanced ovarian cancer. Reduction in tumor burden not only palliates symptoms but theoretically improves the effect of adjuvant therapy. Bulky tumors often have poor blood supply to significant portions of the cell mass, which makes chemotherapy less effective. The role of cytoreductive surgery in patients with stage IV disease is uncertain, but the procedure is frequently performed to palliate symptoms.

Prognostic Factors

Several factors have been identified that predict clinical outcome. The stage of disease (Table 18-2) and residual volume of tumor following debulking surgery have the strongest predictive value. Hoskins et al. reported that patients with optimal cytoreduction had a median survival of 39 months, compared with 17 months in patients who had suboptimal cytoreduction.

Histologic subtype and tumor grade provide important information in early-stage ovarian cancer, with grade 3 tumors and clear cell histology associated with more aggressive disease. In patients with advanced disease, the effect of tumor grade and histologic subtype are not as strong.

Tumor ploidy and oncogene amplification can be used to identify aggressive neoplasms. Patients with aneuploid tumors typically have higher stage and shorter survival times. Overexpression or amplification of the HER-2/*neu* proto-oncogene also has been associated with a statistically shorter survival.

Management of Stages I and II Disease

Patients with stage I tumors that are well or moderately differentiated require no further therapy if the disease is adequately staged. A poorly differentiated lesion, stages IC or II disease, or a tumor with dense adhesions to adjacent structures warrants adjuvant therapy. Chemotherapy is reserved for these high-risk patients, and several studies have shown improved survival for patients given adjuvant chemotherapy when compared with historic controls. A platinum-based chemotherapy regimen is the standard adjuvant treatment used. External beam and intraperitoneal radiocolloid radiotherapy have not been clearly shown to impact on survival. Young et al. compared intraperitoneal radioactive phosphorous (^{32}P) colloid with single-agent oral melphalan and found similar 5-year survival and relapse rates for the two treatments; approximately 80% of the patients survived 5 years. The Gynecologic Oncology Group (GOG) is currently comparing cisplatin and cyclophosphamide with intraperitoneal ^{32}P.

Management of Stage III Disease

In stage III patients, survival is strongly influenced by volume of residual disease. Chemotherapy is recommended following debulking surgery. Platinum-based combination chemotherapy is currently favored based on the higher response rates seen in patients with advanced disease receiving platinum-containing regimens. Carboplatin and cisplatin produce similar response rates, disease-free intervals, and survival rates. Carboplatin is less nephrotoxic, neurotoxic, and emetogenic than cisplatin; myelosuppression is the dose-limiting toxicity of carboplatin. The dose intensity of platinum-based chemotherapy may influence survival, as several studies have demonstrated a prolongation of median survival time with increasing dose intensity. The decreased toxicity of carboplatin makes it better suited to dose intensity regimens than cisplatin. Although Taxol is currently approved only for use in recurrent ovarian cancer, several studies are presently examining its use as primary treatment in conjunction with platinum. The dose-limiting toxicity of Taxol is neutropenia, and therefore cisplatin rather than carboplatin is used. There are conflicting data on the optimal number of courses of chemotherapy, with the majority of patients treated in the United States receiving six courses.

Second-look laparotomy following chemotherapy has been widely practiced for patients who have no clinical evidence of disease. This procedure is a detailed inspection of the peritoneal cavity for evidence of gross and microscopic disease. Patients considered eligible for second-look laparotomy should have a normalized CA-125 level and no detectable disease on physical examination or radiographic studies. The second-look laparotomy itself has not influenced survival, however, and presently is most commonly used only in a protocol setting. Gross disease is present in approximately one-third of patients at second-look surgery. In the absence of obvious tumor, multiple biopsies are done throughout the peritoneal cavity to search for microscopic disease. Approximately 45% of patients undergoing second-look laparotomy will have no surgically detectable disease. Unfortunately, one-half of these patients will nevertheless have relapses and ultimately die of their disease. Even in a protocol setting, many centers are using laparoscopy rather than laparotomy for second-look surgery because of its decreased morbidity and recovery time.

Management of Stage IV Disease

Patients with stage IV disease are typically treated in a manner similar to that for stage III disease: initial cytoreductive surgery followed by adjuvant chemotherapy. While this may palliate symptoms of disease, no clear survival benefit has been demonstrated. No study has been able to show a statistical difference in outcome of stage IV patients with optimal versus suboptimal cytoreductive surgery. The 5-year survival in both groups is less than 5%, and cytoreductive surgery does not prolong progression-free survival. Optimal management of these patients has yet to be defined. Possible options include chemotherapy alone, traditional management with cytoreductive surgery followed by adjuvant chemotherapy, or neoadjuvant chemotherapy followed by debulking surgery.

Management of Recurrent Disease

When recurrent ovarian cancer is detected, treatment decisions should take into account the length of time between completion of chemotherapy and recurrence. Platinum-treated patients with a disease-free interval longer than 6 months have a 40% chance of responding to reinduction therapy with platinum chemotherapy. Patients who have persistent disease after platinum chemotherapy, progressive disease during chemotherapy, or a relapse within 6 months of completion of chemotherapy are considered to have platinum-resistant disease. These patients are candidates for second-line chemotherapy. The most promising second-line agent to date is paclitaxel (Taxol), which is currently being investigated in multiple studies as a front-line chemotherapeutic agent. The response rate to Taxol in platinum-resistant ovarian cancer patients is approximately 30%. Other second-line agents that have been studied include melphalan, altretamine, etoposide, ifosfamide, and 5-fluorouracil; response rates are 25% or less. Hormonal therapy has also been attempted, with an approximately 18% total response rate.

Palliative cytoreductive surgery for recurrent ovarian cancer is generally not done except perhaps in patients with a long disease-free interval and/or localized recurrent disease amenable to surgical resection.

The majority of patients with progressive ovarian cancer die of complications from bowel obstruction and inanition. Large-bowel obstructions can be effectively decompressed with a loop colostomy. However, patients with small-bowel obstructions, which are more common, usually present with multifocal areas of involvement. Rarely do these patients respond to surgical therapy. Total parenteral nutrition,

Table 18-3. Serum tumor markers in malignant germ cell tumors of the ovary

Histology	Alpha-fetoprotein	Human chorionic gonadotropin
Dysgerminoma	−	+/−
Endodermal sinus tumor	+	−
Immmature teratoma	+/−	−
Mixed germ cell tumor	+/−	+/−
Choriocarcinoma	−	+
Embryonal carcinoma	+/−	+
Polyembryoma	+/−	+

Source: WJ Hoskins, CA Perez, RC Young (eds). *Principles and Practice of Gynecologic Oncology.* Philadelphia: Lippincott, 1992

although expensive, has prolonged life in some patients with a nonfunctional bowel. This is not commonly used but may be tried on an individual basis. Percutaneuous gastrostomy tube placement offers small-bowel decompression and minimizes chronic nausea and vomiting.

BORDERLINE EPITHELIAL TUMORS

Borderline epithelial ovarian neoplasms represent a subset of ovarian cancers that have a much better prognosis than do higher-grade lesions. These lesions have histologic features that separate them from high-grade lesions, and they are seen in women who are younger than the average age for high-grade ovarian cancer. Even when disease is widely disseminated throughout the abdominal cavity, the 5-year survival rate may approach 50%. Patients with stage III and stage IV disease should undergo aggressive cytoreductive surgery. Prospective studies have been unable to show any impact on survival with adjuvant therapy following cytoreductive surgery. However, despite these results, such a treatment regimen continues to be frequently used.

GERM CELL TUMORS

Germ cell tumors account for 2–3% of ovarian cancers and almost always occur in young women. Patients frequently present with a large palpable mass and often have pain caused by torsion of the tumor. Preoperative evaluation should include serum evaluation of human chorionic gonadotropin (HCG) and alpha-fetoprotein (AFP) levels (Table 18-3). These markers can then be used in following response to postoperative chemotherapy.

The majority of germ cell tumors are unilateral. Surgical management involves removing the affected ovary and closely inspecting the contralateral ovary, without biopsy if it appears normal. Maximum efforts are made to conserve the contralateral ovary in these patients because of their age and fertility considerations. Chemotherapy has proved quite effective against these neoplasms; thus, conservation of the contralateral ovary is justified if it appears normal, even if there is disease spread beyond the affected ovary. The two most common therapeutic regimens used for metastatic or high-risk germ cell neoplasms are bleomycin, etoposide, and cisplatin (BEP), and vincristine, dactinomycin, and cyclophosphamide (VAC). The BEP regimen is currently favored because of a higher response rate in initial studies.

SEX CORD–STROMAL TUMORS

Sex cord–stromal tumors arise from the mesenchyme of the embryonic gonad and represent approximately 2% of all ovarian cancers. The most common histologic subtypes seen are granulosa cell tumors and Sertoli-Leydig cell tumors. Less frequently encountered is the sex cord tumor with annular tubules (SCTAT), which is associated with Peutz-Jeghers syndrome. Granulosa cell tumors usually occur in the perimenopausal years; however, these lesions can occur as early as the teen-age years. Sertoli-Leydig cell tumors typically occur in the third decade of life, but later occurrences are seen. Because these tumors may have hormonal activity, estrogenic or androgenic symptoms frequently lead to the diagnosis. Amenorrhea, oligomenorrhea, dysfunctional uterine bleeding, or hirsutism may cause the patient to see her physician for evaluation.

Patients with sex cord–stromal tumors typically present with unilateral stage 1 disease. Because of the rarity of these tumors, no large experience is available on which to base chemotherapeutic recommendations. Adjuvant chemotherapy is often given for large stage I tumors or when extraovarian spread is noted.

Management of the Unsuspected Ovarian Mass Found at Laparotomy

The finding of an unsuspected ovarian mass at the time of exploratory laparotomy or laparotomy for an unrelated condition can pose a therapeutic dilemma to the surgeon. Treatment will depend on several factors, including the size and consistency of the mass, whether it is bilateral, whether other structures are grossly involved, and the age of the patient.

OVARIAN MASSES IN WOMEN OF CHILDBEARING AGE

An unsuspected mass found in a young patient is likely to be benign in origin but still may require removal. The most common ovarian masses in women of childbearing age are those related to normal cyclical ovarian function; these are not actual neoplastic growths. Women not on oral contraceptives, hormones, or medications that suppress ovarian function can have either an asymptomatic or symptomatic corpus luteum. This is the normal ovarian response after ovulation. However, the corpus luteum can sometimes become cystic or even hemorrhagic. A hemorrhagic corpus luteum can present as an acute abdomen with peritoneal signs and free blood in the abdomen. This in itself may lead to laparotomy. Oversewing the bleeding area without oophorectomy or cystectomy is frequently the only treatment that is required. It is important to do pregnancy testing in these patients prior to surgery as the surgery may result in loss of function of the corpus luteum, which supports the pregnancy for the first trimester. In pregnant patients, postoperative support with progesterone therapy can be used to carry the pregnancy through the critical period.

Ovulating patients can also present with functional ovarian cysts. These are usually asymptomatic but can cause lower abdominal or pelvic pain; however, signs of an acute abdomen are rare. A simple cyst up to 5 cm in diameter found incidentally at the time of surgery in an ovulating patient can be safely followed. If it is only a functional cyst, it should disappear after the patient's next menstrual period. Resolution can be evaluated with physical examination alone or in conjunction with pelvic ultrasound. Functional cysts are more common in patients who have anovulatory cycles, such as patients with polycystic ovarian syndrome or obese patients.

Neoplastic growths, both benign and malignant, also can occur in young patients. In a patient taking oral contraceptives, any cyst on the ovary should be considered neoplastic, as these patients should not have corpus luteums or functional cysts. Ovulatory patients also can develop neoplasms. Most of the neoplastic growths in young patients are benign. Benign cystic teratomas, or dermoids, are one of the most common benign tumors seen in young patients. These cystic masses may be of any size and are usually unilateral; however, 1–15% are bilateral. Treatment is cystectomy of the involved ovary with close inspection of the contralateral ovary. For even large dermoids, a cystectomy can usually be performed. The remainder of the ovary, even if it is stretched out after removal of the cyst, can be left behind and will usually function normally. Other common benign neoplasms in young patients include epithelial cystadenomas (serous, mucinous, or endometrioid). These are usually treated with unilateral oophorectomy if the other ovary appears normal. Endometriomas, or the so-called chocolate cyst of endometriosis, are also seen in young patients. These patients may have a history of endometriosis, chronic pelvic pain, or other obvious endometriomas in the pelvis or abdominal cavity, which may aid in the diagnosis. The treatment for endometriomas may be either cystectomy or oophorectomy, depending on the amount of ovarian involvement.

In any patient for whom the diagnosis is unclear by examination and/or after consultation with a gynecologist, the

Table 18-4. Staging procedure for the unsuspected ovarian mass

1. Collection of ascitic fluid for cytology
2. Peritoneal washings from cul-de-sac and paracolic gutters for cytology
3. Omentectomy
4. Random biopsies of peritoneal surfaces and diaphragm
5. Lymph node sampling from para-aortic and iliac chains, along with any enlarged lymph nodes within the abdomen or pelvis
6. Biopsy of any suspicious intra-abdominal findings

safest procedure is excision of the involved ovary with frozen-section diagnosis to rule out malignancy. Malignant neoplasms are uncommon in young women (<40 years of age). The most frequently seen malignant tumors in young women and girls are those of germ cell or stromal origin. They are usually unilateral and may be multicystic or contain solid components. Treatment of these tumors is described above. Malignant epithelial tumors are particularly uncommon in young women; however, if a multiseptated or solid mass is found unexpectedly at the time of laparotomy, suggesting an epithelial tumor, the involved ovary should be removed and frozen-section diagnosis obtained. Epithelial tumors are more likely than other types to involve both ovaries, so in all but the very earliest grade I tumors, bilateral oophorectomy is recommended (Table 18-4).

OVARIAN MASSES IN POSTMENOPAUSAL WOMEN

The risk of an ovarian mass being malignant begins to increase at 40 years of age and rises steadily thereafter. Therefore the finding of an unsuspected ovarian mass in a postmenopausal woman is a more ominous sign. Benign lesions can also occur. The most common benign lesions in patients older than 40 years are epithelial cystadenomas (serous, mucinous, and endometrioid). Dermoid cysts also can occur but are a much less frequent finding than in younger patients.

The most common malignant neoplasms in older patients are malignant epithelial tumors, with germ cell and stromal cell tumors occurring only rarely.

Treatment of an unsuspected ovarian mass in a postmenopausal patient includes oophorectomy on the involved side. If frozen-section analysis cannot rule out malignancy, both ovaries should be removed and a staging procedure performed, if technically feasible. Consultation with a gynecologic oncologist should be obtained if at all possible.

CONCLUSIONS

An unsuspected mass on the ovary at the time of surgery should be considered a significant finding, and appropriate consultation and/or removal of the tumor with frozen-section diagnosis should be undertaken in all cases except for simple

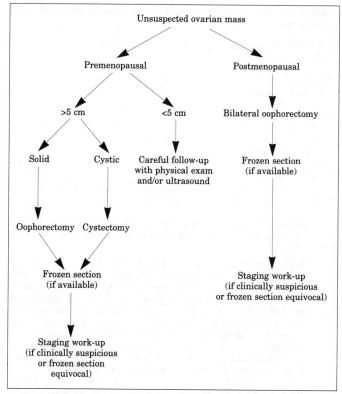

Fig. 18-1. Management of the unsuspected ovarian mass found at the time of laparotomy.

functional cysts in young premenopausal patients. If frozen-section analysis is not immediately available, the lesion should still be removed and sent for permanent section pathologic diagnosis (assuming the remainder of the pelvic and abdominal organs are normal). It must be understood that the patient may need additional definitive surgery at a later time if the lesion is found to be malignant (Fig. 18-1).

Endometrial Carcinoma

EPIDEMIOLOGY

Since 1972, epithelial carcinoma of the uterus has been the most common gynecologic pelvic malignancy in the United States. With over 31,000 cases expected in 1994, endometrial carcinoma accounts for approximately 13% of all malignancies in women and ranks fourth in frequency behind breast, lung, and colon carcinomas. While endometrial carcinoma is primarily a postmenopausal disease, with a median

Table 18-5. Characteristics and relative risks for endometrial carcinoma

Characteristic	Relative risk
Nulliparity	2.0
Late menopause	2.4
Chronic disease	
Diabetes mellitus	2.8
Hypertension	1.5
Obesity	
>30 lbs	3.0
>50 lbs	10.0
"Bloody" menopause	4.0
Unopposed estrogen	9.5
Complex atypical hyperplasia	29.0

Source: WJ Hoskins, CA Perez, RC Young (eds). *Principles and Practice of Gynecologic Oncology.* Philadelphia: Lippincott, 1992.

age at onset of 63 years, up to 25% of cases occur in pre-menopausal women, with 5% occurring in patients younger than 40 years.

Endometrial cancer is a highly curable disease, attested to by the less than 5,900 deaths from disease expected in 1994. This relatively low rate of disease-related mortality is partly a result of limited disease at presentation (75% of tumors are limited to the uterus) and the ability to identify the preinvasive or early invasive condition from symptomatology (unexpected vaginal bleeding). In addition, the role of unopposed estrogen exposure in the development of this disease is understood and generally known among treating physicians. Less well known but now incorporated into treatment strategies are the findings elucidated from surgical staging (FIGO, 1988) that can direct adjuvant treatment to patients at high risk for microscopic metastatic disease. Despite our improved understanding of the natural history of the disease and refinement of strategies for adjuvant therapy, however, little progress has been made in the treatment of metastatic disease, and recurrence continues to be a lethal event.

ETIOLOGY

Although the true etiology of endometrial cancer is not known, insight into the mechanisms of disease is often gained by examining the phenotypes of affected individuals. Study of these individuals has suggested at least two distinct etiologic mechanisms, as endometrial carcinomas have been identified in atrophic, normal, and hyperestrogenized endometrium.

The first and largest subgroup of affected individuals demonstrate a chronic estrogenized status—both from endogenous and exogenous sources. Table 18-5 lists the demonstrated risk factors for endometrial carcinoma and the relative risks for developing the disease. Many of these risk factors reflect an individual's exposure to chronic estrogen therapy. For

Table 18-6. Classification of endometrial hyperplasia

Hyperplastic lesion	Progressing to cancer (%)
No cellular atypia	
Simple (cystic)	1
Complex (adenomatous)	3
Cellular atypia	
Simple (cystic)	8
Complex (adenomatous)	29

Source: WJ Hoskins, CA Perez, RC Young (eds). *Principles and Practice of Gynecologic Oncology*. Philadelphia: Lippincott, 1992

example, nulliparity, early menarche, and late menopause represent long-term exposure to endogenous estrogen. The relationship of uterine cancer to obesity is most likely due to the increased conversion of androstenedione to estrone in fat stores. The role of diabetes, hypertension, and other medical diseases in the development of uterine carcinoma is less clear but may reflect the anovulatory state frequently seen in these patients or direct effects of the disease processes on hormonal metabolism. Women in this group tend to present with preinvasive, early-stage, well-differentiated lesions of common epithelial histologies, which are associated with an overall better prognosis.

The second and less common group of women with endometrial carcinoma present with higher-grade lesions, commonly with atypical histologic subtypes such as clear cell carcinoma or serous carcinoma. These tumors have more aggressive clinical courses, and patients present with more advanced lesions. These lesions commonly coexist with atrophic endometria and are more likely to be deeply invasive. The tumors appear to have no early presenting signs or preinvasive states.

While hyperplastic conditions have been identified in the endometrium, their direct role as a preinvasive state, similar to the role of cervical hyperplasia, has been debated. Endometrial hyperplasia is a condition in which epithelial glandular growth occurs, with an increase in the number and size of glands. These glands enlarge, develop irregular outlines and intraluminal bridges, and may demonstrate mitoses, nuclear enlargement, and prominent nucleoli. Lesions with extensive glandular crowding and cellular atypia can be difficult to distinguish from well-differentiated adenocarcinomas.

Morrow et al. followed 170 women with varying degrees of endometrial hyperplasia without treatment and studied the frequency with which they developed endometrial carcinoma. The results from this study are summarized in Table 18-6. With the background incidence of carcinoma being approximately 1%, it can be appreciated that only certain hyperplastic lesions are truly "preinvasive." In general, hyperplastic lesions are highly treatable with intermittent progestogen therapy after appropriate diagnostic evaluation.

Table 18-7. International Society of Gynecologic Pathologists' histologic classification scheme

Endometrioid adenocarcinoma
    Papillary
    Secretory
    Ciliated cell
    Adenocarcinoma with squamous differentiation
Mucinous carcinoma
Serous carcinoma
Clear cell carcinoma
Squamous carcinoma
Undifferentiated carcinoma
Mixed types
Miscellaneous carcinoma
Metastatic carcinoma

Source: WJ Hoskins, CA Perez, RC Young (eds). *Principles and Practice of Gynecologic Oncology*. Philadelphia: Lippincott, 1992.

Table 18-8. Typically presenting histologic pathologies in endometrial carcinoma

Histology	Cases (%)
Adenocarcinoma	75
Adenosquamous	18
Papillary serous	6
Clear cell	1

Source: Adapted from C Morrow, B Bundy, R Kurman, et al. Relationship between surgical-pathological risk factors and outcome in clinical stage I and II carcinoma of the endometrium: A Gynecologic Oncology Group study. *Gynecol Oncol* 40:55, 1991.

PATHOLOGY

The International Society of Gynecologic Pathologists has proposed a classification scheme for carcinomas arising in the endometrium (Table 18-7). The most commonly reported tumor histologies are listed in Table 18-8. The differentiation of a carcinoma is expressed as its grade, with well-differentiated lesions designated grade 1 and poorly differentiated lesions grade 3. Atypical histologies such as serous carcinoma, clear cell carcinoma, and ciliated cell carcinoma are difficult to grade because their growth patterns are architecturally limited. In these lesions, nuclear grade is more important. Flow cytometric studies of endometrial lesions reveal that approximately 60% have diploid characteristics. A lesion in which two or more cell types each make up 30% or more of the tumor is classified as a mixed-cell type. An example of this is adenosquamous carcinoma.

CLINICAL PRESENTATION AND DIAGNOSTIC WORK-UP

Symptoms of endometrial carcinoma are related principally to the exophytic growth of the primary lesion. Unexpected vaginal bleeding or discharge can be identified in more than 90% of patients and, outside of more vague complaints such as pelvic pressure or pelvic pain, is usually the symptom that prompts patients to seek medical attention.

The classic method of diagnosing endometrial cancer is the fractional dilatation and curettage. This procedure, which separately evaluates the endocervix and the endometrium, not only provides adequate tissue for diagnosis but also allows evaluation of the uterus and adnexa under anesthesia. Endometrial aspiration, which can be performed in the office setting, has largely replaced dilatation and curettage as the initial diagnostic survey because, in over 85% of cases, it provides appropriate information to formulate a plan of clinical management. However, if insufficient information is obtained with endometrial aspiration, formal evaluation with a dilatation and curettage is mandatory.

Once the diagnosis of endometrial carcinoma is confirmed, the patient should undergo a thorough evaluation. A complete physical examination of potential metastatic sites, such as lymph nodes and extrapelvic structures, is important. Chest radiography and barium enema x-ray study are helpful. Additional procedures that have been advocated are IV pyelography, CT, and MRI. These studies can provide, preoperatively, information regarding the extent of disease in the pelvis and at metastatic sites. Proctosigmoidoscopy and cystoscopy can provide information regarding local tumor involvement of the bowel and bladder. In the majority of cases, however, radiographic studies provide little additional information than will be obtained at the time of surgery. Nevertheless, in medically inoperable cases or in cases with extensive metastatic disease, these tests can help focus radiotherapy and identify measurable lesions to follow during adjuvant therapy.

STAGING

Since 1988, staging of endometrial carcinoma has required information obtained at the time of surgery (surgical staging). Prior to this, information from clinical examination and fractional dilatation and curettage was used for staging (clinical staging). Results from two large, prospective, surgical staging trials performed by the GOG provided sufficient evidence of the importance of surgical findings in clinical management and prognosis to justify changing the staging scheme. The FIGO (1988) surgical staging scheme is listed in Table 18-9. Under these guidelines, the surgical approach requires a total extrafascial (type I) hysterectomy, bilateral salpingo-oophorectomy, cytologic washing of the peritoneal cavity, and a thorough abdominal-pelvic exploration. Obvious nodules need to be sampled. In addition, certain patients will require peritoneal biopsies (random), omental biopsies, and pelvic and para-aortic lymph node biopsies to complete staging. Our usual approach is to open the uterus at the time of the hysterectomy. If a grade I or II tumor

Table 18-9. FIGO (1988) staging classification of endometrial carcinoma

Stage I (5-year survival: 75–100%)
Endometrial cancer in this stage means carcinoma confined to the corpus uteri.
   IA: Tumor limited to the endometrium
   IB: Myometrial invasion less than 50%
   IC: Myometrial invasion more than 50%

Stage II (5-year survival: up to 60%)
Endometrial cancer in this stage means the cancer has involved the corpus and the cervix but not outside the uterus (results from dilatation and curettage do not influence stage).
   IIA: Endocervical gland involvement only
   IIB: Cervical stromal invasion

Stage III (5-year survival: up to 50%)
Endometrial carcinoma in this stage means extension outside the uterus but confined to the true pelvis or para-aortic area.
   IIIA: Tumor invades the uterine serosa and/or adnexa, and/or
         positive peritoneal cytology
   IIIB: Vaginal metastases
   IIIC: Metastases to the pelvic and/or para-aortic lymph nodes

Stage IV (5-year survival: up to 20%)
Distant metastases or involvement of the adjacent pelvic organs classifies this stage.
   IVA: Tumor invasion of the bowel or bladder mucosa
   IVB: Distant metastases including intra-abdominal and or
         inguinal lymph nodes

Grade scheme
I: 5% or less of a nonsquamous or nonmorular solid growth pattern
II: 6–50% of a nonsquamous or nonmorular solid growth pattern
III: More than 50% of a nonsquamous or nonmorular solid growth pattern

invades less than 33% of the myometrium grossly without involvement of the lower uterine segment, no sampling is performed. All other cases undergo complete surgical staging.

PROGNOSTIC FACTORS

The degree to which surgical findings influence clinical management is based largely on their individual association with the probability of microscopic nodal metastases. The recommendations on adjuvant therapy are based on these estimates. The most discriminatory prognostic factor for the presence of nodal metastases are myometrial invasion and tumor grade. These two factors are not wholly independent. In general, as grade increases, the depth of myometrial invasion increases. In the GOG studies, more than 75% of grade 1 lesions were limited to the endometrium or superficial myometrium, whereas 60% of grade 3 lesions invaded at least 50% of the myometrium. However, of the two factors, myometrial depth is more influential. For example, only 1% of patients with endometrial involvement only will have nodal metastases, regardless of grade. However, the incidence of pelvic node metastases increases to 25% with deeply invasive tumors.

MANAGEMENT

Low-Risk Disease

Relatively few malignancies have more treatment options than does endometrial carcinoma, especially for localized disease (limited to the uterus), which accounts for more than 75% of all lesions. Most of the treatment alternatives use some form of postoperative adjuvant therapy. Figure 18-2 outlines one treatment approach. Patients are assigned to various risk groups based on uterine and extrauterine risk factors for recurrence found during staging surgery. Based on the criteria for the operative technique outlined above, a patient can be assigned by surgicopathologic findings at the time of staging.

Patients presenting with low-risk disease—less than 10% myometrial invasion with grade 1 or 2 (stage IA) tumors—have less than a 1% chance of microscopic nodal involvement and need no adjuvant radiotherapy. In the GOG trials, no recurrences were identified among 91 stage IA patients, and the 5-year disease-free survival rate was 100%.

Intermediate-Risk Disease

Patients identified as having features that fall into the intermediate risk category represent a cohort for whom the benefits of adjuvant therapy have not been established. While adjuvant radiotherapy in this subgroup may be effective in controlling disease recurrence in the field of treatment, its effect on overall recurrence and the survival rates has not been defined.

When myometrial invasion is limited (<50%) in low-grade lesions, the greatest risk is for local recurrence. Some investigators have argued that this risk is too low to warrant adjuvant therapy; however, others have demonstrated that vaginal cuff irradiation has a low risk-to-benefit ratio and is very effective in controlling recurrence in this area. One study by Aalders et al. demonstrated that while vaginal cuff irradiation was superior to whole pelvic irradiation in controlling vaginal cuff recurrence, survival was no different.

Patients who present with deeper invading tumors; those with grade 3 or atypical histologic subtypes such as clear cell, serous, and undifferentiated cell carcinomas; patients with

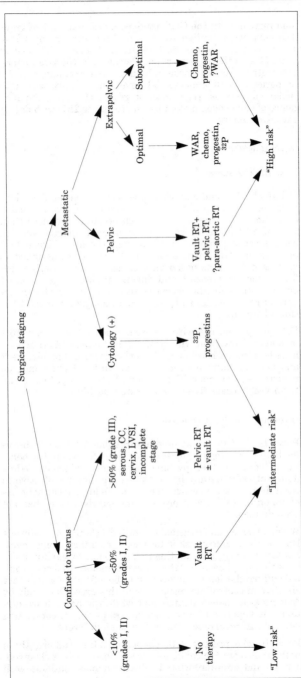

Fig. 18-2. Surgical staging and treatment options for endometrial cancer. (WAR = whole abdominal radiation; 32P = intra-abdominal radio-colloid treatment; CC = clear cell; LVSI = lymphatic and/or vascular space involvement; RT = radiotherapy.)

extensive lymphatic–vascular space invasion; and incompletely staged patients with other intermediate risk factors constitute a group of patients who collectively have up to a 40% chance of microscopic lymphatic metastases. For this group, most physicians will recommend some form of adjuvant therapy. The amount, type (with or without chemotherapy), and duration are debatable.

As shown in Fig. 18-2, one approach for this subgroup is pelvic radiotherapy (40–45 Gy).

Many investigators have become cognizant of the natural history of the atypical histologies in this disease. Because patterns of spread and recurrence have resembled those for epithelial ovarian carcinomas, investigators have tried to improve long-term survival with chemotherapy. Several single-agent and combination regimens have been studied and are closely based on active agents in the treatment of ovarian carcinoma. To date, outside of limited data on whole abdominal radiotherapy, very little progress has been made in adjuvant or prophylactic therapy.

Patients who have been incompletely staged, especially those with low- or intermediate-risk factors, represent a special problem for treating physicians. Since one of the greatest predictors of para-aortic node involvement is pelvic node involvement, the absence of this information makes the decision of whether to administer para-aortic radiation difficult. The morbidity of para-aortic irradiation is well described, and such treatment is not indicated if the risk for involvement is low. However, many patients who have incomplete staging may receive whole pelvic irradiation.

One of most controversial findings in patients with otherwise limited disease at the time of surgery is positive peritoneal cytology. While the independent significance of this finding was questioned in earlier studies, several larger, more recent studies have confirmed its importance. Treatment options range from no adjuvant therapy to hormonal therapy to whole abdominal radiotherapy. One technique that has been advocated is the use of the radiocolloid ^{32}P. The solution is administered into the peritoneal cavity via a transperitoneal catheter. The isotope is a pure beta emitter with a maximum energy of 1.71 MeV penetrating an average depth of 3–5 mm. This treatment appears ideal for treating any microscopic residual disease, assuming adequate intra-abdominal distribution. However, survival data are difficult to interpret because no controlled trials have been performed.

Progestin therapy has been found to be effective in the setting of positive cytology. Progestins are administered either PO or IM for 6–12 months. Data from Piver et al. have shown that persistent use in patients found at second-look laparoscopy to have positive cytology can reverse this finding. However, further controlled data are needed to elucidate the primary role of adjuvant therapy in this setting.

Table 18-10. Active chemotherapeutic agents, single and combination, and their response rates in endometrial carcinoma

Regimen	Overall response (%)
Single	
Doxorubicin	38
Cisplatin	42
Cytembena	33
Carboplatin	28
Megace	25
Combination	
PAC	56
PAC/Meg	60
PA	60
AC	45
AC/Meg	27
VAC	31

PAC = cyclophosphamide, doxorubicin, cisplatin; Meg = megestrol acetate; PA = cisplatin, doxorubicin; AC = cyclophosphamide, doxorubicin; VAC = vinblastine, cisplatin, doxorubicin.

High-Risk Disease

Metastatic disease, either in the abdomen or in the lymphatics, is a poor prognostic finding and adjuvant therapy directed at the volume and location of residual disease is warranted. Patients with disease limited to the pelvic and/or para-aortic nodes are candidates for adjuvant radiotherapy, with curative intent, because tumoricidal doses can be delivered to these areas as long as bulky disease is not present. The 5-year disease-free survival rate among patients with positive para-aortic nodes who were treated with para-aortic irradiation was 36% in the GOG trial. Patients with metastatic disease in the pelvic nodes but with negative para-aortic nodes should receive pelvic radiotherapy that covers the common iliac nodes.

Patients with intra-abdominal metastatic disease may benefit from adjuvant therapy if "optimal debulking" can be performed. The predominant modality of treatment for patients with metastatic disease is chemotherapy. Many single-agent and multiagent cytotoxic chemotherapeutic regimens have been studied. The most active agents against endometrial therapy are listed in Table 18-10. With recent refinements in technique, interest has been renewed in whole abdominal irradiation for patients with no residual disease or optimally cytoreduced residual disease; this is currently the subject of a prospective GOG trial.

Inoperable Patients

Despite the fact that endometrial cancer patients, in general, are elderly, have chronic medical problems, and are perhaps less tolerant to therapy, more than 89% can undergo primary surgery and staging procedures. For those who are inoperable, however, curative radiotherapy can be administered as a sole modality. Grigsby et al. reported on this sub-group and achieved 5-year survival rates of up to 75% for clinical stage I and 50% for clinical stage II disease.

Recurrent Disease

Modalities for the treatment of recurrence include radiotherapy, surgery, hormonal therapy, and single-agent or combination chemotherapy. Patients with a pelvic recurrence who have not received radiotherapy as part of their primary therapy can undergo pelvic irradiation with or without vaginal cuff irradiation. Even with distant disease, local control, especially of vaginal symptoms, can be achieved. The rare patient with a central recurrence after radiation and surgery may be salvaged with pelvic exenteration. While no large series exists for evaluation, long-term salvage rates for these patients are about 35%—generally lower than for similar procedures performed for recurrent cervical cancer.

Patients with demonstrated estrogen and/or progesterone receptors can be successfully palliated with high-dose hormonal therapy. PO or IM progestin therapy with or without tamoxifen can achieve objective responses in up to 70% of estrogen/progesterone-receptor–positive patients. Unfortunately, responses are short (4–6 months), and progression is noted in most patients within 1 year.

Chemotherapy produces response rates similar to those in patients with metastatic disease. One peculiar observation is that use of a previously active agent for reinduction of remission is often met with poor response rates. For example, when platinum agents are used for primary treatment, response rates are 35–45%. However, when platinum agents are used as second-line therapy, the response rate falls to less than 10%. Because of limited options and the aggressive nature of recurrent disease, physicians are urged to enter patients with recurrent endometrial cancer into clinical trials.

Cervical Carcinoma

EPIDEMIOLOGY

Carcinoma of the uterine cervix is considered a preventable disease in the majority of cases. Knowledge of the natural history of this disease, an improved understanding of the preinvasive stage, and the widespread availability of cervical cytology screening programs have contributed to this. For more than 30 years, cervical carcinoma has steadily decreased in incidence, and since 1972, it has been less common than either endometrial or ovarian cancer. Despite these trends, more than 15,000 new cases are expected in 1994, with more than 4,600 deaths from the disease, indicating that even today, more than one-third of women in this country are not undergoing routine Pap smear screening.

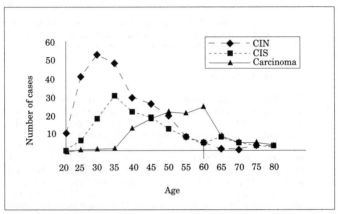

Fig. 18-3. Age at presentation distribution of cervical dysplasia, carcinoma in situ, and carcinoma.

NATURAL HISTORY

Most investigators support the theory that carcinoma of the cervix arises from dysplastic epithelium over a period of years. Cervical dysplasia is a condition of graded intraepithelial cellular atypia. Lesions begin in the transformation zone between the nonkeratinized squamous epithelium of the cervix and the columnar cells of the endocervix. Progressive metaplasia from constant exposure to the vaginal environment, with its low pH, occurs over the life of the individual. Etiologic agents that are not completely understood initiate transformation of these cells to malignant phenotypes causing "dysplasia." Figure 18-3 shows the incidence curves for the various dysplastic lesions and cancer by age at onset. Untreated mildly dysplastic lesions—cervical intraepithelial neoplasia (CIN)—generally require 5–8 years to progress to carcinoma in situ (CIS) and another 1–5 years to develop into cancer. This rather long latency period allows effective treatment during the preinvasive state, ultimately preventing carcinoma development.

Women with cervical cancer have consistently been found to have higher frequencies of lower socioeconomic class, early age at first intercourse, history of multiple sexual partners, and multiparity. Association of cervical cancer to a viral agent (human papillomavirus [HPV]) has been predicated by epidemiologic studies of affected individuals. Spread effectively through sexual contact, this virus is highly prevalent in the United States, with more than 10–12 million affected women. HPV is isolated in about 60% of cervical cancers. With more than 60 subtypes described and more than 20 of these subtypes affecting the anogenital tract specifically, the implication of this virus in the etiology of cervical cancer has gained acceptance.

Table 18-11. Diagnostic work-up for carcinoma of the uterine cervix

General
History
Physical examination, including bimanual pelvic and rectal
    examinations
Diagnostic procedures
Cytologic smears (Papanicolaou) if not bleeding
Colposcopy
Conization (subclinical tumor)
Punch biopsies (edge of gross tumor, four quadrants)
Dilatation and curettage
Cystoscopy, rectosigmoidoscopy (stages IIB, III, IVA)
Radiographic procedures
Standard
    Chest radiography
    IV pyelography
    Barium enema (stage III, IVA, and earlier stages if there are
        symptoms referable to colon or rectum)
Complementary
    Lymphangiography
    Computed tomography or magnetic resonance imaging
Laboratory studies
Complete blood count
Blood chemistry
Urinalysis

Source: CA Perez. Uterine Cervix. In CA Perez, LW Brady (eds), *Principles and Practice of Radiation Oncology* (2nd ed). Philadelphia: Lippincott, 1992.

PATHOLOGY

Carcinomas of the cervix are predominantly squamous cell carcinomas (85–90%); adenocarcinomas are less frequent (10–15%) but are increasing in frequency. Whether this trend represents a true increase in disease or reflects the improved ability to identify and treat squamous lesions during the preinvasive stage is not known. Adenocarcinoma, adenosquamous carcinoma, and small-cell variants are seen, and cervical lymphomas, both primary and secondary, have been described. The natural history of the two major groups suggests that adenocarcinomas are more aggressive and present at a more advanced stage than squamous lesions, for tumors of the same stage and size.

CLINICAL PRESENTATION AND DIAGNOSTIC WORK-UP

The most common symptom at presentation is vaginal bleeding. This sometimes can be profuse but most commonly takes the form of spotting, usually postcoitally. Postmenopausal or irregular bleeding also may occur. Lesions that are exophytic or associated with infection are more likely to present as acute bleeding or a heavy vaginal discharge. More advanced lesions may present as pain, both in the pelvis and in the lower extremities or upper back, lower extremity edema, or a mass in a node-bearing region.

Table 18-11 outlines the diagnostic work-up for a patient suspected of having cervical cancer. On general physical examination, the supraclavicular and groin areas should be carefully palpated for metastatic disease. On pelvic examination, a speculum is placed to inspect the cervix and vagina. Grossly exophytic lesions may be biopsied at this point to establish the diagnosis. Other cancerous lesions will expand the cervix and harden its texture to palpation; this should be noted during a digital examination. Evaluation for disease outside the cervix or direct extension from the cervix can be done with a rectovaginal examination. This is the only way to evaluate the cervix in postmenopausal women in whom the vaginal anatomy may be altered or to evaluate an endocervical primary tumor. Rectovaginal evaluation also provides information on parametrial spread and enlarged obturator node groups.

The diagnosis of cervical carcinoma must be made histologically. Outpatient biopsy can be easily performed in patients with gross lesions. However, patients with a suggestion of carcinoma on a Pap smear must undergo colposcopic evaluation to direct biopsies or to explain the cytologic result. If a suspicious area is identified by colposcopy, biopsies may be directed to this area to confirm the diagnosis. Cervical conization and endocervical curettings may be necessary to establish the diagnosis.

STAGING

Carcinoma of the uterine cervix has remained a clinically staged disease since its description. No evidence of improved survival has been demonstrated by performing surgical staging procedures, which in some cases have only increased treatment complication rates. FIGO has provided guidelines and accepted procedures for staging patients. All patients newly diagnosed with cervical cancer should be examined jointly by a gynecologic oncologist and a radiotherapist to assess disease status and formulate a treatment plan. Information from the physical examination and other clinical data are used in the FIGO clinical staging system for cervical carcinoma (Table 18-12).

PROGNOSTIC FACTORS

Several patient and tumor features have been related to the clinical course of this disease. Table 18-13 lists the major factors that influence prognosis. In patients with disease limited to the cervix (stage I), lymphatic vascular space involvement, tumor size, and depth of stromal invasion are most important in predicting lymphatic metastases, disease-free survival, and overall survival. Survival in patients with more extensive disease (stages II–IV) is heavily influenced by the presence of pelvic and para-aortic lymphatic metastases, tumor volume, age, and performance status in addition to stage.

Table 18-12. Staging of cervical carcinoma

Cervical cancer is clinically staged pretreatment with the use of *only* the core tests listed in Table 18-11. Biopsies or findings subsequent to initiation of therapy may influence therapy and/or prognosis but do not alter the stage.

Stage I: 5-year survival rate: 65–90% (adenocarcinoma: 70–75%)
Stage I is carcinoma strictly confined to the cervix; extension to the corpus does not advance the stage.
   IA: Preclinical invasive carcinoma
   IA1: Minimal microscopic stromal invasion
   IA2: Tumor with invasive component 5 mm or less in depth taken from the base of the epithelium and 7 mm or less in horizontal spread
   IB: All grossly visible tumors, limited to the cervix
Stage II: 5-year survival rate: 45–80% (adenocarcinoma: 30–40%)
Stage II means carcinoma extends beyond the cervix but has not extended to the pelvic wall. The carcinoma involves the vagina but not as far as the lower third.
   IIA: Tumor invades the upper two-thirds of the vagina in addition to the cervix; no obvious parametrial involvement
   IIB: Clinical parametrial involvement but not to the sidewall
Stage III: 5-year survival: up to 61% (adenocarcinoma: 20–30%)
Stage III means either the carcinoma has extended to the pelvic wall or the tumor involves the lower third of the vagina. All cases with hydronephrosis or nonfunctioning kidney are included, unless hydronephrosis is known to be due to another cause.
   IIIA: Involvement of the lower one-third of the vagina
   IIIB: Extension to the pelvic wall, hydronephrosis or nonfunctioning renal unit (does not require fixation to the side wall)
Stage IV: 5-year survival: <15%
Stage IV means the carcinoma has extended beyond the true pelvis or has clinically involved the mucosa of the bladder of rectum. Bullous edema of the bladder as such does not permit a case to be allotted to stage IV.
   IVA: Spread involves direct extension to the bladder/rectum or other adjacent pelvic organs
   IVB: Distant metastatic spread

Table 18-13. Major prognostic factors of survival in patients with cervical carcinoma

Age
Stage
Tumor volume
Tumor grade
Histologic type
Lymphatic spread
Lymph vascular invasion
Performance status
Her-2/*neu* and c-*myc* oncogene overexpression
Tumor aneuploidy

MANAGEMENT

In general, surgery or radiotherapy is equally effective for early-stage, small-volume disease. Younger patients may be better served by surgery, providing the opportunity for ovarian preservation and avoiding the vaginal atrophy and stenosis associated with radiotherapy. The value of adjuvant treatments such as chemotherapy for patients with more advanced disease is uncertain; clinical trials are appropriate for patients with stage III or IV disease or with lymph node involvement.

Stage IA: Microinvasion

Treatment strategies for early microinvasive disease (stage IA) often are heavily influenced by the need to preserve fertility. Often, lesions in this stage are identified in younger patients in whom effective conservation of the uterus is desired.

Since 1974, the Society of Gynecologic Oncology (SGO) has defined microinvasion as any nonconfluent lesion with invasion less than 3 mm deep and without lymphatic vascular space invasion. The distinction is made because lymphatic metastases are identified in up to 8% of cases with 5 mm of invasion (microinvasion by FIGO definition) and far less than 1% by the SGO definition. Therefore, under the SGO rules governing microinvasion, the following treatments are considered equivalent standard therapies:

1. Total hysterectomy. Oophorectomy is optional and usually not done in younger patients.

2. Intracavitary radiation alone (inoperable patients). Lymphatic metastases are rare, so no pelvic radiation portal is required. One or two brachytherapy insertions (tandem and ovoids) to achieve a 100–125 Gy vaginal surface dose is recommended.

3. Conization. Cone margins must be negative for neoplasia. It must be used only in special cases when fertility preservation is a concern.

Stages IB and IIA

Either radiotherapy or radical hysterectomy and bilateral pelvic lymphadenectomy, in experienced hands, results in cure rates of 75–90% for patients with small-volume, stage IB/IIA disease. The choice of treatment depends on patient factors, tumor characteristics, and available local expertise. The size of the primary tumor is an important prognostic factor and should be carefully evaluated in choosing optimal therapy. Most squamous cell lesions smaller than 4–5 cm are considered for surgery. For adenocarcinomas larger than 3 cm, survival data suggest the primary treatment should be radiotherapy. Patients found to have small-volume para-aortic nodal disease and controllable pelvic disease may be cured with pelvic and para-aortic irradiation. Local control with postoperative radiotherapy may be enhanced by resection of macroscopically involved pelvic nodes. Treatment of unresected para-aortic nodes with extended field radiation leads to long-term disease control in those patients with small-volume (<2 cm) nodal disease below L3.

Standard treatment options include:

1. Radiotherapy: External beam pelvic irradiation (40–45 Gy over 4–5 weeks) combined with two or more intracavitary applications. Empiric irradiation of the para-aortic nodes versus combined chemotherapy is being evaluated in patients with large-volume (>5 cm) primary tumors.

2. Radical hysterectomy (class III) that includes bilateral pelvic lymphadenectomy: The uterus and parametrial tissue, upper vagina, and uterosacral ligaments are removed en bloc. Patients identified as having more than two bilateral microscopically positive pelvic nodes are usually treated with adjuvant radiotherapy. While pelvic control is probably enhanced with this treatment, the effect on survival is not proved.

3. Total hysterectomy (class I) after pelvic radiotherapy: Primarily indicated for patients in whom the tumor responds slowly to radiotherapy or in whom vaginal anatomy precludes optimal brachytherapy.

Stages IIB Through IVA

The treatment of choice for advanced lesions (stage IIB/IVA) is radiotherapy. Survival and local control rates are superior in patients with smaller tumor burdens. For instance, unilateral, medial parametrial disease responds far better than bilateral, fixed pelvic disease, which in turn is more responsive than lesions involving the lower third of the vagina. A standard pelvic field is used. Parametrial and side wall boost doses are occasionally needed to treat grossly positive or radiation refractory node-bearing tissues. Extended field radiation in patients with positive pelvic nodes and unresected para-aortic nodes has been shown to improve long-term disease control. Pelvic and/or para-aortic radiotherapy is followed by two brachytherapy applications. Several agents have been used to enhance the cytotoxic effects of radiation. Currently under investigation are hydroxyurea, 5-fluorouracil, and cisplatin.

Treatment options include:

1. Radiotherapy with radiosensitizing cytotoxic agents.

2. Radiation and chemotherapy (sequential or concurrent), neoadjuvant chemotherapy, altered radiation fractionation, and template brachytherapy.

3. Total pelvic exenteration, which may be indicated in patients without parametrial disease but with direct rectal or bladder invasion (stage IVA).

Table 18-14. Recurrence sites for carcinoma of the uterine cervix

Site	Percent (%)
Pelvis	43
Uterine	27
Other distant	14
Lung	8
Lower vagina	6
Bone	2

Stage IVB

Treatment of stage IVB metastatic disease is best done with chemotherapy. Radiotherapy is often given for palliation of the central disease. Response rates to primary chemotherapy can be as high as 40%, but progression-free intervals are short (5–6 months). The most active agents are platinum alone or in combination with other agents, ifosfamide, and mitomycin C. A number of phase II clinical trials are currently available for this cohort of patients.

Recurrent Disease

As seen in Table 18-14, the most common site of recurrence is the pelvis. Symptoms of recurrent cervical cancer are nonspecific. Pain in the pelvis or lower extremities, edema of the lower extremities, and bleeding are the most common symptoms at presentation and often indicate tumor involvement of the pelvic musculature. Radiographic evaluation with biopsies should be used to document recurrent disease. In patients who have not been previously irradiated, radiotherapy can be used to treat recurrent disease. Patients with small central recurrences after radiotherapy who are free of pelvic side wall involvement can be cured by exenterative procedures (up to 40%). Unfortunately, less than 3% of treated patients have such recurrences. In most patients, therefore, treatment includes chemotherapy.

As for metastatic disease, single-agent or combination therapy has only modest success in recurrent disease. In general, response rates for recurrent disease are poorer than for untreated metastatic disease. Chemotherapy agents with the most success are cisplatin and platinum analogues, ifosfamide, mitoxantrone, etoposide, vincristine, bleomycin, methotrexate, and 5-fluorouracil. Overall response rates are 20–30%, with progression-free intervals of 4–6 months; most patients die of their disease within 12 months because of recurrence.

Since recurrence of cervical cancer is a lethal event in most cases, continued efforts to identify better treatment strategies and more effective chemotherapy are paramount.

Table 18-15. Follow-up protocol posttreatment for carcinoma of the uterine cervix

Physical exam
    Year 1: every 3 months
    Year 2: every 4 months
    Years 3–5: every 6 months
    Year 5+: annually
Pap smear: every visit
Radiographic
    Chest radiograph: annually
    IV pyelogram: For patients with hydronephrosis
    Computed tomography/magnetic resonance imaging: for locally
        advanced disease

SURVEILLANCE

More than 75% of all recurrences are identified within 24 months of completion of treatment. It is during this interval that surveillance for treatment failure should be heightened. An example of a follow-up protocol is presented in Table 18-15.

Patients treated with radiotherapy require careful attention to vaginal health for continued sexual function and ability to evaluate central disease response. This is accomplished with the use of vaginal estrogen cream (half an applicator-full, three times weekly) and vaginal dilators or regular intercourse. Estrogen replacement therapy is not contraindicated on the basis of the carcinoma and should be initiated during the external beam irradiation. (As little as 3 Gy of radiation can obliterate ovarian function.)

Assessment of response to radiotherapy can be difficult, as tumor is replaced by fibrous connective tissue, especially in locally advanced cases. This is further complicated by the fact that tumor regression can continue for up to 12 weeks after completion of therapy. A high index of suspicion is warranted in radiotherapy-treated patients, and careful attention to alterations in symptoms may help identify recurrent disease.

Follow-up evaluation is additionally important in identifying treatment complications. For tumors treated with either surgery or radiation, the complication rate is about 2%. The most common complications following radical hysterectomy are related to denervation of the pelvic viscera. Bladder dysfunction (usually temporary) and constipation are treatable but disturbing issues for patients. Self-catheterization is taught to all patients undergoing this procedure. Less common is vesicovaginal fistula (<3% of cases). Gastrointestinal side effects are most common following radiotherapy. Treatment-related diarrhea is usually self-limiting. Short-term effects appear within 6 months–2 years after completing radiotherapy. Subintimal endarteritis is the pathologic process promulgating mucosal thinning and friability and leading to enteritis and hemorrhagic cystitis. Chronic diarrhea with electrolyte imbalance, dehydration, and bowel perforation are long-term events complicating a minority of cases.

Vulvar Cancer

EPIDEMIOLOGY AND ETIOLOGY

Vulvar cancer is quite uncommon, accounting for only 4–5% of all tumors of the female genital tract. The cause of vulvar cancer is probably multifactorial and may be preceded by vulvar intraepithelial neoplasia (VIN). However, the progression of VIN to carcinoma is not as clear as that of CIN to carcinoma. Risk factors for developing vulvar cancer are advanced age, low socioeconomic status, hypertension, obesity, diabetes, previous neoplasm of the lower genital tract, and, in some countries, chronic granulomatous venereal diseases. As in cervical cancer, HPV particles, most commonly type 16, have been identified in some vulvar neoplasms; however, the association of HPV and vulvar cancer is not as strong as for cervical cancer. Immunosuppressed patients are also at a higher risk for developing vulvar cancer.

PATHOLOGY

Approximately 85% of all vulvar cancers are squamous cell carcinomas. The second most common malignancy of the vulva is malignant melanoma, which accounts for 10% of vulvar tumors. The less common tumor types are basal cell carcinoma, verrucous carcinoma, Merkel's cell tumors, transitional cell carcinoma, adenosquamous carcinoma, and vulvar Paget's disease. Tumors may also arise in the Bartholin's gland (approximately 50% are squamous carcinomas and 50% adenocarcinomas).

Rarely, sarcomas can arise on the vulva. The most common of these is leiomyosarcoma. Others include malignant fibrous histiocytoma, malignant rhabdoid tumor, and epithelioid sarcoma. Other rare tumors of the vulva include malignant schwannoma and yolk sac tumors.

Metastases to the vulva are most commonly from tumors of the genital tract—that is, the vagina, cervix, endometrium, and ovary. However, metastases from breast, stomach, kidney, and lung cancers and choriocarcinoma have been reported.

CLINICAL PRESENTATION AND DIAGNOSTIC EVALUATION

The usual presenting symptom for patients with vulvar cancer is a lump, sore, or mass on the vulva. Patients usually give a long history of vulvar itching and/or irritation. Patients also may present with bleeding, discharge, or dysuria. In developed countries, more than half of patients present with early-stage lesions; however, in less developed areas, patients may present with a large mass in the groin.

Table 18-16. FIGO (1989) staging of vulvar carcinoma

Stage	Clinical findings
0	Carcinoma in situ; intraepithelial carcinoma
I	Tumor confined to the vulva or perineum; ≤2 cm in greatest dimension; no nodal metastasis
II	Tumor confined to the vulva or perineum; >2 cm in greatest dimension; no nodal metastasis
III	Tumor of any size with adjacent spread to the urethra, vagina, or anus with unilateral regional lymph node metastasis
IVA	Tumor invades the upper urethra, bladder mucosa, rectal mucosa, pelvic bone, or bilateral regional node metastasis
IVB	Any distant metastasis, including pelvic lymph nodes

Physical examination usually reveals a raised lesion that may be fleshy, ulcerated, leukoplakic, or warty in appearance. The most common site is the labia majora, but the labia minora, clitoris, and perineum may also be primary sites. Only 5% of cases are multifocal.

Any lesion or abnormality on the vulva should be biopsied to rule out carcinoma. This may be done by punch biopsy or, for smaller lesions, excisional biopsy. Physician delay in diagnosis is especially common for lesions with a warty appearance; therefore, before treating any confluent "warts" on the vulva, a biopsy should be done to exclude carcinoma. As vulvar cancer is often associated with malignancies or premalignant conditions of the rest of the lower genital tract, it is important that all vulvar cancer patients have an evaluation, including colposcopy, of the entire vulva, vagina, and cervix prior to treatment.

STAGING AND PROGNOSTIC FACTORS

Until 1989, vulvar cancer was staged clinically. Now a FIGO surgical staging system is used (Table 18-16). Clinical staging allows evaluation of nodal disease only by palpation, which is inaccurate in predicting involvement as much as 50% of the time. Surgical staging takes into account the prognostic significance of lymph node status and acknowledges the inability to diagnose groin node metastases by palpation alone. However, because the staging system has only recently been changed, most reports in the current literature are based on the older clinical staging system.

Vulvar cancer can spread by direct extension to adjacent organs, via lymphatics to the regional lymph nodes, or via the bloodstream to distant organs. Spread to lymph nodes is usually from the inguinal to the pelvic nodes, especially the iliac nodes. The overall incidence of lymph node metastasis in vulvar cancer is about 30%. The incidence of pelvic lymph node metastases is about 5%, and such metastases virtually never occur without involvement of more than three unilateral groin nodes. Hematogenous spread is less common but can result in metastases to such organs as the liver, lungs, and bone.

Table 18-17. Lymph node metastasis by stage in vulvar carcinoma (by 1969 FIGO staging)

Stage	Incidence of lymph node metastasis (%)
I	10
II	26
III	65
IV	90
Overall	30

Table 18-18. Incidence of lymph node metastasis correlated with depth of invasion in stage I vulvar carcinoma

Depth of invasion	Percent positive groin nodes
≤1 mm	0
1.1–2.0 mm	6.6
2.1–3.0 mm	8.2
3.1–4.0 mm	22.0
4.1–5.0 mm	25.0
>5 mm	27.5
Total	10.7

Factors associated with regional lymph node involvement and prognosis of vulvar cancer include size of the lesion, depth of invasion, histologic subtype, and lymphatic and vascular invasion. Patients with stage II disease have a poorer prognosis, with a 5-year survival rate of 77% versus 90% for those with stage I disease. Lymph node involvement also correlates with stage of disease (Table 18-17), with stage I associated with a 10% incidence of lymph node metastasis and stage IV 90%. Depth of stromal invasion in stage I lesions also correlates well with the incidence of lymph node metastasis (Table 18-18), with those lesions invading less than 1 mm into the stroma having less than a 1% risk of lymph node involvement.

MANAGEMENT

The traditional treatment for vulvar cancer has been radical vulvectomy with bilateral groin dissection, often including bilateral pelvic lymph node dissection. This treatment, although effective, is associated with a high morbidity rate, including high rates of wound breakdown secondary to the removal of large amounts of skin and soft tissue, prolonged hospitalization, and poor cosmetic result often leading to psychological problems. Because of these difficulties, during the 1980s significant changes were made in the management of vulvar cancer, including the following:

1. Vulvar conservation for patients with unifocal lesions and an otherwise normal vulva.

2. Elimination of routine pelvic lymphadenectomy.

3. Omission of groin dissection for patients with stage I tumors with less than 1 mm of stromal invasion.

Table 18-19. Five-year survival correlated with stage for patients with vulvar cancer treated with curative intent

FIGO stage (1969)	5-year survival (%)
I	90.4
II	77.1
III	51.3
IV	69.7

4. Use of separate groin incisions for groin dissection.

5. Omission of contralateral groin dissection in patients with lateral lesions and negative ipsilateral nodes.

6. Use of preoperative radiotherapy in patients with advanced disease.

7. Use of postoperative radiation in patients with multiple positive groin nodes to decrease the incidence of recurrence in the groin.

The most important consideration is individualization of treatment to best fit each patient.

The overall prognosis of vulvar cancer is good, with a 5-year survival rate of 70% for patients with operable disease (Table 18-19). For patients with negative groin nodes, the 5-year survival rate is 90%, but it drops to 50% for patients with positive nodes. The number of positive groin nodes is the most important prognostic factor.

Stage I Lesions

Most stage I lesions are now treated with a radical local excision of the area involved by cancer. This excision, regardless of the size of the lesion, should be to the level of the urogenital diaphragm. Lateral and deep margins should clear the tumor by at least 1 cm. If the surrounding vulva is involved with extensive VIN, radical vulvectomy may still be indicated to remove all abnormal areas. Early lesions in the clitoral area are often best treated with radiotherapy because of the psychosexual sequelae associated with removing the clitoris.

Stage I lesions with less than 1 mm of stromal invasion have been found to have an insignificant risk of lymph node metastasis, and therefore groin dissection may be omitted in this group of patients. Patients with lateral stage I lesions should have unilateral groin dissection for removal of the ipsilateral lymph nodes. If these nodes are negative for metastatic disease, it is not necessary to do bilateral groin dissection, as the risk of positive contralateral nodes is less than 1% in this setting. For patients with positive ipsilateral groin nodes, however, therapy is more extensive. The risk of positive pelvic nodes and positive contralateral groin nodes increases with the number of ipsilateral groin nodes that are positive. Patients with two or more positive ipsilateral groin nodes, which is unusual for stage I tumors, are best treated with adjuvant pelvic and bilateral groin irradiation. This treatment has been shown to increase survival and decrease groin recurrences.

Stage II and Early Stage III Lesions

In general, the treatment for patients with stage II and early stage III lesions is radical vulvectomy and bilateral inguinal-femoral lymphadenectomy, although more conservative surgery, such as described for stage I, is being done in some centers, including the University of Texas M. D. Anderson Cancer Center. A review of such conservative surgery for these lesions from the University of California at Los Angeles suggests that the risk of local recurrence in conservatively treated patients is very low provided the tumor-free surgical margin is at least 1 cm. However, most stage II and early stage III lesions are still being treated with more extensive procedures.

Large Stage III and Stage IV Lesions

For patients with locally advanced disease—that is, cancer involving the anus, rectum, rectovaginal septum, or urethra—standard radical vulvectomy is usually not adequate to remove the lesion. Over the past 30 years pelvic exenteration has been a popular treatment for such lesions. However, the morbidity and mortality for such a procedure can be quite high, and more recently, as with the earlier stage lesions, the trend has been toward less radical approaches. Newer treatments include preoperative irradiation of the involved areas to shrink the tumor prior to surgical removal. Preoperative radiotherapy involves external irradiation of the vulva and may also include intracavitary brachytherapy if indicated by the involvement of such tissues as the rectovaginal septum. In 1987, Boronow reported the use of such treatment in 37 patients with locally advanced disease, citing a 5-year survival rate of 75.6%.

For patients with enlarged (clinically involved) groin nodes, the traditional treatment has been en bloc radical vulvectomy, bilateral inguinal-femoral lymphadenectomy, and at least ipsilateral pelvic lymphadenectomy. These patients are likely to receive postoperative irradiation, and because irradiation after full groin dissection can cause debilitating leg edema, modifications of therapy have been studied. One modification is removing all enlarged groin nodes through a separate incision and sending them for frozen-section diagnosis. If the nodes are positive for metastatic disease, a full lymphadenectomy is not performed, but the patient receives full pelvic and groin irradiation as soon as the groin incision is healed. If the nodes are negative for metastatic disease, a full groin dissection is performed. Some centers will also obtain a preoperative CT scan of the pelvis and remove any enlarged pelvic nodes seen on it through an extraperitoneal approach. Studies from the 1980s have shown that a modified approach can result in less morbidity without decreasing survival. Chemotherapy has been used only for recurrent disease, but the integration of chemotherapy into the management of advanced vulvar squamous carcinoma deserves further study.

Recurrences

Local recurrence following definitive surgery occurs in about 30% of patients. Risk of recurrence correlates most closely with the number of positive groin nodes, and risk of local recurrence also correlates closely with adequacy of surgical margins (>1 cm). Local recurrences may be potentially successfully treated with further wide radical excision or radiation. Regional and distant recurrences are more difficult to manage. Radiation and surgery may be used for groin recurrences, but for recurrence at distant sites, chemotherapy should be offered. For recurrent squamous carcinoma of the vulva, some data about the efficacy of chemotherapy are available. Doxorubicin and bleomycin have been shown to have some activity as single agents. Several combinations, all including bleomycin, have been tried, with some activity seen against inoperable disease. Some studies have also looked at the efficacy of chemotherapy in combination with radiotherapy, with some responses.

Radiation Therapy

Radiation therapy has been shown to improve tumor control and survival in patients with loco-regionally advanced disease and in decreasing the extent and morbidity of curative surgery. Techniques commonly used for treatment of vulvar carcinoma involve methods to include the lower pelvic and inguinal nodes and the vulva while minimizing the dose to the femoral heads. Gross disease in the groins or vulva can be treated with en face electron fields and in some cases, interstitial implants may be used to boost the dose. Acute radiation reactions include moist desquamation, which is induced with doses of 35–45 Gy, and may be treated with local care. If the vulva receives more than 45–50 Gy, a break in treatment may be required. Long-term complications of radiation may include leg edema, especially when combined with groin dissection, and femoral head fractures. Femoral head fractures can be minimized by limiting the dose to this area to less than 35 Gy.

Vaginal Cancer

EPIDEMIOLOGY AND ETIOLOGY

Primary carcinoma of the vagina is a very rare malignancy, accounting for only 1–2% of all gynecologic malignancies. Most vaginal neoplasms are not primary vaginal cancers but metastatic lesions, often from the cervix or vulva. The peak incidence of primary vaginal cancer is in the 50s through 80s, with a mean age of 60–65 years.

Potential risk factors include low socioeconomic status, history of genital warts, chronic vaginal discharge or irritation, a previous abnormal Pap smear, early hysterectomy, and vaginal trauma. Previous irradiation for cervical carcinoma may or may not be a risk factor.

Women who have been prenatally exposed to diethylstilbestrol (DES) are at an increased risk for developing an otherwise rare vaginal tumor, clear cell adenocarcinoma. The risk for exposed patients has been estimated to be between 0.14 and 1.4 per 1,000, with the greatest risk found in those exposed during the first 16 weeks of gestation. The median age at tumor diagnosis in DES-exposed patients is 19 years.

PATHOLOGY

Squamous cell carcinomas account for 80–90% of all primary vaginal cancers. They are most often located in the upper posterior wall of the vagina. To define a malignancy as vaginal in origin, there must be neither a cervical nor vulvar cancer present at the time of diagnosis or within 10 years prior to the diagnosis. Histologically, these tumors are similar to squamous cell neoplasms at other sites. They are assigned a grade according to cytologic and histologic features, but grade does not correlate well with prognosis.

Malignant melanoma is the second most common cancer of the vagina, accounting for 3–5% of all vaginal neoplasms. It occurs most frequently in the lower third of the vagina. Rare verrucous carcinomas and small-cell carcinomas also can occur in the vagina, as can smooth muscle tumors, rhabdomyosarcomas, and other sarcomas. Malignant lymphoma localized in the female genital tract is also seen; it presents as a mass, with the overlying mucosa intact.

Clear cell adenocarcinomas of the vagina are by far most common in DES-exposed women. These patients often have adenosis of the vagina, which occurs mainly in the upper one third of the vagina, as do the clear cell adenocarcinomas. Most of these lesions are exophytic and superficially invasive. Microscopically, they may be tubulocystic, papillary, or solid. The tubulocystic pattern is associated with a better prognosis and is the most common type.

CLINICAL PRESENTATION AND DIAGNOSTIC WORK-UP

The most common presenting symptom of patients with vaginal cancer is abnormal vaginal bleeding, which occurs in 50–75% of cases. It may take the form of postcoital spotting or dysfunctional bleeding. Vaginal discharge also may occur. Pelvic pain and dysuria usually occur only when the disease is more advanced and has spread to adjacent organs.

Physical examination with careful inspection and palpation

Table 18-20. Clinical staging of vaginal cancer

AJCC	FIGO	Characteristics
Tx		Primary tumor cannot be assessed
Tis	0	Carcinoma in situ (intraepithelial)
T1	I	Confined to vaginal mucosa
T2	II	Submucosal infiltration into the parametrium, not extending to the pelvic wall
	IIA	Subvaginal infiltration, not into the parametrium
	IIB	Parametrial infiltration, not to the pelvic side wall
T3	III	Tumor extending to the pelvic side wall
T4	IV	Tumor extending to bladder or rectum or metastasis outside true pelvis

of the vagina are integral in the clinical evaluation. Exfoliative cytology is usually helpful in diagnosing squamous lesions. Colposcopy with application of acetic acid can also be useful, with biopsies of any abnormal areas.

Upon the diagnosis of invasive cancer, a metastatic evaluation should be performed. This should include chest radiography, IV urography, cystoscopy, proctoscopy, and, if indicated, barium enema x-ray and CT scan or MRI.

STAGING AND PROGNOSTIC FACTORS

Patients are staged using the FIGO or American Joint Committee on Cancer (AJCC) staging system (Table 18-20). Carcinomas in situ are superficial tumors that have not penetrated the basement membrane of the mucosal layer; they tend to be multicentric. Stage I lesions, although confined to the vaginal mucosa, may spread to involve more than one vaginal wall.

The most important prognostic factor in vaginal cancer is the clinical stage, which correlates with the depth of tumor penetration into the vaginal wall or surrounding tissues. Nonepithelial tumors, such as sarcoma and melanoma, have a poorer prognosis.

MANAGEMENT

In general radiotherapy is the preferred treatment for most vaginal cancers. However, management of these patients is complex and requires individualization of treatment. Typical radiotherapy techniques incude:

1. External irradiation: Similar to that used for cervical cancer, external irradiation should be delivered through anterior-posterior opposed portals that encompass the vagina to the introitus and the pelvic lymph nodes to the upper common iliac chain. Portals of 15 × 15 cm at the skin are usually adequate. For tumors involving the middle or lower third of the vagina, elective treatment of the inguinal and femoral lymph nodes with modifications of standard pelvic portals is recommended.

Table 18-21. Overall survival by stage for vaginal carcinoma

Stage	5-year survival (%)
0	95
I	80
IIA	50
IIB	40
III	35
IV	10

2. Brachytherapy: Intracavitary therapy is accomplished with vaginal cylinders, using the largest possible diameter to improve the mucosa-to-tumor dose ratio. Lesions in the upper third of the vagina can be treated with the same intracavitary applicators used for cervical carcinoma. In using any type of vaginal applicator, it is important to know not only the tumor dose but also the surface dose of radiation. For some thicker tumors, interstitial therapy with ^{137}Cs, ^{226}Ra, or ^{192}Ir needles can also be used.

Surgical procedures are usually reserved for the treatment of irradiation failures, nonepithelial tumors, and stage I clear cell adenocarcinomas in young women.

Survival rates of patients with vaginal cancer with adequate treatment range from 20 to 80%, depending on the stage of disease (Table 18-21). Survival rates of patients with stage I and II clear cell adenocarcinoma of the vagina have been reported to be as high as 92% and 88%, respectively. Decreased survival is associated with tumor size greater than 2 cm, invasion deeper than 3 mm, and a predominant histologic pattern other than tubulocystic. Survival rates of patients with tumors of other cell types range from less than 10% to about 35%.

Carcinoma in Situ

Carcinoma in situ can be managed by surgical excision or laser vaporization of involved areas. The advantage of surgical excision is that it allows for histologic review of the area removed to rule out underlying invasive cancers. With multiple biopsies of all involved areas prior to treatment, though, laser vaporization may also be safely used and may produce a better functional result. Occasionally, an intracavitary application device that delivers 65–80 Gy of radiation to the involved vaginal mucosa is used to treat carcinoma in situ; however, this procedure may cause vaginal fibrosis and stenosis. Topical chemotherapy with 5-fluorouracil has also been used in various regimens.

Stage I

Except for lesions involving the upper vaginal fornices, radiotherapy is the usual treatment for stage I lesions. Superficial lesions may be treated with an intracavitary cylinder to provide a 60- to 70-Gy mucosal dose to the whole vagina, with an additional 20–30 Gy boost to the tumor area. For thicker lesions, a single-plane implant may be combined with an intracavitary cylinder to increase the dose to the tumor to 80–100 Gy and decrease the dose to the entire vaginal mucosa. External beam irradiation is usually used only for aggressive lesions to supplement intracavitary and interstitial therapy.

For lesions in the upper vaginal fornices, surgical treatment with radical hysterectomy (removal of the uterus and parametrial tissue), pelvic lymphadenectomy, and partial vaginectomy may be adequate therapy.

Stage IIA

Stage IIA tumors are usually treated with external radiation, with 45–50 Gy delivered to the pelvis and parametrium. In addition, intracavitary and/or interstitial therapy is used to deliver 50–60 Gy more to 0.5 cm beyond the deep margin of the tumor.

Stages IIB, III, and IV

Advanced tumors of the vagina are treated with 40 Gy of whole pelvis external radiation and a 50- to 60-Gy total parametrial dose, with midline shielding. Intracavitary and/or interstitial radiation is also used to deliver a total tumor dose of 75–80 Gy to the vaginal lesion and 65 Gy to the parametrial and paravaginal extensions.

Recurrent Disease

Recurrences in the vagina after irradiation can be effectively treated with surgery, ranging from wide local excision, to partial vaginectomy, to a posterior or total pelvic exenteration. Because vaginal cancer is such a rare disease and chemotherapy is generally used as salvage therapy only, little information is available about the efficacy of chemotherapy against this disease. Among drugs that have undergone phase II studies in squamous vaginal carcinomas, only doxorubicin has shown any activity. Combinations of drugs and drugs combined with radiation have also been studied, but because of small patient numbers, no definitively active combinations have been identified.

Clear Cell Adenocarcinomas

Surgery for vaginal clear cell carcinoma requires removal of most of the vagina with reconstructive procedures. A radical hysterectomy and pelvic lymph node dissection are also necessary to remove the parametria and paracolpium to the pelvic side wall. Some cases of early cancers have been treated with intracavitary irradiation with good results and preservation of ovarian function. For extensive lesions that are not amenable to surgery, radiotherapy, as described above for advanced-stage squamous neoplasms, is indicated.

Nonepithelial Tumors

Melanoma and sarcoma are treated primarily with radical surgical resection. Rhabdomyosarcoma is treated with a combination of surgery, radiation, and chemotherapy.

Complications

The most commonly reported minor complications of treatment for vaginal cancer are fibrosis of the vagina and small areas of mucosal necrosis (10% of patients) following radiotherapy. The most commonly reported major complications are proctitis, rectovaginal fistulae, and vesicovaginal fistulae.

Selected References

OVARIAN CANCER

Alberts DS, Green S, Hannigan E, et al. Improved therapeutic index of carboplatin plus cyclophosphamide vs. cisplatin plus cyclophosphamide: Final report by the Southwest Oncology Group of a phase III randomized trial in stage III and IV ovarian cancer. *J Clin Oncol* 10:706, 1992.

Hoskins WJ. Surgical staging and cytoreductive surgery of epithelial ovarian cancer. *Cancer* 71(Suppl):1534, 1993.

Hoskins WJ, Perez CA, Young RC. *Principles and Practice of Gynecologic Oncology*. Philadelphia: Lippincott, 1992.

Piver MS, Malfetano J, Decker TR, et al. Five-year survival for stage IC or stage I grade 3 epithelial ovarian cancer treated with cisplatinum-based chemotherapy. *Gynecol Oncol* 46:357, 1992.

Slamon DJ, Godolphin W, Jones LA, et al. Studies of *Her-2/neu* protooncogene in human breast in ovarian cancer. *Science* 224:707, 1989.

Young RC, Decker DG, Wharton JT, et al. Staging laparotomy in early ovarian cancer. *JAMA* 250:3072, 1983.

Young RC, Walton LA, Ellenberg SS, et al. Adjuvant therapy in stage I and II epithelial ovarian cancer. Results of two prospective randomized trials. *N Engl J Med* 322:1021, 1990.

ENDOMETRIAL CANCER

Aalders J, Abeler V, Kolstad P, et al. Postoperative external irradiation and prognostic parameters in stage I endometrial carcinoma. Clinical and histopathologic study of 540 patients. *Obstet Gynecol* 56:419, 1980.

Creasman W. Prognostic significance of hormone receptors in endometrial cancer. *Cancer* 71:1467, 1993.

Grigsby P, Kuske R, Perez C, et al. Medically inoperable stage I adenocarcinoma of the endometrium treated with radiotherapy alone. *Int J Radiat Oncol Biol Phys* 13:483, 1987.

Morrow C, Bundy B, Kurman R, et al. Relationship between surgical-pathological risk factors and outcome in clinical stage I and II carcinoma of the endometrium: A Gynecologic

Oncology Group study. *Gynecol Oncol* 40:55, 1991.

Piver M, Recio F, Baker T, et al. A prospective trial of progesterone therapy for malignant peritoneal cytology in patients with endometrial carcinoma. *Gynecol Oncol* 47:373, 1992.

Turner D, Gershenson D, Atkinson N, et al. The prognostic significance of peritoneal cytology for stage I endometrial cancer. *Obstet Gynecol* 74:775, 1989.

CERVICAL CANCER

Alberts DS, Kronmal R, Baker LH, et al. Phase II randomized trial of cisplatin chemotherapy regimens in the treatment of recurrent or metastatic squamous cell cancer of the cervix: A Southwest Oncology Group study. *J Clin Oncol* 5:1791, 1987.

Buxton EJ, Meanwell CA, Hilton C, et al. Combination bleomycin, ifosfamide, and cisplatin chemotherapy in cervical cancer. *J Natl Cancer Inst* 81:359, 1989.

Coia L, Won M, Lanciano R, et al. The Patterns of Care Outcome Study for cancer of the uterine cervix: Results of the Second National Practice Survey. *Cancer* 66:2451, 1990.

Delgado G, Bundy B, Zaino R, et al. Prospective surgical-pathological study of disease-free interval in patients with stage IB squamous cell carcinoma of the cervix: A Gynecologic Oncology Group study. *Gynecol Oncol* 38: 352, 1990.

Eifel PJ, Morris M, Oswald MJ, et al. Adenocarcinoma of the uterine cervix: Prognosis and patterns of failure in 367 cases. *Cancer* 65:2507, 1990.

Rotman M, Choi K, Guze C, et al. Prophylactic irradiation of the para-aortic lymph node chain in stage IIB and bulky stage IB carcinoma of the cervix: Initial treatment results of RTOG 7920. *Int J Radiat Oncol Biol Phys* 19: 513, 1990.

Sevin BU, Nadji M, Averette HE, et al. Microinvasive carcinoma of the cervix. *Cancer* 70:2121, 1992.

VULVAR CANCER

Barnhill DR, Hoskins WJ, Metz P. Use of the rhomboid flap after partial vulvectomy. *Obstet Gynecol* 7:123, 1979.

Boronow RC, Hickman BT, Reagan MT, et al. Combined therapy as an alternative to exenteration from locally advanced vulvovaginal cancer. II. Results, complications and dosimetric and surgical considerations. *Am J Clin Oncol* 10:171, 1987.

Burke TW, Stringer CA, Gershenson DM, et al. Radical wide excision and selective inguinal node dissection for squamous carcinoma of the vulva. *Gynecol Oncol* 38:328, 1990.

Federation Internationale de Gynecologic et d'Obstetrique (FIGO), 1989 meeting, Rio de Janeiro.

Hacker NF. Vulvar Cancer. In JS Berek, NF Hacker (eds), *Practical Gynecologic Oncology*. Baltimore: Williams & Wilkins, 1989.

Hacker NF, Berek JS. Vulvar Cancer. In CM Haskell (ed), *Cancer Treatment* (3rd ed). Philadelphia: Saunders, 1990.

Hacker NF, Eifel P, McGuire W, Wilkinson EJ. Vulva. In WJ Hoskins, CA Perez, RC Young (eds), *Principles and Practice of Gynecologic Oncology*. Philadelphia: Lippincott, 1992.

Hacker NF, Leuchter RS, Berek JS, et al. Radical vulvectomy and bilateral inguinal lymphadenectomy through separate groin incisions. *Obstet Gynecol* 58:574, 1982.

Heaps JM, Fu YS, Montz FJ, et al. Surgical-pathologic variables predictive of local recurrence in squamous cell carcinoma of the vulva. *Gynecol Oncol* 38:309, 1990.

VAGINAL CANCER

Brinton LA, Nasca PC, Mallin K, et al. Case-control study of in situ and invasive carcinoma of the vagina. *Gynecol Oncol* 38:49, 1990.

Daw E. Primary carcinoma of the vagina. *J Obstet Gynecol Br Commonwealth* 78:853, 1971.

Herbst AL, Green TH Jr., Ulfelder H. Primary carcinoma of the vagina. *Am J Obstet Gynecol* 106:210, 1970.

Herbst AL, Ulfelder H, Poskanzer DC. Adenocarcinoma of the vagina: Association of maternal stilbestrol therapy with tumor appearance in young women. *N Engl J Med* 284:878, 1971.

Perez CA, Bedwinek JM, Breaux SR. Patterns of failure after treatment of gynecologic tumors. *Cancer Treat Symp* 2:217, 1983.

Perez CA, Camel HM, Galakatos AE, et al. Definitive irradiation in carcinoma of the vagina: Long term evaluation of results. *Int J Radiat Oncol Biol Phys* 15:1283, 1988.

Perez CA, Gersell DJ, Hoskins WJ, McGuire WP. In WJ Hoskins, CAPerez, RC Young (eds), *Principles and Practice of Gynecologic Oncology*. Philadelphia: Lippincott, 1992.

Underwood RB, Smith RT. Carcinoma of the vagina. *JAMA* 217:46, 1971.

Oncologic Surgical Emergencies

Andrew M. Lowy and Derrick J. Beech

It is beyond the scope of this text to discuss all the common surgical emergencies that can occur in patients with cancer. This chapter focuses on emergencies in the patient with a known malignancy, particularly those problems specific to cancer patients, whether related to neoplastic disease or the complications of its treatment.

Intestinal Perforation

Gastrointestinal (GI) perforation in the cancer patient may occur as a result of a benign condition, from primary or metastatic tumor, or from a treatment-related complication. The clinical presentation of a perforated viscus is rarely subtle. The patient complains of severe abdominal pain, and physical examination reveals marked tenderness. As the peritonitis worsens, abdominal distention from reflex ileus becomes apparent. Clinically, there is evidence of hypovolemia from third-space fluid loss, marked by thirst, tachycardia, and low urine output. Free intraperitoneal air on upright films of the chest and abdomen confirm the diagnosis. Aside from routine blood tests and an electrocardiogram, little other work-up is required, as GI perforation demands surgical exploration in nearly all cases.

In a series by Ferrara et al., GI perforation occurred in organs uninvolved by tumor 66% of the time, most commonly due to peptic ulcer disease and diverticulitis. Neutropenic enterocolitis can progress to perforation when medical therapy is unsuccessful. Non-Hodgkin's lymphoma is most frequently associated with tumor-related perforation, which often results from tumor necrosis following chemotherapy. Tumors metastatic to the bowel may cause perforation. The most commonly involved tumors include melanoma and carcinoma of the lung and breast.

At operation, the area of perforation should be resected if possible. A conservative approach to reestablishing bowel continuity is prudent, especially in the setting of poor nutrition and generalized debilitation present in many patients with cancer. Ostomies are easily reversed at a subsequent procedure if the patient does well. In contrast, anastomotic leak has dire consequences. Pyloric exclusion may be used to protect difficult duodenal anastomoses. The use of gastrostomy and feeding jejunostomy tubes eliminates the problems associated with nasogastric intubation and allows for early enteral feeding. Copious irrigation of the peritoneal cavity should be performed. Monofilament and retention sutures, as well as delayed primary skin closure, may help reduce the incidence of wound infection, dehiscence, and evisceration. For benign conditions, such as perforated duodenal ulcer, standard surgical therapy should be carried out. Aggressive

Postoperative nutritional support with enteral feeding, when possible, or with IV hyperalimentation is crucial to recovery.

Intra-Abdominal Hemorrhage

Tumors are rarely the source of intra-abdominal hemorrhage even in the known cancer patient. More frequent scenarios include bleeding because of severe thrombocytopenia and coagulopathy or as a complication of an invasive procedure. Peptic ulcer disease and gastritis, the most common causes of bleeding in unselected series, are the leading culprits in 54–75% of patients with cancer. GI lymphomas and metastatic tumors are the most common lesions to initiate massive hemorrhage. Because tumors are responsible for spontaneous hemorrhage in a minority of patients, the same systematic approach to diagnosis and treatment should be undertaken as in those patients without malignant disease. While resuscitation with crystalloid and blood products is underway, the diagnostic work-up to define the site and etiology of bleeding should begin. Bleeding proximal to the ligament of Treitz is marked clinically by hematemesis or blood per nasogastric aspirate. Such signs should be followed by prompt upper endoscopy.

Bright red blood per rectum should initiate investigation of a colonic or rectal source. In such cases, proctoscopy or sigmoidoscopy is an expedient initial diagnostic maneuver. Angiography and nuclear red cell scans are often needed to localize colonic and small bowel bleeding sites. Extraluminal hemorrhage should be suspected when there is significant blood loss without hematemesis, melena, or hematochezia. The retroperitoneum is the most frequent site of occult intra-abdominal hemorrhage. If suspected, it is best evaluated with a computed tomography (CT) scan.

Therapy for intra-abdominal hemorrhage is initially directed at resuscitation and correction of any existing coagulopathy. A history of aspirin or nonsteroidal anti-inflammatory use within 1 week must raise suspicion of platelet dysfunction, and a bleeding time should be obtained. When the site and source of bleeding is identified, specific therapy is instituted. Under controlled conditions, invasive therapies such as endoscopic coagulation and angiographic embolization may be attempted. The timing of surgical intervention is based on the rate and volume of blood loss, the underlying pathology, and the patient's overall health status.

Intestinal Obstruction

Bowel obstruction is the source of considerable morbidity in the cancer patient. Adhesions and radiation enteritis are the most common benign causes of intestinal obstruction and are present in approximately one-third of cancer patients presenting with obstruction. Primary or metastatic malignancy is responsible in 60% of cases. Intra-abdominal malignancies most often implicated include carcinoma of the colon, ovary, and stomach. Melanoma along with carcinoma of the lung and breast are the most common extra-abdominal malignancies associated with bowel obstruction.

In most cases, the approach to diagnosis and treatment of obstruction in patients with cancer should be similar to that for patients with benign disease. A malignant etiology of obstruction or diffuse carcinomatosis should not be assumed based on a history of cancer alone. After a complete history, physical exam, and plain x-rays of the abdomen, the site of obstruction (small versus large bowel) needs to be delineated. Colonic obstruction should be excluded first by use of Hypaque enema. An upper GI series of tests is helpful to visualize the site(s) and degree of obstruction, particularly in patients with partial or recurrent small-bowel obstruction. Laparotomy is indicated immediately for patients presenting with obstruction and abdominal tenderness, leukocytosis, fever, or persistent tachycardia. A trial of nasogastric suction and IV fluids is reasonable in the stable patient with small-bowel obstruction. In patients with malignant obstruction, bowel strangulation and infarction are uncommon. Large-bowel obstruction will require surgical intervention in most cases. Ten to 28% of patients may resolve their obstruction with conservative measures alone.

At surgery, relief of obstruction may be accomplished by lysis of adhesions, resection, intestinal bypass, or creation of ostomies. In cases of radiation enteritis, gentle handling of the bowel is imperative. Short segments of involved bowel may be resected, but long segments are best treated with bypass. In some patients, none of these options are viable due to the extent of neoplastic disease. In such cases, placement of gastrostomy and feeding jejunostomy tubes are indicated. The gastrostomy tube, in particular, provides significant palliation by relieving emesis and the need for a nasogastric tube. Morbidity and mortality after bowel obstruction depends on the etiology of the obstruction and the stage of malignancy. Reported perioperative mortality rates of 9–19% are nearly equivalent to mortality rates in unselected series. Cancer patients with benign causes of obstruction certainly benefit from operation. Unfortunately, if malignant obstruction is present, only 35% of patients will gain lasting relief of symptoms after surgical treatment. In the patient with known carcinomatosis, operation is usually futile and perioperative mortality exceeds 40%. When this diagnosis is established preoperatively, placement of a percutaneous endoscopic gastrostomy (PEG) tube for palliation is indicated.

Pseudo-Obstruction

Small- and large-bowel ileus is a common problem in patients with cancer. Narcotic analgesics, electrolyte derangements from chemotherapeutic agents, radiation therapy, and prolonged bedrest may all contribute to decreased bowel motility. The treatment of pseudo-obstruction involves relief of the underlying cause. Bowel rest, often with nasogastric suction, cessation of narcotics, correction of electrolyte imbalance, and treatment of infection results in improvement for most patients. In cases of colonic pseudo-obstruction refractory to conservative therapy, colonoscopic decompression is indicated. It may be repeated if dilatation recurs. Surgery is indicated for recurrence following repeat colonoscopy. Surgical therapy usually consists of tube cecostomy placement.

Neutropenic Enterocolitis

The terms *neutropenic enterocolitis, typhlitis, necrotizing enteropathy*, and *ileocecal syndrome* have all been used to describe a clinical entity characterized by febrile neutropenia, abdominal distension, right-sided abdominal pain, tenderness, and diarrhea. The syndrome most often occurs in patients undergoing chemotherapy for hematologic malignancy, though it may also be seen in patients with solid tumors. Signs and symptoms characteristically develop after prolonged neutropenia (7 days or more). The initial presentation, consisting of right-sided abdominal pain, tenderness, and fever, often suggests appendicitis. The presence of significant watery diarrhea may mimic pseudomembranous colitis, but all conditions associated with acute abdominal pain must be considered in the differential diagnosis. The diagnosis is made clinically, often by exclusion of other pathologic causes. Serial examinations by the same examiner are critical to proper diagnosis and treatment. Abdominal films characteristically reveal an ileus pattern with some dilation of the cecum. Pneumatosis is an inconsistent finding. The CT findings in neutropenic enterocolitis are nonspecific, consisting mainly of bowel wall thickening and edema. The CT scan is often more valuable in ruling out other pathologic conditions. Complete work-up should include stool cultures for bacteria, fungus, and *Clostridium difficile* toxin.

The severity of neutropenic enterocolitis varies and therapy must be individualized. Medical treatment including bowel rest, nasogastric suction, broad-spectrum antibiotics, and IV hyperalimentation is successful in many cases. While granulocyte transfusion has never been proved effective, granulocyte colony-stimulating factors, which shorten the neutropenic period, will likely improve outcome. Surgical intervention is indicated in cases of perforation, uncontrolled hemorrhage, sepsis, and progression of symptoms on medical therapy. Right hemicolectomy with ileostomy is the operation of choice in most cases.

Biliary Obstruction from Metastatic Disease

Biliary obstruction by tumors metastatic to the hilum of the liver or portal lymph nodes is an uncommon but troublesome problem in the cancer patient. A variety of tumor types, including lymphoma, melanoma, and carcinoma of the breast, colon, stomach, lung, and ovary, may cause such obstruction. Evaluation is best performed with CT scan, which provides information on the biliary tree as well as the remainder of the abdomen. In a series of 12 patients with biliary obstruction from metastases, 11 patients had disease either in other intra-abdominal sites or in extra-abdominal locations. Thus, the prognosis for patients with biliary obstruction from metastatic disease is poor. The 60-day mortality in this group has been reported to be as high as 67%. Thus, treatment should be directed at the palliation of jaundice and the prevention of cholangitis. Drainage of the biliary tree is best accomplished by endoscopic retrograde cholangiopancreatography (ERCP) and biliary stenting. If this approach is unsuccessful, percutaneous transhepatic drainage is indicated. Surgery should be reserved for low-risk patients in whom the suspicion of metastatic disease is low.

Anorectal Disease

Anorectal disease is commonplace in patients with cancer. Treatment-related alterations in bowel habits predisposes patients to anal fissure, hemorrhoids, and perianal sepsis. Pain and bleeding are the most common symptoms of anorectal pathology. Physical examination should include careful visual inspection, palpation, and digital rectal exam. If the diagnosis is not readily apparent on bedside examination, examination under anesthesia should be performed. This eliminates patient discomfort and allows anoscopy and proctoscopy to be performed. Most anorectal disorders may be treated conservatively with good result. This includes stool softeners or antidiarrheal medications, local analgesics, and sitz baths. Perianal infection should be treated with IV antibiotics that have activity against GI flora. If suppuration or fluctuance is noted, then surgical drainage is indicated.

Catheter Infection

The use of indwelling vascular access catheters is now standard practice in cancer care. Catheter-based infection is a major source of morbidity. When catheter infection is suspected, a careful examination of the access site should be performed. Erythema, induration, and suppuration are signs of site infection requiring immediate catheter removal. Bacteremia and sepsis from catheter infection should be documented by blood cultures drawn from both the catheter and peripheral sites. Coagulase-negative staphylococci are the most common pathogen isolated in catheter-based infection, though numerous gram-positive, gram-negative, and fungal species may also be responsible. More than 80% of catheter-based infections can be treated effectively with a 10- to 14-day course of IV antibiotics. Antibiotic therapy should be given through the infected catheter and rotated between ports when multilumen catheters are present. Persistence of positive blood cultures or signs of systemic sepsis, particularly in the neutropenic patient, necessitates immediate catheter removal. Patients with vascular grafts or implanted prostheses should not be treated initially with antibiotics; immediate catheter removal is indicated in these patients once an infection has been documented.

Cardiovascular Emergencies

SUPERIOR VENA CAVA SYNDROME

Obstruction of the superior vena cava results in a constellation of signs and symptoms collectively known as the superior vena cava syndrome (SVCS). Impedance to caval outflow may result from external compression by neoplastic disease, fibrosis secondary to inflammation, or thrombosis. At one time, common etiologies of SVCS included granulomatous disease and syphilitic aortitis. With improvements in antimicrobial therapy, these diseases are now rare, and malignant disease is present in 87–97% of patients with SVCS. Lung cancer and lymphoma are the tumors most frequently associated with SVCS. An increasingly common cause of SVCS is thrombosis secondary to indwelling central venous catheters and cardiac pacemakers. Treatment of SVCS is predicated on establishing the underlying cause of caval obstruction, as this guides therapy and determines prognosis. It is no longer acceptable to begin empiric treatment such as mediastinal radiation without a pathologic diagnosis. Appropriate therapy directed at a specific tumor type can result in meaningful palliation and even cure for patients presenting with SVCS.

Pathophysiology

The superior vena cava is the primary conduit for venous drainage of the head, neck, upper extremities, and upper thorax. It is a thin-walled, compliant vessel surrounded by more rigid structures, including the mediastinal and paratracheal lymph nodes, trachea and right mainstem bronchus, pulmonary artery, and aorta. As such, the superior vena cava is susceptible to external compression by any space-occupying lesion. Obstruction of caval outflow results in venous hypertension of the head, neck, and upper extremities, which in turn is responsible for the characteristic clinical presentation of SVCS.

Presentation

In most cases, obstruction of the superior vena cava does not occur acutely, and the signs and symptoms of SCVS develop gradually. The most common symptoms include dyspnea and feelings of facial fullness, which are present in 63% and 50% of patients, respectively. The common physical findings include facial edema, venous engorgement of the neck and chest wall, cyanosis, and plethora. Symptoms worsen when the patient bends forward or reclines. Obstruction of the superior vena cava becomes a true emergency when associated laryngeal edema results in significant airway compromise or in cases of severely elevated intracranial pressure.

Evaluation

In the absence of airway compromise or elevated intracranial pressure, the patient with SVCS should be thoroughly evaluated to determine the etiology of caval obstruction. This evaluation begins with a careful history and physical examination. A prior history of malignancy, heavy smoking, or symptoms such as cough, fever, and night sweats should be noted. On physical examination it is important to carefully examine all lymph node basins and to note the presence of a pacemaker or central venous catheter. A chest radiograph will reveal an abnormality in 84% of patients with SVCS, although the findings are often nonspecific. The test of choice to evaluate SVC obstruction is CT of the chest with IV contrast. Magnetic resonance imaging (MRI) is an excellent alternative for the patient with renal insufficiency or contrast allergy. The CT scan will readily define the etiology of the obstruction (external compression versus thrombosis). It also provides anatomic detail regarding the presence of a tumor mass and can be used to guide a percutaneous biopsy. When superior vena cava thrombosis is demonstrated without evidence of malignancy, thrombolytic therapy and/or anticoagulation should be initiated. If the CT scan demonstrates external compression of the superior vena cava by neoplastic disease, efforts should be directed at obtaining a tissue diagnosis. Minimally invasive techniques for tissue diagnosis include sputum cytology, CT-guided percutaneous biopsy, bronchoscopy, lymph node biopsy, and bone marrow biopsy. Invasive procedures such as mediastinoscopy and thoracotomy should be considered if all initial measures are inadequate for diagnosis. Such invasive procedures can be performed safely in most patients with SVCS and are preferable to proceeding with nonspecific therapy.

Therapy

When the etiology of SVCS is due to malignant disease, treatment is based on tumor type. In the past, patients with SVCS were treated with mediastinal radiation on an emergent basis. This often frustrated later attempts at tissue diagnosis as radiation-induced tissue necrosis begins within 72 hours of treatment. It is now recognized that the symptoms of SVCS may be temporized by using diuretics and head elevation. Steroids have been used to reduce inflammation, though their effectiveness has never been adequately demonstrated. Only those patients with impending airway obstruction or severely elevated intracranial pressure should be considered for emergent radiation therapy. Even in such cases, intubation, mechanical ventilation, and the use of osmotic diuretics can provide time for a tissue diagnosis to be obtained. When a tissue diagnosis is secured, tumor-specific therapy is begun. Small-cell lung cancer and lymphoma are best treated with combination chemotherapy; radiation may be used for consolidation. In a series of 56 patients with small-cell lung cancer, SVCS resolved in all 23 patients treated with chemotherapy alone, 64% of those treated with radiation therapy alone, and 83% of those treated with combination therapy. Non–small-cell lung cancer is most often treated with radiation therapy. One commonly used fractionation schedule provides high-dose (3–4 Gy/day) treatment for 3 days followed by conventional dose fractionation (1.8–2.0 Gy/day) to a total of 50–60 Gy. On such a treatment schedule, 70% of patients will respond within 2 weeks.

Patients with SVCS secondary to catheter-induced thrombosis may be successfully treated with thrombolytic agents followed by systemic anticoagulation. Thrombolytic agents are most effective when patients are treated within 5 days of the onset of symptoms. Alternatively, systemic anticoagulation followed by catheter removal will often result in gradual recanalization of the vessel and resolution of symptoms.

Surgical intervention consisting of innominate vein–right atrial bypass is generally reserved for patients with benign causes of superior vena cava obstruction. The use of balloon angioplasty and expandable metal stents are under investigation as palliative modalities for SVCS refractory to more standard therapy.

Summary

Identification of the etiology of superior vena cava obstruction represents the most important step toward improving outcome. Cases of catheter-induced thrombosis should be treated with systemic anticoagulation and/or thrombolytic therapy. Currently, malignant disease is the most common cause of SVC obstruction. In such cases, the SVCS is most effectively treated by tumor-specific therapy, whether it be chemotherapy, radiotherapy, or multimodality in nature.

PERICARDIAL TAMPONADE

Pericardial tamponade in the cancer patient most often results from malignant obstruction of pericardial lymphatics, leading to the accumulation of pericardial fluid. Both primary neoplasms of the heart and metastatic lesions may incite development of pericardial effusions. Metastatic disease to the pericardium is the prevailing etiology of pericardial effusion and tamponade. Carcinoma of the lung and breast, lymphoma, leukemia, and melanoma are the most commonly associated malignancies. Radiation-induced effusions may also occur in the cancer patient.

Pathophysiology

The pericardial sac normally contains 20 ml of fluid at a mean pressure below that of right and left ventricular end-diastolic pressure. With the gradual accumulation of pericardial fluid, this pressure will rise until the intrapericardial pressure equals or surpasses that of ventricular end-diastolic pressure. At this point, diastolic filling is compromised and cardiac output falls. The development of pericardial tamponade depends on the rate and volume of pericardial fluid accumulation, as well as the compliance of the pericardial sac. A pericardial effusion as small as 150 ml may induce tamponade. In cases of more gradual accumulation, effusions may reach 1–2 liters.

Presentation and Diagnosis

The symptoms of pericardial tamponade are often vague. Frequent complaints include chest pain, anxiety, and dyspnea. Clinical signs include tachycardia, diminished heart sounds, jugular venous distention, pulsus paradoxus, and ultimately shock. The electrocardiogram reveals low voltage throughout all leads, with sinus tachycardia. Two-dimensional echocardiography will best demonstrate the presence of pericardial fluid and is the test of choice for the stable patient with suspected pericardial tamponade.

Therapy

The treatment of pericardial tamponade is removal of the pericardial effusion, which may be accomplished in the emergent setting at the bedside via needle pericardiocentesis. A drainage catheter may then be inserted into the pericardial space over a guidewire. If the patient is stable, pericardiocentesis under echocardiographic guidance will help minimize complications. Removal of a small amount of fluid results in dramatic and immediate improvement for the patient in extremis. Without additional treatment, malignant pericardial effusions will often recur. Thus, the drainage catheter should be left in place to assess the rate of fluid accumulation. The options for preventing reaccumulation include tetracycline sclerosis, surgery, and radiation therapy. The instillation of 500–1,000 mg of tetracycline into the pericardial sac induces an inflammatory response, with subsequent fibrosis and obliteration of the pericardial space. Multiple instillations are usually necessary. Treatment should be repeated until the drainage is less than 25 ml in 24 hours to achieve optimal results. Successful control of effusions with this technique is obtained in 86% of treated patients. Surgical options include subxiphoid pericardiotomy, window pericardiectomy, and complete pericardiectomy. In most cases, the subxiphoid approach is preferred. It avoids thoracotomy and can be performed under local anesthesia. Multiple series have documented a recurrence rate of 7% using this technique. Complete pericardiectomy should be reserved for patients with radiation-induced effusions. Radiation therapy is useful in the stable patient with a malignant effusion secondary to lymphoma. Treatment is given in 2- to 3-Gy fractions to a total dose of 20–40 Gy.

Summary

Outcome after treatment of pericardial tamponade is related to tumor type. The median survival ranges from 3.5 months for patients with lung cancer to as long as 18.5 months in patients with breast cancer. Thus, the presence of a malignant pericardial effusion does not preclude meaningful survival.

Metabolic Emergencies

HYPERCALCEMIA

Hypercalcemia is the most common metabolic complication of malignancy, occurring in approximately 10% of cancer patients. Cancer is the leading cause of hypercalcemia among hospitalized patients. Tumors most commonly associated with hypercalcemia include carcinomas of the breast, lung, and kidney and multiple myeloma. Patients with parathyroid carcinoma characteristically present with intractable hypercalcemia.

Pathophysiology

Although more than 80% of patients with hypercalcemia have bone metastasis, there is no correlation between the extent of bony involvement and the degree of hypercalcemia. Current data suggest that even in the presence of bony metastasis, hypercalcemia is mediated by tumor-induced humoral factors. Parathyroid hormone (PTH)-related protein, osteoclast-activating factor, prostaglandins, and numerous other cytokines may play a role in the development of hypercalcemia in patients with malignancies.

Parathyroid Hormone and PTH-Like Protein

Calcium homeostasis is normally a tightly regulated process. Serum calcium level is primarily controlled by PTH, 1,25-dihydroxyvitamin D_3, and calcitonin. The effect of these hormones on bone, intestine, and kidneys is primarily to ensure that the net absorption of calcium by the GI tract is balanced with the amount excreted by the kidney (150–250 mg/day). Under normal conditions the serum calcium level is maintained between 8.5 mg/dl and 10.5 mg/dl. Approximately 45% of calcium exists in the ionized, metabolically active form, with the remaining calcium being protein bound. In the past, it was thought that hypercalcemia associated with malignancy was the result of ectopic parathyroid hormone. However, current studies examining the PTH-specific mRNA from tumors have failed to confirm the presence of ectopic PTH. Most cases of hormonally mediated hypercalcemia in cancer patients result from the activity of a PTH-like protein. PTH-related protein affects the kidney and bone in a manner similar to PTH (enhancement of renal tubular resorption of calcium). In contrast to hyperparathyroidism, patients with hypercalcemia secondary to PTH-related protein have impaired production of 1,25-dihydroxyvitamin D_3 and show no evidence of renal bicarbonate wasting. This mechanism is particularly prevalent in solid tumors, especially epidermoid carcinomas.

Osteoclast-Activating Factor

OAF is responsible for hypercalcemia in patients with multiple myeloma and lymphoma. This osteolytic polypeptide stimulates osteoclast proliferation and the release of lysosomal enzymes and collagenase. Despite the potent osteolytic activity of OAF in vitro, patients with elevated OAF levels do not always develop hypercalcemia unless there is associated renal insufficiency. Several osteotrophic factors (OAF, colony-stimulating factor, gamma-interferon) are involved in the development of hypercalcemia in patients with lymphoma due to human T cell lymphotrophic virus (HTLV). Transforming growth factor, epidermal growth factor, interleukin-1, platelet-derived growth factor, tumor-derived hematopoietic colony-stimulating factors, tumor necrosis factor (TNF) (particularly TNF-β), and lymphotoxin are all potent inducers of bone resorption in vitro and may have a role in the hypercalcemia of malignancy.

Clinical Presentation

There are multiple organ systems involved in the constellation of symptoms caused by hypercalcemia. These symptoms are nonspecific, with the severity being directly related to the degree of calcium elevation. Neuromuscular symptoms often predominate, with the initial manifestations of fatigue, weakness, lethargy, and apathy progressing to profound mental status changes and psychotic behavior if left untreated.

Renal tubular dysfunction can occur secondary to hypercalcemia and is manifested by the development of polydipsia, polyuria, and nocturia. Polydipsia and polyuria are among the earliest symptoms of hypercalcemia and are due to a reversible defect in renal tubular concentrating ability, similar to nephrogenic diabetes insipidus. Severe volume contraction occurs, resulting in a decreased glomerular filtration rate, thus potentiating serum calcium elevation. Patients with prolonged hypercalcemia may progress to permanent renal tubular damage with renal tubular acidosis, glucosuria, aminoaciduria, and hypophosphaturia.

Nausea, vomiting, anorexia, obstipation, ileus, and abdominal pain are among the GI symptoms that may occur with hypercalcemia.

The role of calcium as a neurotransmitter makes the myocardium particularly prone to hypercalcemia-induced toxicity. Acute hypercalcemia can slow the heart rate and shorten ventricular systole. With moderate elevation of the calcium level the QT interval is shortened, and atrial and ventricular arrhythmias may occur. Electrocardiographic changes seen with elevated serum calcium levels include bradycardia, prolonged PR interval, shortened QT interval, and widened T waves. Under extreme circumstances, sudden death from cardiac arrhythmias can occur when the serum calcium rises acutely.

Diagnostic Evaluation

Critical laboratory studies in the work-up of patients with hypercalcemia include serum calcium, phosphate, alkaline phosphatase, PTH, electrolytes, blood urea nitrogen (BUN), total protein, albumin, and creatinine levels. In patients with severe hypoalbuminemia, the ionized calcium level is a more accurate measure of the effective calcium level. Severely malnourished, protein-depleted patients may show an elevated ionized calcium level without an increase in total calcium. Also, abnormal calcium binding to paraprotein without an elevation in the ionized calcium can be seen in patients with multiple myeloma. Elevated immunoreactive PTH levels in association with hypophosphatemia suggest ectopic PTH secretion. Hypercalcemia secondary to malignancy usually has an acute onset, high serum calcium level (>14 mg/dl), low serum chloride level, and elevated or normal serum phosphate and bicarbonate levels. These laboratory findings help differentiate hypercalcemia due to cancer from that secondary to hyperparathyroidism, which is associated with an elevated serum calcium in the presence of decreased serum phosphate and bicarbonate levels.

Treatment

Prompt identification and treatment of hypercalcemia is essential. Symptomatic patients with hypercalcemia and/or those patients with a serum calcium level of 14 mg/dl or greater need medical emergency treatment. IV hydration with restoration of intravascular volume increases glomerular filtration rate and is the mainstay of hypercalcemia management. Diuretics that block calcium resorption in the ascending loop of Henle and augment renal calcium excretion (e.g., furosemide) may be helpful after intravascular volume repletion has taken place. The initial dose of furosemide in patients without renal impairment is 40 mg given as an IV bolus, followed by 40–80 mg every 2–4 hours as needed. Ethycrynic acid (50 mg IV or 0.5–1.0 mg/kg) can occasionally serve as an alternative to furosemide; however, thiazide diuretics may potentiate hypercalcemia and should never be used.

Plicamycin (Mithracin) is an effective inhibitor of bone resorption that generally induces a decline in serum calcium within

6–48 hours. Plicamycin is an antitumor antibiotic with limited antineoplastic activity but excellent reduction in bone resorption when used at doses of 25 µg/kg/day by IV infusion. The toxicities of plicamycin include thrombocytopenia, hypotension, and hepatic and renal insufficiency. These toxicities are rare when the dose is restricted to less than 30 µg/kg/day.

Intravenous phosphates are effective in lowering serum calcium. The usual dose is 1.5 g over 6–8 hours in the emergent treatment of hypercalcemia. The use of intravenous phosphate in the treatment of symptomatic hypercalcemia is currently controversial due to the potential complications of renal failure and soft tissue calcification from an acute increase in the systemic calcium-phosphate complex. Oral phosphates may also be used to treat hypercalcemia. Doses of 0.5–3.0 g/day may be highly effective in reducing the serum calcium. The major side effects of this therapy (diarrhea and nausea) limit the utility of the oral route for phosphate administration in the emergency setting. Diphosphonates (biphosphonates) block osteoclastic bone resorption with significant reduction of serum calcium levels. Etidronate disodium is the only diphosphonate approved for use in the United States. A typical dose regimen is 7.5 mg/kg/day IV for several days followed by 20 mg/kg/day PO. Ralston et al. evaluated 39 patients with hypercalcemia of malignancy (serum calcium >11.2 mg/dl). All patients evaluated underwent aggressive saline diuresis along with randomly assigned treatment with diphosphonate, plicamycin, or corticosteroids and calcitonin. All three therapeutic regimens produced significant decreases in serum calcium. The regimen containing corticosteroids produced the most rapid reduction in serum calcium level; however, the calcium level rarely decreased to the normal range. Diphosphonates produced a more sustained and complete reduction in the serum calcium level although the onset of action was slower. Plicamycin effectively lowered the serum calcium level, but this effect was transient, with approximately half of the patients studied showing an increase in the serum calcium level by day 9 of treatment.

Gallium nitrate, a new agent used in the treatment of hypercalcemia, is a potent inhibitor of bone resorption, with profound effects in reducing serum calcium in patients with malignant disease and hyperparathyroidism. Hydroxyapatite is rendered less soluble and more resistant to cell-mediated resorption when gallium nitrate is incorporated into bone. Gallium nitrate causes impairment in osteoclast acidification of bone matrix by decreasing transmembrane proton transport. This agent may also enhance bone formation by stimulating bone collagen synthesis and by increasing calcium incorporation into bone. These actions result in a net reduction of serum calcium. The dose of gallium nitrate is 100–200 mg/m^2/day via continuous IV infusion given for a total of 5–7 days. Normal serum calcium levels are seen in 80–90% of patients. Nephrotoxicity, the dose-limiting factor, may be minimized by pretreatment IV hydration.

HYPONATREMIA/SYNDROME OF INAPPROPRIATE ANTIDIURETIC HORMONE

Significant neurologic dysfunction can occur when the serum sodium level abruptly falls or when it decreases to levels below 115–125 mg/dl. Mental status changes, seizures, coma, and ultimately death may result if therapeutic intervention is not urgently instituted. The syndrome of inappropriate antidiuretic hormone (SIADH) may be associated with cancers of the prostate, adrenal glands, esophagus, pancreas, colon, and head and neck; carcinoid tumors; and mesotheliomas. Small-cell carcinoma of the lung is the most common malignancy associated with SIADH.

Pathophysiology

Dilutional hyponatremia occurs due to excessive water resorption in the collecting ducts. This increase in intravascular volume leads to increased renal perfusion along with a significant decrease in proximal tubular absorption of sodium. In the presence of renal insufficiency, there is increased ADH secretion and excessive water reabsorption from the collecting ducts, resulting in a significant dilutional hyponatremia.

Clinical Evaluation

Patients with mild hyponatremia frequently complain of anorexia, nausea, myalgia, headaches, and subtle neurologic symptoms. When the onset of hyponatremia is rapid or the absolute serum sodium level falls below 115 mg/dl, patients develop more severe neurologic dysfunction. Alterations in mental status can range from lethargy to confusion and coma. Seizures and psychotic behavior can occur at critically low serum sodium levels. Physical findings in patients with profound hyponatremia include alterations in mental status, pathologic reflexes, papilledema, and, occasionally, focal neurologic signs.

Diagnostic Evaluation

Laboratory data and diagnostic studies should aid the clinician in determining the etiology of hyponatremia. Pseudohyponatremia, or dilutional hyponatremia, due to hyperproteinemia, hyperglycemia, or hyperlipidemia can be ruled out by serum protein electrophoresis, serum glucose, and serum lipid determinations. The possibility of drug-induced hyponatremia should also be considered. Chemotherapeutic agents such as vincristine and cyclophosphamide, as well as mannitol, morphine, diuretics, and abrupt withdrawal of steroids, may contribute to hyponatremia.

A detailed history and physical examination along with meticulous evaluation of the patient's intake and output will aid in determining whether the patient's intravascular volume is adequate and will eliminate the possibility of water toxicity as the cause of hyponatremia. Laboratory investigation should include measurement of serum and urine electrolytes and creatinine. A typical finding in patients with SIADH is that the urine sodium concentration is inappropriately high for the level of hyponatremia. Also, the urine osmolality is greater than plasma osmolality, and the urine is never maximally diluted. Other significant findings might include a low BUN, hypouricemia, and hypophosphatemia due to a decreased proximal tubular resorption of these compounds. Chest radiograph and brain CT scan should be done if pathology of the pulmonary or central nervous system (CNS) is suspected.

Treatment

Ideally, therapy for SIADH should be directed toward the underlying cause. In the case of small-cell lung cancer, effective multidrug chemotherapy will usually result in resolution of hyponatremia. SIADH resulting from CNS metastasis may improve with the use of corticosteroids and radiation therapy. If the etiology of SIADH cannot be identified, then the therapy for patients with severe hyponatremia is water restriction. A restriction of free water to 500–1,000 ml per day should correct the hyponatremia within 5–10 days. If no improvement is seen in the serum sodium level with restriction of free water after this time period, then demeclocycline should be used. Demeclocycline is an ADH antagonist that produces a dose-dependent, reversible nephrogenic diabetes insipidus. The recommended initial dose of demeclocycline is 600 mg daily (given in two or three divided doses). The potential adverse effect of nephrotoxicity with demeclocycline is usually seen only when extremely high doses are used (1,200 mg/day). Since this agent is secreted in urine and bile, dose adjustments must be made in patients with renal or hepatic insufficiencies.

When severe hyponatremia produces seizures or coma, 3% hypertonic saline or normal saline infusion with IV furosemide should be used. The rate of serum sodium correction should be limited to 0.5–1.0 mEq/liter/hour to minimize the risk of CNS toxicity.

HYPOGLYCEMIA

Insulin-producing islet cell tumors are the prototypical lesions associated with hypoglycemia. The non–islet cell tumors most often associated with hypoglycemia include hepatomas, adrenocortical tumors, and tumors of mesenchymal origin. Mesenchymal tumors comprise more than 50% of non–islet cell neoplasms seen in association with hypoglycemia. Of these, mesothelioma, fibrosarcoma, neurofibrosarcoma, and hemangiopericytoma are most commonly associated with hypoglycemia.

Pathophysiology

The mechanism of hypoglycemia resulting from insulin-secreting islet cell tumors involves the unregulated and inappropriate excess secretion of insulin. In contrast, the serum insulin level is normal with non–islet cell tumors. Substances with nonsuppressible insulin–like activities (NSILAs) have been detected in patients with malignancy-associated hypoglycemia. Two classes of compounds have been isolated based on molecular weight and ethanol solubility. The low molecular weight compounds consist of IGF-I, IGF-II, somatomedin A, and somatomedin C. IGF-I and IGF-II share similar amino acid sequences with proinsulin; however, they do not react with anti-insulin antibodies. The metabolic activity of these compounds is only 1–2% that of insulin. Approximately 40% of cancer patients with symptomatic hypoglycemia have elevated plasma levels of NSILAs. This supports the role of NSILA in hypoglycemia of malignancy.

Increased glucose use may account for the hypoglycemia seen in association with large tumors. Hepatic glucose production(700 g/day) may fall short of daily glucose requirements in the presence of tumors weighing over 1 kg (which use 50–200 g/day of glucose). Defects in the usual counter-regulatory mechanism of glucose control may also account for malignancy-induced hypoglycemia. Cancer-related hypoglycemia usually develops gradually. It does not allow the usual increase in counter-regulatory hormones seen with hypoglycemia from other etiologies.

Clinical Evaluation

Symptoms of hypoglycemia include excessive fatigue, weakness, dizziness, and confusion. In malignancy-associated hypoglycemia, neurologic symptoms usually predominate and may progress to seizures and coma if left untreated. These more severe neurologic complications are usually associated with serum glucose levels below 40–45 mg/dl.

Diagnostic Evaluation

Before concluding that cancer is the etiology of hypoglycemia, all other potential causes must be excluded. Exogenous insulin or oral hypoglycemic agents, adrenal insufficiency, pituitary insufficiency, ethanol abuse, and malnutrition are among the common causes of hypoglycemia. Measurement of fasting and late-afternoon serum glucose levels will aid in determining if hypoglycemia is due to an islet cell or non–islet cell tumor. Patients with insulinomas have increased insulin levels, with fasting glucose levels below 50 mg/dl. This finding is quite different from that of non–islet cell tumors, in which there is a normal or low insulin level associated with hypoglycemia. Also, because insulinomas produce large amounts of proinsulin, they tend to have an elevated proinsulin to insulin ratio.

Treatment

Under ideal circumstances, complete extirpation of the tumor is the optimal therapeutic intervention for hypoglycemia secondary to solid tumors. In the case of an insulinoma, simple enucleation or subtotal pancreatectomy will frequently provide cure. These tumors are usually benign, with excellent results from simple tumor resection. Diazoxide may be beneficial in patients with insulin-secreting tumors by inhibiting insulin secretion. For the same reason, this drug is not effective in the treatment of non–islet cell tumors. Radiation therapy may at times reduce tumor bulk and provide palliation of hypoglycemia. Diet modification should be the second line of therapy when resection is not possible. Frequent feedings between meals and nightly can reduce the occurrence of hypoglycemic attacks. Corticosteroids and growth hormone may at times provide temporary relief. Glucagon injections subcutaneously can also be used as an aid in glucose regulation.

TUMOR LYSIS SYNDROME

Tumor lysis syndrome occurs when there is rapid cell turnover and increased release of intracellular contents into the bloodstream. This syndrome is characterized by hyperuricemia, hyperkalemia, hyperphosphatemia, and hypocalcemia. Occasionally this syndrome occurs spontaneously in patients with lymphomas and leukemia; however, it is more common after cytotoxic chemotherapy-induced rapid cell lysis. The rapid release of intracellular contents can overwhelm the excretory ability of the kidneys, and electrolyte levels can become dangerously elevated. Patients with large, bulky tumors that are sensitive to cytotoxic chemotherapy are particularly prone to this syndrome, as are patients undergoing treatment for Burkitt's and non-Hodgkin's lymphoma, acute lymphoblastic leukemia, acute nonlymphoblastic leukemia, and chronic myelogenous leukemia in blast crisis. Although rare, tumor lysis syndrome can occur after treatment of small-cell lung cancer, metastatic breast cancer, and metastatic medulloblastoma. Tumor lysis syndrome occurs not only with cytotoxic chemotherapy but also following radiation and hormonal therapy (e.g., tamoxifen, steroids, interferon).

Pathophysiology

As mentioned above, the metabolic abnormalities associated with tumor lysis syndrome include hyperuricemia, hyperkalemia, and hyperphosphatemia with hypocalcemia. The pathologic processes seen with this syndrome are due to the propensity of uric acid, xanthine, and phosphate to precipitate in the renal tubules. This can impair renal excretory function and cause further serum elevation of these metabolites. Renal insufficiency usually does not develop from the metabolic derangements alone; a combination of low urine flow rates and elevated serum metabolites is usually required to precipitate renal dysfunction. Thus, oliguric patients are at significantly higher risk of developing renal failure during rapid cellular lysis.

Hyperkalemia results from the release of intracellular contents and is further perpetuated by renal insufficiency. The potential toxicities of potassium elevation are life threatening and require urgent intervention. Signs of cardiac toxicity are evident by the characteristic electrocardiographic changes seen with potassium levels above 6 mEq/liter. Loss of P waves, peaked T waves, widened QRS complex, and depressed ST segments indicate severe hyperkalemia effects that may progress to heart block and diastolic cardiac arrest if left untreated.

Hyperphosphatemia can also result from rapid tumor lysis and is usually accompanied by hypocalcemia. The mechanism of hypocalcemia in tumor lysis syndrome is thought to be due to the formation of calcium-phosphate salts that precipitate in the soft tissues. Hyperphosphatemia is further exacerbated by the formation of these calcium-phosphate complexes in renal tubules causing progressive renal insufficiency.

Treatment

Preventive measures can be taken to minimize the toxicities of tumor lysis. Patients should undergo vigorous IV hydration before initiating potentially toxic chemotherapeutic agents. Another important preventive measure is to alkalinize the urine during the first 1–2 days of cytotoxic treatment. These measures counteract hyperuricemia by increasing the solubility of uric acid. Allopurinol has also been shown to effectively decrease the formation of uric acid and reduce the incidence of uric acid nephropathy. In patients with large, bulky tumors that are known to have a high growth fraction, allopurinol should be administered before chemotherapeutic intervention.

An electrocardiogram should be obtained in patients with hyperkalemia or hypocalcemia, and continuous cardiac monitoring should be instituted. Hyperkalemia should be treated with the standard measures for acutely lowering the serum potassium level. These include IV administration of insulin and glucose, loop diuretics, and/or bicarbonate. Calcium should be used to acutely counteract cardiac toxicities if the patient is not on digitalis. Regardless of the measures used to acutely lower the serum potassium, an oral or rectal sodium-potassium exchange resin should be given to lower the total body potassium load (15 g sodium polystyrene sulfonate [Kayexalate] PO every 6 hours).

If there is evidence of worsening renal function with poor resolution of the metabolic abnormalities, hemodialysis should be considered.

Spinal Cord Compression

Spinal cord compression is the second most common neurologic complication of cancer. Autopsy studies suggest that 5% of patients with malignancies have evidence of spinal cord involvement, with the annual incidence estimated at 18,000 new cases in the United States this year. Spinal cord compression can produce paralysis and loss of sphincter control if left untreated. Early recognition and diagnosis is essential. Patients who present early with minimal neurologic deficits have a more favorable prognosis. Unfortunately, close to 80% of patients are unable to walk at the time of presentation.

PATHOPHYSIOLOGY

The mechanism of spinal cord compression usually involves extradural metastatic lesions of the vertebral body or neural arch. Tumor expansion occurs posteriorly, resulting in anterior compression of the dural sac. Rarely, metastasis can occur in intradural locations without bony involvement. Paraspinal tumors can also cause cord compression by penetrating through the intervertebral foramen.

Most of the data regarding spinal cord compression in malignancy is extrapolated from animal models. If spinal cord compression develops gradually, decompression can be delayed without impairing the return of neurologic function; however, rapid cord compression requires immediate therapeutic intervention to avoid irreversible neurologic deficits.

Spinal cord edema plays a significant role in the development of neurologic injury. Siegal et al. demonstrated in a rat model that edema in the compressed spinal cord segment was associated with a consistent elevation of prostaglandin estradiol (PGE_2), a mediator of inflammation and edema.

CLINICAL PRESENTATION

Although spinal cord compression can occur as the initial manifestation of disease, most patients who develop malignant spinal cord involvement have been previously diagnosed with cancer. The interval from primary diagnosis to epidural cord compression varies with the type of tumor involved. Lung cancer has an aggressive presentation, with epidural cord compression developing within a few months after diagnosis of the primary lesion. In contrast to lung cancer, patients with carcinoma of the breast have been reported to manifest spinal cord compression as long as 20 years after their initial presentation.

The distribution of spinal cord segments involved—cervical 10%, thoracic 70%, lumbosacral 20%—reflects the number of vertebrae in each anatomic segment. More than 90% of patients present with localized back pain, which may be exacerbated by movement, recumbency, coughing, sneezing, or straining. The pain due to cord compression can be radicular in distribution. Pain is usually present for several weeks before neurologic symptoms develop. Left untreated, weakness and numbness occur, usually beginning in the toes and ascending to the level of the lesion. Autonomic dysfunction usually occurs late in the disease process. The onset of urinary retention and constipation represents an ominous sign indicating possible progression to irreversible paraplegia if left untreated.

Physical examination may reveal tenderness to palpation over the involved vertebrae. Straight leg raise and neck flexion may produce pain at the level of the involved vertebrae. Weakness, spasticity, abnormal reflexes, and extensor plantar response (Babinski's sign) may be evident on physical examination. A palpable urinary bladder or decreased anal sphincter tone suggests autonomic involvement and an advanced stage of disease.

DIAGNOSTIC EVALUATION

Patients with signs of impending neurologic deficits and signs of impending paralysis should undergo emergency evaluation and treatment. Based on the history and physical examination, dexamethasone should be given (10 mg IV followed by 4 mg every 6 hours). Rapid radiographic assessment should then take place. More than two-thirds of patients with cord compression have radiographic evidence of bony abnormalities on plain films of the spine. Radiographic findings suggestive of a spine metastasis include erosion and loss of vertebral pedicles, partial or complete collapse of vertebral bodies, and paraspinal soft tissue masses. The finding of normal spine radiographs does not exclude the possibility of epidural metastases. For instance, patients with lymphoma typically have normal spine radiographs even in the presence of epidural tumors.

Currently, MRI is the initial study of choice in evaluating patients with suspected spinal cord compression after plain radiographs have been obtained. The MRI has several advantages over the standard myelogram. Lumbar puncture, which is required for a myelogram, is associated with significant morbidity in the presence of a space-occupying lesion and potential bleeding complications in patients with coagulopathies. This procedure is eliminated with the use of MRI. Also, MRI is less invasive and requires less time to perform than myelography. MRI is useful in defining the extent of tumor involvement and designing portals for radiation therapy or for planning operative intervention.

MRI gives excellent delineation of extradural versus intradural lesions. Gadolinium (Gd-DPTA) contrast is usually not required for extradural lesions, but optimal imaging of extramedullary and intramedullary intradural lesions requires the use of this agent. If the MRI results in equivocal or negative findings, then myelography with or without CT scan should performed.

TREATMENT

Early intervention is essential in the management of malignant spinal cord compression. There is a clear correlation between the functional status at the time of presentation and the posttreatment outcome. Less than 10% of patients who present with paraplegia become ambulatory after treatment. Radiotherapy and/or surgical intervention are the standard treatment modalities. Typically, 3000 cGy is given in 300- to 500-cGy dose fractions, with excellent resolution of pain and neurologic symptoms.

Laminectomy is effective in managing patients with epidural masses but has limited use if the pathologic process is anterior to the spinal cord. In select cases surgical resection may provide symptomatic relief, but careful patient selection is essential.

Chemotherapy may play a role in managing patients with epidural cord compression from lesions that are sensitive to certain agents; however, the role of chemotherapy in an adjuvant setting or as primary treatment has not clearly been defined.

Selected References

Alt B, Glass NR, Sollinger H. Neutropenic enterocolitis in adults. Review of the literature and assessment of surgical intervention. *Am J Surg* 149:405, 1985.

Armstrong BA, Perez CA, Simpson J, et al. Role of irradiation in the management of superior vena cava syndrome. *Int J Radiol Oncol Biol Phys* 13:531, 1987.

Annest LS, Jolly PC. The results of surgical treatment of bowel obstruction caused by peritoneal carcinomatosis. *Am Surg* 45:718, 1979.

Bear HD, Turner MA, Parker GA, et al. Treatment of biliary obstruction caused by metastatic cancer. *Am J Surg* 157:381, 1989.

Besarob A, Caro JF. Mechanism of hypercalcemia in malignancy. *Cancer* 41:2276, 1978.

Boss GR, Seegimiller JE. Hyperuricemia and gout: Classification complications and management. *N Engl J Med* 300:1459, 1979.

Delaney TF, Oldfield EH. Spinal Cord Compression. In VT DeVita, S Hellman, SA Rosenberg (eds), *Cancer: Principles and Practice of Oncology* (4th ed). Philadelphia: 1993.

Einzig AI. Hypercalcemia in Malignancies. In JP Dutcher, PH Wiesnik (eds), *Handbook of Hematologic and Oncologic Emergencies.* New York: Plenum, 1987.

Escalante CP. Causes and management of superior vena cava syndrome. *Oncology* 7:61, 1993.

Ferrara JJ, Martin EW, Carey LC. Morbidity of emergency operations in patients with metastatic cancer receiving chemotherapy. *Surgery* 92:605, 1982.

Gallick HL, Weaver DW, Sachs RJ, et al. Intestinal obstruction in cancer patients. An assessment of risk factors and outcome. *Am Surg* 8:434, 1986.

Gray BH, Olin JW, Graor RA, et al. Safety and efficacy of thrombolytic therapy for superior vena cava syndrome. *Chest* 99:54, 1991.

Gregory JR, McMurtrey MJ, Mountain CF. A surgical approach to the treatment of pericardial effusion in cancer patients. *Am J Clin Oncol* 8:319, 1985.

Helms SR, Carlson MD. Cardiovascular emergencies. *Semin Oncol* 16:463, 1989.

Henderson JE, Shustic C, Kremer R, et al. Circulating concentrations of parathyroid hormone-like peptide in malignancy and hyperparathyroidism. *J Bone Miner Res* 5:105, 1990.

Kahn CR. The riddle of tumour hypoglycemia revised. *Clin Endocrinol Metab* 9:335, 1980.

Kemeny N, Brennan MF. The surgical complications of chemotherapy in the cancer patient. *Curr Probl Surg* 24:607, 1987.

Kim RY, Spenser SA, Meredith RF, et al. Extradural spinal cord compression. Analysis of factors determining functional prognosis. *Radiology* 176:279, 1990.

Lightdale CJ, Kurtz RC, Boyle CC, et al. Cancer and upper gastrointestinal tract hemorrhage: Benign causes of bleeding demonstrated by endoscopy. *JAMA* 226:139, 1973.

Massaferri EL, O'Dorisio TM, LoBuglio AF. Treatment of hypercalcemia associated with malignancy. *Semin Oncol* 5:141, 1978.

Osteen RT, Guyton S, Steele G, et al. Malignant intestinal obstruction. *Surgery* 87:611, 1980.

Maddox AM, Valdivieso M, Lukeman J, et al. Superior vena cava obstruction in small cell bronchogenic carcinoma: Clinical parameters and survival. *Cancer* 52:2165, 1983.

Millard PR, Jerrome DW, Millward-Sadler GH. Spindle-cell tumours and hypoglycemia. *J Clin Pathol* 29:520, 1976.

Mundy GR. The hypercalcemia of malignancy revised. *J Clin Invest* 82:1, 1988.

Mundy GR, Martin JT. The hypercalcemia of malignancy: Pathogenesis and management. *Metabolism* 31:1247, 1982.

Press OW, Livingston R. Management of malignant pericardial effusion and tamponade. *JAMA* 257:1088, 1987.

Ralston SH, Gardner MD, Drybrugh FJ, et al. Comparison of aminohydroxypylidene diphosphonate, mithramycin, and corticosteroids/calcitonin in treatment of cancer associated hypercalcemia. *Lancet* 2:907, 1985.

Schwartz EE, Goodman LR, Haskin ME. Role of CT scanning in the superior vena cava syndrome. *Am J Clin Oncol* 9:71, 1986.

Sheperd FA, Morgan C, Evans WK, et al. Medical management of malignant pericardial effusion by tetracycline sclerosis. *Am J Cardiol* 60:1161, 1987.

Siegal T, Shohami E, Siegal TG. Indomethacin and dexamethasone treatment in experimental spinal cord compression. Part II. Effect on edema and prostaglandin synthesis. *Neurosurgery* 22:334, 1988.

Silverman P, Distelhorst CW. Metabolic emergencies in clinical oncology. *Semin Oncol* 16:504, 1989.

Stellato TA, Zollinger RM Jr, Shuck JM. Metastatic malignant biliary obstruction. *Am Surg* 53:385, 1987.

Stellato TA, Shenk RR. Gastrointestinal emergencies in the oncology patient. *Semin Oncol* 16:521, 1989.

Theologides A. Neoplastic cardiac tamponade. *Semin Oncol* 5:181, 1978.

Ushio Y, Posner R, Posner JB, Shapiro WR. Experimental spinal cord compression by epidural neoplasms. *Neurology* 27:422, 1977.

Warrell RP Jr, Bockman RS, Coonley CJ, et al. Gallium nitrate inhibits calcium resorption from bone and is effective treatment for cancer-related hypercalcemia. *J Clin Invest* 73:1487, 1984.

Yoachim J. Superior Vena Cava Syndrome. In VT DeVita, S Hellman, SA Rosenberg (eds), *Cancer: Principles and Practice of Oncology* (4th ed). Philadelphia: Lippincott, 1993.

Nutrition in Cancer Patients

Paula M. Termuhlen

Cancer patients face unique problems that can result in nutritional depletion during the perioperative period. For example, cancer cachexia is a well-described condition in which the abnormal metabolic priorities of the patient (host) and tumor alter the body's usual protein and energy requirements. Furthermore, tumors of the head and neck or gastrointestinal tract often compromise nutrition by interfering with ingestion, digestion, and absorption. Preoperative and postoperative chemotherapy and radiation therapy can adversely affect the integrity and function of the alimentary tract, contributing to the difficulty of maintaining adequate nutrition.

Nutrition plays a key role in the recovery and rehabilitation of cancer patients. Adequate protein, calories, and essential micronutrients help maintain a reasonable quality of life for these patients. Surgeons caring for cancer patients must be knowledgeable about the general principles of nutritional assessment and the unique nutritional problems of cancer patients if optimal recovery from treatment is to be achieved.

Cancer Cachexia

Cachexia of malignancy, a nutritional problem unique to cancer patients, is a syndrome of progressive involuntary weight loss and intractable anorexia. Without effective intervention, cancer cachexia will result in death. The physical and biochemical features of this syndrome include tissue wasting, skeletal muscle atrophy, myopathy, anergy, anemia, and glucose intolerance. In addition, patients are unable to absorb and use nutrients adequately.

Not all tumors produce the same degree of cachexia, and much variation is observed among individual patients. Greater weight loss is associated with a tumor in a visceral organ (e.g., pancreas or stomach) than with a tumor in a nonvisceral organ (e.g., breast). Based on common indices of nutritional assessment, protein-calorie malnutrition exists preoperatively in up to 50% of cancer patients. Cancer cachexia may also have prognostic significance: Patients who have no weight loss at the time of surgery demonstrate lower morbidity and higher survival rates than patients who have had moderate to severe weight loss, regardless of tumor type.

ANOREXIA

The etiology of cancer cachexia is multifactorial, but the most obvious contributing factor is anorexia due to the presence of a malignancy or to its treatment. Many patients report altered taste perception that contributes to decreased food intake; however, this alteration appears to be an individual phenomenon unrelated to specific tumor types or sites. Adjuvant therapy, such as chemotherapy and radiation therapy, often causes nausea and vomiting and thus food aversion. In addition, radiotherapy can cause mucosal damage, malabsorption, and diarrhea, all of which contribute to reduced oral intake.

SUBSTRATE UTILIZATION

Aside from anorexia, other causes of cancer cachexia are abnormal host carbohydrate, protein, and lipid metabolism. Studies have shown that even with adequate caloric intake, specific substrate utilization is abnormal and insufficient for adequate nutritional support.

Glucose

Glucose intolerance and insulin resistance are often found in cancer patients, and studies have documented abnormal glucose clearance in patients with many different tumors, including lung and colorectal cancers. A diabetes-like state develops in patients with cachexia that is a result of accentuated gluconeogenesis in the liver. Tumors can augment gluconeogenesis by the increased peripheral release of metabolic substrates such as lactate. In addition, unidentified mediators cause increased gluconeogenesis in the liver by the induction of associated enzymes. The increase in gluconeogenesis contributes to nutritional depletion by causing host energy to be used inefficiently in futile metabolic cycles.

Protein

Depletion of protein in cachectic patients manifests as skeletal muscle atrophy, visceral organ atrophy, and hypoalbuminemia. Protein wasting results from altered nitrogen metabolism, which causes patients with cancer to be unable to adapt to decreased food intake as well as nonstressed patients suffering from simple starvation. Even when cancer patients are given supplemental nutrition, such as total parenteral nutrition, whole-body protein turnover rates remain elevated. Studies in animals suggest that tumors use nitrogen released from tissues at the expense of the malnourished host. There is evidence of decreased protein synthesis and increased protein breakdown in skeletal muscle, which contribute to tissue wasting in patients. Hypoalbuminemia is consistently found in cancer patients and is most likely related to increased albumin turnover. Overall, hepatic production of proteins appears increased in cancer patients, but this is offset by increased turnover in the peripheral body cell mass.

Lipids

Lipid metabolism is also abnormal, resulting in depletion of lipid stores and hyperlipidemia. Increased turnover of lipid stores plays a role because glucose infusions in weight-losing patients fail to suppress lipolysis. Hyperlipidemia results from a decrease in the amount of lipoprotein lipase, which transports triglycerides from blood into adipose tissue. Abnormally high or even normal serum insulin levels appear to not promote fat storage in cancer patients and thus contribute to the hyperlipidemia.

METABOLIC RATE

The abnormal carbohydrate, protein, and lipid metabolism of the host is accompanied by an inability to adjust the metabolic rate to food intake. Although some patients with weight loss have documented hypermetabolism, this finding is inconsistent in large studies, varying among individual patients and tumor types. Host- and tumor-secreted factors have been the focus for identifying the mechanism of the metabolic changes in cancer cachexia. To date, no tumor-produced substance having a systemic effect has been isolated. However, factors secreted by the host as part of the immune response to a tumor appear to play a role in cancer cachexia.

The cytokine tumor necrosis factor (TNF) has not only local immune effects but also systemic effects that produce clinical results similar to those seen in cachexia. TNF, also known as cachectin, has a cytotoxic effect on tumors and inhibits lipoprotein lipase, resulting in hyperlipidemia. Receptors for TNF are found ubiquitously but particularly in the liver, adipose tissue, and muscle cells, which are key sites for abnormal metabolism in cancer patients. In healthy volunteers, TNF has been shown to increase temperature and heart rate as well as peripheral protein turnover. One theory is that cytokines such as TNF released by the immune system in response to a tumor promote an acute-phase response that reroutes nutrients from the periphery to the liver. Ultimately, this response becomes unregulated, resulting in anorexia and abnormal carbohydrate, protein, and lipid metabolism.

Preoperative Assessment of Nutritional Status

Malnutrition, as commonly manifested by weight loss, exists in more than 50% of cancer patients. Traditionally, malnourished patients without cancer who have undergone major operative procedures have had higher rates of morbidity (e.g., poor wound healing, increased wound infection rates, prolonged postoperative ileus) than their well-nourished counterparts. That finding is perhaps due to the fact that underlying the malnutrition is a depressed immune system, which is often found in cancer patients as well.

Cancer patients should undergo a thorough preoperative nutritional assessment, and high-risk patients should be identified. Many nutritional assessment techniques exist. Most are based on a complete history and physical examination as well as documentation of changes in weight over time. Other studies include anthropomorphic studies, measurements of serum albumin and transferrin, tests of immune function by assessment of delayed cutaneous hypersensitivity, and estimates of energy expenditure. However, for most patients nutritional status can be adequately assessed through a comprehensive history and physical examination.

Preoperatively, malnourished patients should have a full nutritional assessment including an estimate of the patient's basal energy expenditure (BEE), which can be calculated indirectly by the Harris-Benedict equation:

Male: $BEE = 66.5 + 13.7(wt) + 5(ht) - 6.7$ (age)

Female: $BEE = 66.5 + 9.6(wt) + 1.8(ht) - 4.7$ (age)

where wt = weight in kilograms, ht = height in centimeters, and age is in years.

The metabolic cart assessment, based on a patient's carbon dioxide production, is a clinical method of determining energy expenditure that gives a more personalized assessment but is cumbersome, time consuming, and expensive.

Preoperative Nutritional Supplementation

It has been difficult to establish a clear benefit to short-term preoperative nutritional supplementation in terms of decreased morbidity and mortality. However, there is some evidence to suggest a benefit to severely malnourished patients if preoperative nutritional supplementation is given for at least 7–10 days. More thorough preoperative nutritional supplementation should be considered for the nutritionally high-risk patient who may be grossly underweight (<80% of standard weight for height) or grossly overweight (>120% of standard weight for height). A recent weight loss of 12% or more of usual body weight is particularly important because patients with acute-onset protein-calorie malnutrition and associated hypoalbuminemia have a higher mortality rate than those with a marasmic or adapted form of protein-calorie malnutrition that has occurred over a longer period of time. Alcoholic patients are also at high risk for being nutritionally depleted, as are patients with malabsorptive syndromes, short gut, gastrointestinal fistulas, renal failure requiring dialysis, abscesses, and large healing wounds. In addition, patients with systemic infections and associated fever have increased metabolic needs that place them at high risk for the complications associated with nutritional depletion. Stopping oral intake and providing only IV solutions perioperatively for hydration adds additional risk. Although the use of preoperative nutritional support remains controversial except in severely malnourished patients, the use of postoperative nutritional supplementation is a key therapeutic modality in helping patients recover.

Postoperative Nutritional Supplementation

ACUTE PHASE

Postoperative nutritional support can be divided into two phases: acute and chronic. Patients recovering from a major operative procedure will need nutritional supplementation until they demonstrate the ability to obtain full nourishment independently. Both enteral and parenteral means of support are available. It has been recognized that enteral feeding should be used whenever possible, and many patients have enteral feeding tubes placed at the time of operation so that feeding can begin early in the postoperative period. If enteral feeding is unable to meet the patient's nutritional needs, then parenteral feeding should be instituted, alone or in conjunction with enteral feeding. In general, the goals for nutritional support are approximately 25 kcal and 1.5 g of protein per kilogram of body weight per day.

CHRONIC PHASE

The chronic phase of postoperative nutritional support is related to the longer-term consequences of a particular operation and adjuvant therapy. Many operative procedures produce prolonged inability to obtain adequate nutrition orally. These include pancreaticoduodenectomy with prolonged gastric emptying, esophagectomy with gastric stasis and regurgitation, and gastrectomy with dumping syndrome. Patients undergoing operations in the head and neck region are also at particular risk for inadequate oral nutrition. For most of these patients, an enteral feeding tube can be placed into the jejunum during the operation and used for long periods. Patients are often discharged with feeding tubes in place. Thus, a patient's quality of life is enhanced by the ability to manage himself or herself outside a hospital. Beyond supplying sufficient protein and calories, supplementation may need to include vitamins, iron, and pancreatic enzymes.

Nutritional Complications of Adjuvant Therapy

Additional nutritional problems can arise with adjuvant therapy. Patients may receive chemotherapy or radiotherapy as part of their treatment plan either before or after surgery, or both. These therapies have various adverse effects. Mucosal inflammation and pain are the initial postradiotherapy complaints that prevent patients from obtaining adequate nutrition. Such late effects as loss of taste, fibrosis, stricture formation, obstruction, and fistulization also may occur. Each chemotherapeutic agent has its own systemic side effects, although many agents produce nausea and vomiting as well as fluid and electrolyte imbalances.

Future Considerations

Studies are underway to address the unique nutritional needs and metabolic abnormalities of cancer patients. Specific amino acids such as glutamine and arginine seem to be easily utilized by the intestine and promote more efficient nitrogen retention during stress. Arginine also seems to enhance immune function and is a potentially fruitful target for research. A promising enteral product includes supplemental arginine, RNA, and omega-3 fatty acids as part of its formula. Each of these substances individually stimulates the immune system. In one clinical trial, fewer infections and wound complications, in addition to shorter hospital stays, were documented in cancer patients who underwent major operative procedures and received this product compared with patients who received a common standard enteral product as part of their nutritional support.

Future nutritional research in cancer patients will continue to focus on providing optimal nutrition in a safe and efficacious fashion. In addition, therapeutic nutritional intervention with substrates that stimulate the immune system may provide yet another modality for improving the general health of cancer patients. Furthurmore, advances in molecular biology may someday result in the development of highly sophisticated products that combine nutrient substrates and antineoplastic pharmacologic agents in synergistic formulations designed to control or eradicate tumor cells while maintaining adequate nutrition.

Selected References

Buzby GP, Mullen JL, Matthews DC, et al. Prognostic nutritional index in gastrointestinal surgery. *Am J Surg* 139:160, 1980.

Daly JM, Lieberman MD, Goldfine J, et al. Enteral nutrition with supplemental arginine, RNA, and omega-3 fatty acids in patients after operation: Immunologic, metabolic, and clinical outcome. *Surgery* 112:56, 1992.

Daly JM, Redmond HP, Lieberman MD, et al. Nutritional support of patients with cancer of the gastrointestinal tract. *Surg Clin North Am* 71:523, 1991.

Heys SD, Park KGM, Garlick PJ, et al. Nutrition and malignant disease: Implications for surgical practice. *Br J Surg* 79:614, 1992.

Kern KA, Norton JA. Cancer cachexia. *JPEN J Parenter Enteral Nutr* 12:286, 1988.

McClave SA, Mitoraj TE, Theilmeier KA, et al. Differentiating subtypes (hypoalbuminemic vs. marasmic) of protein calorie malnutrition: Incidence and clinical significance in a university hospital setting. *JPEN J Parenter Enteral Nutr* 16:337, 1992.

Meguid MM, Debonis D, Meguid V, et al. Complications of abdominal operations for malignant disease. *Am J Surg* 156: 341, 1988.

Shike M, Brennan MF. Supportive Care of the Cancer Patient. In VT DeVita, S Hellman, SA Rosenberg (eds), *Cancer: Principles and Practice of Oncology* (3rd ed). Philadelphia: Lippincott, 1989.

Shikova SA, Blackburn GL. Nutritional consequences of major gastrointestinal surgery: Patient outcome and starvation. *Surg Clin North Am* 71: 509, 1991.

Shils ME. Nutrition and Diet in Cancer. In ME Shils, VR Young (eds), *Modern Nutrition in Health and Disease* (7th ed). Philadelphia: Lea & Febiger, 1987

Tchekmedyian NS, Zahyna D, Halpert C, et al. Clinical aspects of nutrition in advanced cancer. *Oncology* 49(Suppl 2):3, 1992.

Pharmacotherapy of Cancer

Phillip B. Ley

A basic understanding of cancer pharmacotherapy and related toxicities is mandatory for the general surgeon to be fully integrated into a multidisciplinary cancer care program. To intelligently discuss surgical options with patients, knowledge of the available adjuvant treatment regimens and their potential for toxicity is essential.

This chapter includes a discussion of basic principles of chemotherapy, an overview of the mechanisms of drug action and drug resistance, and a tabular listing of the drugs available and their places in representative combination chemotherapy protocols used in the treatment of solid tumors most commonly seen by the surgical oncologist. Finally, a summary of cancer pain management and the treatment of chemotherapy-induced emesis is included.

The reader should be aware that a complete discussion of cancer chemotherapy is beyond the scope of this brief overview. The drug and dosage regimens listed have been chosen as representative examples only and do not constitute a listing of all available protocols. For specific prescribing information, the practitioner is advised to consult individual manufacturer package inserts or one of the referenced texts.

Basic Principles of Chemotherapy

Cancer chemotherapeutic agents are the result of drug design and, largely, empiricism. Their use has developed based on an understanding of tumor growth characteristics, the cell cycle, drug mechanisms of action, and drug resistance. It is hoped that new techniques and advances in molecular biology will allow improvements in drug design to extend the possibility of complete chemotherapeutic response and possibly the cure of patients currently deemed beyond salvage.

TUMOR GROWTH AND KINETICS

Kinetic aspects of tumor growth have been well described. Two concepts that underscore our knowledge of the kinetics of tumor growth are Skipper's laws and Gompertzian growth. Skipper's laws apply to cells in the proliferating compartment of a tumor. First, the doubling time of proliferating cells is constant, creating a straight line on a semilog plot. Second, cell kill by a particular drug at a given dose is constant, irrespective of body burden. In most solid tumors, however, only a portion of cells within the tumor—the growth fraction—is proliferating at any given time. This partially accounts for the refractory nature of many solid tumors to chemotherapy.

Human tumors follow a pattern of Gompertzian, rather than straight line, growth. Gompertzian growth describes a cell population decreasing due to cell death and increasing due to proliferation. Also, cell subpopulations may have ceased to proliferate but have not died, further swaying the growth curve from a straight semilog plot. The normal Gompertzian growth curve is sigmoid in shape. Maximum tumor growth rate occurs at about 30% of maximum tumor volume, where nutrient and oxygen supply to the greatest number of tumor cells is optimized. This portion of the curve is also where drug efficacy against a particular tumor may best be estimated.

The cell cycle is an important fundamental concept to understand when designing chemotherapeutic agents and treatment regimens. The cell cycle is divided into five components. The resting or nonproliferating cell is in the G0 phase, entering the active portion of the cycle following stimulation. DNA synthesis occurs during the S phase and is followed by the postsynthetic G2 phase. Mitosis occurs during the M phase and precedes the postmitotic G1 phase.

The cell cycle becomes important in drug selection because the cells in the growth fraction are more susceptible to certain agents. In a broad sense, antineoplastic agents may be classified on the basis of their activity in relation to the cell cycle. Most antimetabolites, etoposide, hydroxyurea, vinca alkaloids, and bleomycin are cell cycle–specific agents that are most effective against tumors with a high growth fraction. In contrast, alkylating agents, antineoplastic antibiotics, fluorouracil, floxuridine, and procarbazine exert their effect independent of the cell cycle and generally show more activity against slow-growing tumors.

DRUG MECHANISMS AND THERAPEUTICS

Knowledge of the basic action mechanisms of chemotherapeutic agents is critical in selecting drugs for an effective chemotherapy combination regimen, minimizing toxicity and drug interactions, and preventing emergence of drug-resistant clones. Agents may damage the DNA template by alkylation, cross-linking, double-strand cleavage by topoisomerase II, intercalation, and blockage of RNA synthesis. Mitosis may be arrested by spindle poisons. Antimetabolites block enzymes necessary for DNA synthesis. Hormonal agents and their antagonists may influence cellular signal transduction, and biologic response modifiers may influence the host's immune response to the tumor alone or in the context of concomitantly administered drugs.

Combination chemotherapy frequently is used in an effort to forestall the development of drug resistance to antineoplastic agents and to achieve synergism with reduced toxicity. The Goldie-Coldman hypothesis assumes that at the time of diagnosis, most tumors possess resistant clones. Multiple mechanisms of drug resistance develop during cancer progression. The most well studied of these involves the *mdr* gene, which codes for membrane-bound P-glycoprotein. P-glycoprotein serves as a channel through which cellular toxins (i.e., chemotherapeutic agents) may be excreted from the cell. Additional mechanisms of drug resistance are decreased drug transport into cells, reduction of drug activation, drug metabolism enhancement, the development of alternative metabolic pathways, drug inhibition of enzyme targets overcome by gene amplification, and impairment of drug binding to target. A single drug may be subject to one or more mechanisms.

Interestingly, normal human cells never develop drug resistance. As a result, several caveats of combination chemotherapy have emerged. Drugs shown to be active as single agents should be chosen, and drugs selected for combined use should have different mechanisms of action. Ideally, drugs with different dose-limiting toxicities should be administered together, although toxicity overlap may necessitate dose reduction, as with myelosuppression. Finally, drug combinations with similar patterns of resistance should be avoided.

Different patterns of chemotherapy administration are used in particular settings with specific goals. Induction chemotherapy is usually high dose and given in combination to induce complete remission. Consolidation is a repetition of an induction regimen in a complete responder to prolong remission or increase the cure rate. Chemotherapy given with an intent similar to that of consolidation but with higher doses than induction or with different agents at high doses is known as intensification. Maintenance regimens are low-dose, long-term protocols intended to delay tumor cell regrowth after complete remission. Induction, consolidation, intensification, and maintenance usually apply to hematologic malignancies but also may describe solid tumor regimens as well.

Neoadjuvant treatment in the preoperative or perioperative period is used more commonly with solid tumors, such as locally advanced breast carcinoma, soft tissue sarcomas of the extremities, and, more recently, rectal carcinoma and squamous cell carcinoma of the head and neck. It is often given in combination with radiotherapy to improve survival, resectability, and organ preservation.

Palliative chemotherapy may be given to control symptoms or, if the toxicity profile is favorable, prolong life for incurable patients. Salvage chemotherapy involves the use of a potentially curative, high-dose protocol in patients failing or recurring after different standard treatment plans have been attempted.

Adjuvant chemotherapy is administered following curative surgery or radiotherapy as a short-course, high-dose regimen to destroy a low number of residual tumor cells. Several factors determine the effectiveness of adjuvant regimens, including tumor burden, drug dose and schedule, combination chemotherapy, and drug resistance. The drug(s) must be active locally against residual cells as well as distantly against clinically occult metastatic deposits. Extensive literature supports the use of adjuvant chemotherapy for breast, colon, rectal, and anal carcinomas and for ovarian germ cell tumors, osteosarcoma, and pediatric solid tumors. No definitive benefit has been reported yet for pancreatic, gastric, and testicular carcinomas or for cervical cancer and melanoma, although investigative adjuvant therapy protocols are ongoing and open for patient enrollment.

Most chemotherapeutic agents exhibit very steep dose-response profiles and have low therapeutic indices, making a high-dose, short-term administration desirable. This can be accomplished through regional dose intensification. One example is intraperitoneal chemotherapy of ovarian or gastric cancer with high risk of peritoneal recurrence, or low-volume intraperitoneal disease, pseudomyxoma peritonei, and peritoneal mesothelioma. Another type of regional dose intensification is intra-arterial therapy, which requires regional tumor confinement and a unique tumor blood supply and is most commonly used in hepatic artery infusion for primary or metastatic liver tumors that are surgically unresectable for cure. Intra-arterial chemotherapy also has been used for brain gliomas and some head and neck tumors. Isolated perfusion of a specific anatomic site, usually the extremities, is one more type of regional dose intensification that allows for the delivery of very high doses to the involved site with little systemic toxicity; it is often combined with hyperthermia. The largest body of literature discusses its use in all stages of melanoma, although limb perfusion for extremity sarcoma has been reported.

Chemotherapeutic Agents

Fundamental knowledge of the drugs available for cancer treatment, their mechanisms of action, general dose ranges, dominant toxicities, and indications for use is important to the general surgeon caring for cancer patients. Table 21-1 lists the available agents and their mechanisms, doses, and toxicities. Specific solid tumors germane to the practice of general surgery and representative chemotherapy combination protocols established for their treatment can be found in Table 21-2.

Management of Cancer Pain

The vast majority of patients with advanced cancer and as many as 60% of patients with any stage of disease experience pain of significant degree. However, cancer pain frequently is undertreated for a multitude of reasons and fears that are largely unfounded. Effective management of cancer pain is achieved best with a multidisciplinary approach including pain specialists, oncologists, nurses, pharmacists, physiatrists, physical and occupational therapists, psychologists, psychiatrists, primary care physicians, social workers, clergy, and hospice caregivers. Open lines of communication are of paramount importance to the successful management of cancer pain.

Table 21-1. Cancer chemotherapeutic agents: Mechanisms, doses, and toxicities

Drug	Dose and schedule	Toxicity
Alkylating agents		Myelosuppression, pulmonary infiltrates
Busulfan	2–6 mg PO daily	pulmonary fibrosis, hemorrhagic cystitis
Chlorambucil	4–10 mg PO daily	alopecia, nausea and vomiting
Cyclophosphamide	1.0–1.5 g/m^2 IV; 50–200 mg PO daily	
Ifosfamide	1.2 g/m^2 IV daily $\times$ 5	
Mechlorethamine	16 mg/m^2 IV	
Melphalan	6–10 mg PO daily; 2–4 mg PO daily maintenance	
Thiotepa	16–32 mg/m^2 IV	
Antimetabolites		Stomatitis, GI tract injury, myelo-
Cytarabine	200 mg/m^2 IV daily $\times$ 5, continuous infusion	suppression, alopecia
Fludarabine	30 mg/m^2 IV daily $\times$ 5	
Floxuridine	16–24 mg/m^2 IV or IA, daily continuous infusion	
Fluorouracil	500 mg/m^2 IV daily $\times$ 3	
6-Mercaptopurine	100 mg/m^2 PO daily	
Methotrexate	2.5–5.0 mg PO daily; 25–50 mg IV weekly; 200 mg–10 g IM with leucovorin	
6-Thioguanine	80 mg/m^2 PO daily	
Antibiotics		
Bleomycin	10 units/m^2 IV or SC daily $\times$ 5–7	Nausea, vomiting, alopecia, ulceration, pulmonary fibrosis
Dactinomycin	2.5 mg/m^2 IV	Stomatitis, GI injury, myelosuppression, alopecia
Daunorubicin	90–180 mg/m^2 IV q3wk. Not to exceed 600 mg/m^2	Stomatitis, alopecia, myelosuppresion; cardiotoxicity at doses >600 mg/m^2
Doxorubicin	50–75 mg/m2 IV q3wk. Continuous infusion reduces cardiac toxicity	Stomatitis, alopecia, myelosuppression; cardiotoxicity at doses >500 mg/m^2
Idarubicin	45–60 mg/m^2 PO q2–4wk; 20–25 mg/m^2 PO daily $\times$ 3. May be given IV.	GI toxicity, alopecia, cardiotoxicty

Table 21-1 (continued).

Drug	Dose and schedule	Toxicity
Mitomycin C	20 mg/m^2 IV q6–8wk	Myelosuppression, GI injury, hypercalcemia
Mitoxantrone	12 mg/m^2 IV daily × 3	Myelosuppression, alopecia, cardiotoxicty
Plicamycin	1 mg/m^2 IV qod × 3	Myelosuppression, hypocalcemia, hepatotoxicity
Mitotic inhibitors		
Etoposide (VP-16)	50–150 mg/m^2 IV daily × 3–5 q3–4wk; 50 mg/m^2 PO daily × 21	Myelosuppression, alopecia, GI toxicity, blisters, neuropathy, anaphylaxis
Taxol*	250 mg/m^2 IV daily × 5	Myelosuppression, stomatitis, neuropathy, anaphylaxis
Vinblastine	2.5–3.7 mg/m^2 IV weekly (not to exceed 18.5 mg/m^2 in adults or 12.5 mg/m^2 in pediatric patients)	Myelosuppression, GI toxicity, neuropathy, blisters, alopecia, hypertension, pulmonary toxicity
Vincristine	1.4 mg/m^2 IV weekly in adults; 2 mg/m^2 IV weekly in pediatric patients	Peripheral neuropathy, GI toxicity, paralytic ileus, SIADH, rash, alopecia, bladder atony
Hormonal agents		
Corticosteroids		Fluid retention, hyperglycemia, hypertension, infection
Dexamethasone	0.5–4.0 mg PO daily. Also available for IV and IM use	
Prednisone	15–100 mg PO daily	
Methyl-prednisolone	10–125 mg IV daily	
Androgens		Fluid retention, masculinization
Fluoxy-mesterone	10–40 mg PO daily	
Methyl-testosterone	50–200 mg PO daily	
Estrogens		Fluid retention, feminization, uterine bleeding, nausea and vomiting
Diethyl-stilbestrol	5 mg PO tid (breast); 1 mg PO daily (prostate)	
Antiestrogens		Hot flashes, nausea and vomiting

Table 21-1 (continued).

Drug	Dose and schedule	Toxicity
Tamoxifen	10 mg PO bid	
LHRH analogues		
Leuprolide	1 mg SC daily	
Antiandrogens		Decreased libido, impotence
Flutamide	250 mg PO tid	
Miscellaneous		
Amino-glutethimide	250–500 mg PO qid	Adrenal insufficiency
Megestrol acetate	40 mg PO qid	
Medroxy-progesterone	100–200 PO daily; 200–600 mg IM twice weekly	
Miscellaneous		
Asparaginase	8,000 IU/m^2 3–7 times weekly for 28 days	GI toxicity, somnolence, confusion, fatty liver
Carmustine	200 mg/m^2 IV	Myelosuppression, emesis
Lomustine	130 mg/m^2 PO	Myelosuppression, emesis
Hydroxyurea	800–1,600 mg/m^2 PO daily	Myelosuppression
Hexamethyl-melamine	100–300 mg/m^2 IV daily	Anorexia, myelosuppression, peripheral neuropathy
Dacarbazine	80–160 mg/m^2 IV daily × 10	Myelosuppression, emesis
Procarbazine	50–200 mg/m^2 PO daily for 10–20 days	Myelosuppression, emesis, neuropathy
Mitotane	2–10 g PO daily	Adrenal insufficiency, emesis, diarrhea, tremors
Streptozocin	500 mg IV daily ×5 q6wk	Hypoglycemia
Cisplatin	40–120 mg/m^2 IV q1–4wk; 20–33 mg/m^2 IV daily × 3–5	Nausea and vomiting, nephrotoxicity, low magnesium, neurotoxicity
Carboplatin	240–500 mg/m^2 IV q28d	Myelosuppression, emesis
Levamisole	50 mg PO q8h for 3 days q2wk with fluorouracil	Rash, arthralgia, myalgia, fever, neutropenia
Leucovorin	10 mg/m^2 PO with fluorouracil	Allergy

GI = gastrointestinal; SIADH = syndrome of inappropriate antidiuretic hormone; LHRH = luteinizing hormone–releasing hormone.
*Taxol is approved for investigational use only in the United States.

Table 21-2. Specific solid tumors with combination chemotherapy regimens

Tumor type	Regimen	Agents
Breast	CMF	Cyclophosphamide
		Methotrexate
		Fluorouracil
	CMFVP	CMF
		Vincristine
		Prednisone
	FAC	Fluorouracil
		Doxorubicin
		Cyclophosphamide
Breast, ER-positive		Tamoxifen
Colorectal, adjuvant		Fluorouracil
		Levamisole
Colorectal, metastatic		Fluorouracil
		Leucovorin
Gastric	EAP	Etoposide
		Doxorubicin
		Cisplatin
	EFP	Etoposide
		Fluorouracil
		Cisplatin
	FAM	Fluorouracil
		Doxorubicin
		Mitomycin C
Pancreatic	SMF	Streptozocin
		Mitomycin C
		Fluorouracil
Head and neck	PFL	Cisplatin
		Fluorouracil
		Leucovorin
	CF	Cisplatin
		Fluorouracil
Lung, small cell	ACE	Doxorubicin
		Cyclophosphamide
		Etoposide
	CAV	Cyclophosphamide
		Doxorubicin
		Vincristine
	PACE	Cisplatin
		Doxorubicin
		Cyclophosphamide
		Etoposide
Lung, non–small cell	CAMP	Cyclophosphamide
		Doxorubicin
		Methotrexate
		Procarbazine
	DOXO/CIS	Doxorubicin
		Cisplatin

Table 21-2 (continued).

Tumor type	Regimen	Agents
	MVP	Mitomycin C
		Vinblastine
		Cisplatin
Melanoma, metastatic	VBD	Vinblastine
		Bleomycin
		Cisplatin
	VDP	Vinblastine
		Dacarbazine
		Cisplatin
		Dacarbazine
Sarcoma, Ewing's	CAV	Cyclophosphamide
		Doxorubicin
		Vincristine
Sarcoma, osteogenic	T-10	Preoperative: methotrexate
		Postoperative: bleomycin, cyclophosphamide, and dactinomycin (BCD)
		Follow-up: methotrexate and doxorubicin
		Maintenance: doxorubicin, cisplatin, BCD
Sarcoma, soft tissue	MAID	Mesna
		Doxorubicin
		Ifosfamide
		DTIC
	CyVADiC	Cyclophosphamide
		Vincristine
		Doxorubicin
		DTIC
	VAC	Vincristine
		Dactinomycin
		Cyclophosphamide
Adrenocortical carcinoma		Mitotane
Neuroendocrine carcinoma		Doxorubicin
		Streptozocin
Neuroblastoma		Doxorubicin
		Cyclophosphamide
		Cisplatin
Liver		Doxorubicin
		Fluorouracil
Wilms' tumor		Dactinomycin
		Vincristine
		Doxorubicin
		Cyclophosphamide

Table 21-2 (continued).

Tumor type	Regimen	Agents
Uterine cervix	BIP	Bleomycin
		Ifosfamide
		Cisplatin
		Mesna
Gestational trophoblastic	DMC	Dactinomycin
		Methotrexate
		Cyclophosphamide
Ovarian	CHAD	Cyclophosphamide
		Hexamethylmelamine
		Doxorubicin
		Cisplatin
Testicular	BEP	Bleomycin
		Etoposide
		Cisplatin
Urinary bladder	MVAC	Methotrexate
		Vinblastine
		Doxorubicin
		Cisplatin
Prostate		Leuprolide
		Flutamide
Renal cell		Aldesleukin
		Interferon-alpha
Lymphoma, non-Hodgkin's	BACOP	Bleomycin
		Doxorubicin
		Cyclophosphamide
		Vincristine
		Prednisone
	CHOP	Cyclophosphamide
		Doxorubicin
		Vincristine
		Prednisone
	COPP	Cyclophosphamide
		Vincristine
		Prednisone
Lymphoma, Hodgkin's	MOPP	Nitrogen mustard
		Vincristine
		Procarbazine
		Prednisone
	ABVD	Doxorubicin
		Bleomycin
		Vinblastine
		Dacarbazine

ER = estrogen receptor.

Cancer pain may be due to direct tumor involvement of bone, nerves, viscera, blood vessels, or mucous membranes and can be postoperative, postradiotherapy, or postchemotherapy. Narcotic use should follow the basic principles of cancer pain management, beginning with an agent that has the potential to provide relief; individualization of the agent, route, dose, and schedule; titration to efficacy; and provision of relief for breakthrough pain. Side effects should be anticipated and treated. Change from one route of administration to another should be done with equianalgesic doses, and the oral route should be used whenever possible. The practitioner should be aware of various adjuncts to pain management, including steroids, antidepressants, anxiolytics, and neuroleptics, as well as neuroablative, neurostimulatory, and anesthetic procedures.

Table 21-3 is a compilation of various nonnarcotic and narcotic analgesic agents for treating cancer pain and includes dose ranges and expected toxicities.

Management of Chemotherapy-Induced Emesis

Since many surgical patients receive neoadjuvant and adjuvant chemotherapy, the general surgeon may be called on to treat chemotherapy-induced emesis, which is often a dose-limiting toxicity that may lead patients to refuse further therapy. Three physiologic areas are included in the pathogenesis of chemotherapy-induced emesis (CIE): (1) the emetic center in the lateral reticular formation of the medulla, (2) vagal and splanchnic afferents from the gastrointestinal tract to the central nervous system, and (3) the chemoreceptor trigger zone in the area postrema of the medulla. Chemotherapeutic agents and their metabolites may trigger the latter two directly.

Three patterns of emesis tend to occur in association with chemotherapy. Acute emesis occurs within 24 hours of chemotherapy. Delayed emesis occurs more than 24 hours after the cessation of chemotherapy administration and is predisposed by female gender, high-dose cisplatin, and prior episodes of acute emesis. Anticipatory emesis may occur prior to retreatment in patients whose prior episodes of emesis were poorly controlled, occurring in up to 25% of patients who received prior chemotherapy. Younger age and history of motion sickness also predispose to CIE. Cisplatin, dacarabazine, mechlorethamine, and high-dose melphalan tend to have a very high incidence of inducing CIE. Carmustine, cyclophosphamide, procarbazine, and high-dose etoposide have a 60–90% incidence rate of causing CIE. Vincristine and chlorambucil, in contrast, have a low incidence of causing CIE.

The treatment of CIE underwent a veritable revolution with the introduction of the first selective serotonin antagonist, ondansetron. IV administration is not necessary in most

Table 21-3. Nonnarcotic and narcotic analgesic agents for treating cancer pain: Dose ranges and expected toxicities*

Drug	Dose and schedule	Equianalgesic dose to 10 mg morphine	Toxicity
Indomethacin	50–75 mg q6h PO	NA	Dyspepsia, allergy, antiplatelet
Diflunisal	500–1,000 mg q12h PO	NA	Dyspepsia, allergy, antiplatelet
Ibuprofen	200–800 mg q6–8h PO	NA	Dyspepsia, allergy, antiplatelet
Codeine	32–65 mg q3–4h PO	NA	Constipation, nausea, sedation
Propoxyphene	65–130 mg q3–4h	NA	Constipation, nausea, sedation
Hydrocodone	5–20 mg q4h	NA	Constipation, nausea, sedation; acetaminophen limits dosing interval
Oxycodone	2.5 mg q4h PO	NA	Constipation, nausea, sedation; acetaminophen and aspirin limit dosing
Morphine	10 mg IM q2–4h; 20–60 mg q2–4h PO	10 mg; 20–60 mg	Constipation, nausea, sedation, respiratory depression
Morphine, slow release	15–60 mg q8–12h PO	20–60 mg	Constipation, nausea, sedation, respiratory depression
Hydromorphone	1.5 mg IM q3–4h; 7.5 mg q3–4h PO	1.5 mg IM; 7.5 mg PO	Constipation, nausea, sedation, respiratory depression
Meperidine	50–125 mg q3–4h IM; 50–300 mg q3–4h PO	75 mg IM; 300 mg PO	Normeperidine accumulation limits chronic use
Levorphanol	1–4 mg IM q3–6h; 2–4 mg q3–6h PO	2 mg IM; 4 mg PO	Long half-life limits use
Methadone	5–15 mg IM q4–6h; 10–20 mg q4–6h PO	10 mg IM; 20 mg PO	Delayed toxicity accumulation
Fentanyl	25–100 mg/hr transdermal q3d	100 mg	

*Narcotic agonist/antagonists such as pentazocine, nalbuphine, and butorphanol generally are avoided for cancer pain therapy.

Table 21-4. Available and commonly used antiemetic agents for chemotherapy-induced emesis

Drug	Dose and schedule	Toxicity
Ondansetron	8–32 mg IV daily; 4–8 mg PO q8h	Headache, constipation
Metoclopramide	2–3 mg/kg IV q2–3h; 10–20 mg PO q8h	Dystonia, akathisia, sedation, diarrhea, extrapyramidal effects
Haloperidol	1–3 mg IV q2–6h; 1–2 mg PO q3–6h	Dystonia, akathisia, hypotension, sedation
Droperidol	0.5–2.0 mg IV q4h	Extrapyramidal effect
Prochlorperazine	5–10 mg PO q3–4h; 25 mg PR q4–6h; 10–20 mg IM q3–6h	Extrapyramidal effect, sedation, dystonia, anticholinergic effects
Chlorpromazine	25–50 mg PO q3–6h	Same as prochloperazine
Dexamethasone	10–20 mg IV daily; 4 mg PO q6–12	Hyperglycemia, euphoria, insomnia, rectal pain
Methylprednisolone	250–500 mg IV daily	Hyperglycemia, euphoria, insomnia, rectal pain
Lorazepam	0.025 mg/kg IV q4–8h; 1–2 mg PO q4–8h	Sedation, amnesia, confusion, hypotension
Diphenhydramine	25–50 mg IV or PO q6h	Anticholinergic effect, sedation
Dronabinol	5–10 mg/m2 PO q3–4h	Dysphoria, confusion, ataxia, hypotension, hallucination

cases of non–cisplatin-induced emesis, since efficacy by oral administration is comparable. High-dose IV metoclopramide has been found effective in treating CIE, though less so than ondansetron, but its extrapyramidal side effects are a major problem. Standard phenothiazines are less effective but serve as useful adjuncts in the treatment of CIE. Corticosteroids, especially dexamethasone and methylprednisolone, act via a mechanism that is still unclear. In combination with other agents, corticosteroids dramatically improve antiemetic efficacy and may reduce the incidence of unwanted side effects by permitting dosage reduction. Lorazepam, a benzodiazepine, is useful in the prevention of anticipatory emesis and may reduce the incidence of dystonic reactions to metoclopramide. Most important, combinations of these agents, specifically ondansetron, dexamethasone, lorazepam, and metoclopramide, increase antiemetic efficacy and reduce troublesome side effects through presumed synergistic activity. Table 21-4 lists available and commonly used antiemetic agents with their dose ranges and the known major side effects.

Selected References

Abramowicz M (ed). Drugs of choice for cancer chemotherapy. *Medical Letter* 35:43, 1993.

DeVita V, Hellman S, Rosenberg S (eds). *Cancer: Principles and Practice of Oncology* (4th ed). Philadelphia: Lippincott, 1993.

Krakoff I. Cancer chemotherapeutic and biologic agents. CA 41:264, 1991.

McEvoy G (ed). *AHFS Drug Information.* Easton, MD: American Society of Hospital Pharmacists, 1992. Pp 522–661.

Pazdur R (ed). *Medical Oncology: A Comprehensive Review.* Huntington, NY: PRR Inc., 1993.

Perry M (ed). *The Chemotherapy Source Book.* Baltimore: Williams & Wilkins, 1992.

Portenoy R. Cancer pain management. *Semin Oncol* 20 (Suppl 1):19, 1993.

Index